T0292790

PSYCHOGENIC DENTURE INTOLERANCE THEORETICAL BACKGROUND, PREVENTION, AND TREATMENT POSSIBILITIES

DENTAL SCIENCE, MATERIALS AND TECHNOLOGY

Additional books in this series can be found on Nova's website at:

https://www.novapublishers.com/catalog/index.php?cPath=23_29&series p=Dental+Science%2C+Materials+and+Technology

Additional e-books in this series can be found on Nova's website at:

https://www.novapublishers.com/catalog/index.php?cPath=23_29&series pe=Dental+Science%2C+Materials+and+Technology

DENTAL SCIENCE, MATERIALS AND TECHNOLOGY

PSYCHOGENIC DENTURE INTOLERANCE THEORETICAL BACKGROUND, PREVENTION, AND TREATMENT POSSIBILITIES

TIBOR KÁROLY FÁBIÁN
AND
PÁL FEJÉRDY

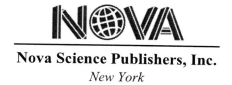

Nova Science Publishers, Inc.
New York

For permission to use material from this book please contact us:
Telephone 631-231-7269; Fax 631-231-8175
Web Site: http://www.novapublishers.com

NOTICE TO THE READER

LIBRARY OF CONGRESS CATALOGING-IN-PUBLICATION DATA

Psychogenic denture intolerance : theoretical background, prevention, and treatment possibilities / Tibor Karoly Fabian and Pal Fejirdy.
    p. ; cm.
 Includes bibliographical references and index.
 ISBN 978-1-62100-608-4 (softcover)
 1. Dentures--Complications--Psychosomatic aspects. I. Fejirdy, Pal, 1945-
II. Title.
 [DNLM: 1. Dentures--adverse effects. 2. Dentures--psychology. 3. Adaptation, Psychological. 4. Psychophysiologic Disorders--prevention & control. 5. Psychophysiologic Disorders--therapy. WU 500 F118p 2010]
 RK656.F33 2010
 617.6'92--dc22
                    2010015627

Published by Nova Science Publishers, Inc. † *New York*

To our Patients and Students

CONTENTS

LIST OF ABBREVIATIONS

AA	arachidonic acid
ACC	interior cingulate cortex
ACSOs	alk(en)yl cystein sulphoxides
ACTH	adrenocorticotrop hormone
ALA	alpha-linolenic acid
APC	antigen presenting cell
ASC	altered state of consciousness
AT	Autogenic Training
BAR	biofeedback assisted relaxation
BDI	BeckDepression Inventory
bis-GMA	bis-phenol-diglycidyl-methacrylate
BMC	bone mineral content
BMD	bone mineral density
BMS	burning mouth syndrome
BSAP	bone specific alkaline phosphatase
BUDA	1,4-butanediol diacrylate
CAM	complementary and alternative medicine
CBCT	cone-beam CT, cone-beam computerized tomography
CBT	cognitive-behavioral therapy
CD3$^+$ cell	collective noun of most kind of T-lymphocytes
CD4$^+$ cell	CD4$^+$ lymphocyte, T-helper cell
CD8$^+$ cell	CD8$^+$ lymphocyte, cytotoxic T-cell,
CD45RO$^+$	CD45RO$^+$ cell, memory T-cell
CGRP	calcitonine gene related peptide
CH	cluster headache
CNS	central nervous system
COX	cyclooxygenase
CPCI	Chronic Pain Coping Inventory
CPH	chronic paroxysmal hemicrania
CRH	corticotrophin-releasing hormone
CSQ	Coping Strategy Questionnaire
CT	computerized tomography

DAS	Dental Anxiety Scale
DC	dendritic cell
DEGDA	diethyleneglycol diacrylate
DFS	Dental Fear Survey
DGLA	dihomogammalinolenic acid
DHA	docosahexaenoic acid
DPD	deoxypyridinoline (marker of bone resorption)
DPT	definitive psychosomatic therapy
DTH	delayed-type hypersensitivity
EC	epicatechin
ECG	epicatechin-3-gallate
EGC	epigallocatechin
EGCG	epigallocatechin-3-gallate
EGDMA	ethylene glycol dimethacrylate
EPA	eicosapentaeoic acid
ER	endoplasmic reticulum
FGF-2	fibroblast growth factor beta-2
FOS	fructooligosaccharide
FPQ-SF	Fear of Pain Questionnaire - Short Form
GABA	gamma-aminobutyric acid
GAG	glycosaminoglycan
GCA	giant cell arteritis
GLA	gamma-linolenic acid
GSR	galvanic skin response
HA	hydroxyapatite
HDDA	1,6-hexanediol diacrylate
HDL	high-density lipoprotein
2-HEMA	2-hydroxyethyl methacrylate
HPA	axis hypothalamic-pituitary-adrenocortical axis
2-HPA	2-hydroxy propyl acrylate
2-HPMA	2-hydroxy propyl metacrylate
HRV	heart rate variability
HSPA	new name of HSP70 (see HSP70)
HSP70	heat shock protein 70, (70 kDa stress proteins)
HSV-2	herpes simplex virus 2
IgA	immunoglobulin A
IgE	immunoglobulin E
IgG	immunoglobulin G
IgM	immunoglobulin M
IGF-I	insulin-like growth factor-I
IGFBP-3	insulin-like growth factor binding protein-3
IL-1β	interleukin-1-beta,
IL-2	interleukin-2
IL-10	interleukin-10
iNOS	inducible nitric oxide synthase
IPT	initial psychosomatic therapy

LA	linoleic acid
LDL	low-density lipoprotein
LLL	low level laser
LLLT	low level laser therapy
MBCT	Mindfulness-Based Cognitive Therapy
MHC	major histocompatibility complex
MMA	methyl methacrylate
MMP	matrix metalloproteinase
MSG	monosodium glutamate
NAS	numerical analogue scale
NFATc1	nuclear factor of activated T cells
NK cell	natural killer cell
NO	nitric oxide
NSAIDs	non-steroidal anti-inflammatory drugs
NST	nucleus of the solitary tract
O_2^-	superoxide radical
OBE	out-of-body experience
OD	occlusal dysesthesia
OHIP	Oral Health Impact Profile
OHRQoL	oral health related quality of life
OHQOL	oral health related quality of life
OMA	oral motor ability
OP	orthopantomography
ORAC	oxygen radical absorbance capacity
OSA	oral stereognostic ability
PCS	Pain Catastrophizing Scale
PDI	psychogenic denture intolerance
PET	positron emission tomography
PEMF	pulsed electromagnetic field
PG	prostaglandin
PGE_2	prostaglandin E_2
PMN cell	polymorphonuclear leukocyte, granulocyte
PMR	progressive muscle relaxation
PMS	premenstrual syndrome
PSI	Psychological Screening Inventory
PSS	Perceived Stress Scale
PUFA	polyunsaturated fatty acid
PVN	paraventricular nuclei
RANKL	receptor activator of nuclear factor-$\kappa\beta$ ligand
rNST	rostral nucleus of the solitary tract (gustatory nucleus)
RCT	randomized controlled trial
RFB	respiratory feedback
ROI	region(s) of interest
RPD	removable partial denture
sAT	standard level Autogenic Training
SCFA	short chain fatty acid

SCL	skin conductance level
SERM	selective estrogen receptor modulator
sIgA	secretory IgA (salivary IgA)
SOC	sense of coherence
SOPA	Survey of Pain Attitudes
SPECT	single photon emission computerized tomography
SRRS	Social Readjustment Rating Scale
SSRI	selective serotonin reuptake inhibitor
STAI-S	Spielberger's State-Trait Anxiety Inventory, State anxiety version
STAI-T	Spielberger's State-Trait Anxiety Inventory, Trait anxiety version
TGF	transforming growth factor
TMD	temporomandibular disorder
TMJ	emporomandibular joint
TNF-αt	umor necrosis factor alpha
TREGDA	triethyleneglycol diacrylate
TREGDMA	triethyleneglycol dimethacrylate
TrP	trigger point
VAS	visual analogue scale
VCO_2	carbon dioxide production
VO_2	oxygen consumption

PREFACE

Psychogenic denture intolerance is a complex and rising problem of dentistry and presents many intricate problems, which are being tackled by various disciplines of both basic and clinical research. Estimations based on the available data and clinical experience indicate that, at least 3-4% of denture wearers suffer from psychogenic symptoms caused by the treatment procedure, insertion or wearing of fixed or removable dentures. No wonder that, there is a high amount of scientific information gathered so far, however data are rather divergent, sometimes even contradictory and there are numerous questions without any available data to answer.

On this account, present work is a selection of scientific data, and as such, it reflects author's opinion and interest. Therefore, majority of the text is dedicated to clinical aspects including clinical manifestations, diagnosis, prevention and treatment possibilities, although numerous aspects of theoretical background and various basic research data will also be introduced. Relevant subject areas of this book include peculiarities of denture-related psychological and psycho-physiological phenomena, background and pathomechanisms of denture induced psychosomatic manifestations, preventive- diagnostic and treatment strategies of premised conditions, basic principles of communication and patient-nurse-dentist interrelationships as well as an introduction in several treatment methods like psychotherapeutic approaches, mind-body therapies, physiotherapies, medicamentous therapies, diet therapy, medicinal herb therapy and complementary/alternative medicine (CAM) methods.

In spite of the clinical significance and theoretical importance a book dedicated exclusively to the phenomena of psychogenic denture intolerance is exceptional (if any) in the market of scientific literature. Therefore, the present book dedicated entirely to this particular disorder may supply a great want. Authors expect that, the principal audience of the present work is made up primarily of university teachers and students of post graduated and/or Ph.D. courses of dental schools. However, any dental practitioners, interested dental graduate students and other professionals working in the orofacial region or psychosomatic medicine may also use this book serviceable. Authors would like to hope that, this collection of data helps the reader to be at home in the psychogenic denture intolerance related research. Authors also hopes that, reader may be inspired to intensify efforts to discover this highly interesting field more deeply, and to form an own opinion reading the cited references, and other available related literature.

Chapter 1

INTRODUCTION

The problem of psychogenic denture intolerance (PDI) stood in the limelight of scientific interest in the second half of the last century. Although early complete denture related studies sometimes missed the point that psychogenic denture intolerance may also develop in relation to other kind of dentures; later on psychogenic problems related to other kinds of dentures (i.e. removable partial dentures and/or fixed dentures) were also analyzed, and lastly a "holistic view" of psychogenic denture intolerance emerged. In this approach, denture intolerance is recognized as a member of the "large family" of orofacial psychosomatic manifestations [*Ross et al. 1953, Schweitzer 1964, Marxkors & Müller-Fahlbusch 1981, Müller-Fahlbusch & Marxkors 1981, Müller-Fahlbusch & Sone 1982, Newton 1984, Demmel & Lamprecht 1996, Wolowski 2000*].

In general, roughly 10 percent of the dental patients may be counted as a *risk patient* for any psychosomatic manifestations [*Doering & Wolowski 2007*], from which more than a third (roughly 3-4 % of all patients with dentures) suffer from psychogenic denture intolerance [*Fábián & Fejérdy 2007*]. This is a not too large but still significant proportion, and the incidence may increase [*Fábián & Fejérdy 2007, Sugawara et al. 1998*]. It should be also considered that, even two or three of such patients may unbalance dentist's entire schedule [*Schweitzer 1964*] and can occupy a large percentage of the dentist's time [*Swoope 1973*]. Moreover, it also gives rise to legal proceedings in certain cases [*Figgener 1996*]. Thus, the importance of psychogenic denture intolerance should not be underestimated, but considered as a rather important and difficult problem of dentistry. (A more detailed introduction to the concept, background and consequences of psychogenic denture intolerance can be found in *Chapter 2*.)

There are various symptoms of psychogenic denture intolerance including pain manifestations, neuromuscular symptoms, immune and inflammatory reactions as well as several other symptoms like cognitive-behavioral symptoms, salivation related problems, halitosis, alterations of taste sensation, alterations of speech, pseudo-neurological symptoms etc. [*Fábián & Fábián 2000; Fábián et al. 2006, 2007*]. Premised symptoms can be triggered due to the preparation, insertion or wearing of fixed and/or removable dentures [*Fábián & Fábián 2000; Fábián et al. 2006, 2007*]. There are various pathways, which can lead to a denture-induced appearance of such symptoms. Some of these pathways are primarily of somatic origin (including also preparative and/or technical causes), whereas others are primarily psychogenic. Pathways of somatic origin are more or less well characterized, whereas much less is known about the *concrete* pathomechanisms of most psychogenic manifestations. However, it is very likely that, pathways of psychogenic manifestations join major somatic pathways at a certain level of pathomechanism. Therefore, besides the most important clinical findings, fundamentals of the pathomechanisms (including recognized psychogenic pathways as well as major somatic pathways) will also be introduced in *Chapter 3*.

One of the most important goals of the diagnosis of PDI is the early recognition (or at least assumption) of the disorder, and the avoidance of further useless invasive dental treatment, especially because aggravation or spread of symptoms following such invasive dental interventions is not uncommon. Early diagnosis (or assumption) of PDI is also crucial for the prevention of symptom chronification which frequently render pain and other symptoms intractable. The most important diagnostic tool for such purposes is collecting detailed patient's history [*Ross et al. 1953, Barsby 1994, Pertes 1998*] and careful evaluation of *all* relevant *psychosocial, medical* and *dental* anamnestic data including their understanding in a context of a *biopsychosocial model* of orofacial disorders [*Engel 1977, Freeman 1999, Bensing 2000, Green & Laskin 2000, Derra 2002, Dworkin & Sherman 2006*]. Careful clinical examination of the oral and orofacial region and general health status as well as X-ray, MRI and other specific examinations are also cornerstones of a proper diagnostic process certainly. Referral to other professionals may also be needed, and especially recommended in the case of pain and other (pseudo)neurological symptoms. Fundamentals of the diagnostic process and the use of premised diagnostic tools will be introduced more detailed in *Chapter 4*.

Prevention is likely to be the most important tool for the management of psychogenic denture intolerance related problems at a *social level*; therefore, prevention of PDI is clearly a scope of *every* dentist's duties. However, there are still very few dentists prepared to recognize risk patients properly and to cope with such patients so far; notwithstanding that, there are more and more dental schools teaching behavioral medicine and behavioral science in the curricula of their undergraduate and/or postgraduate courses [*Piko & Kopp 2004*]. Besides high quality preparative dental skills and technical background, cornerstones of the prevention are screening of risk patients, proper treatment planning, proper communication with the patient, screening of the patient-nurse-dentist interrelationships [*Fábián & Fábián 2000, Fejérdy & Orosz 2007*], as well as prevention of dental fear, prevention of treatment induced pain and prevention of relapse [*Fábián & Fábián 2000, Fábián et al. 2007*]. Maintenance of the mental health of dental team is also crucial for the prevention of PDI [*Fejérdy et al. 2004*]. The most important knowledge in relation with premised fundamental parts of prevention will be introduced in details in *Chapter 5*.

Majority of psychogenic denture intolerance patients refuse to accept psychological background of their symptoms [*Ross et al 1953, Fábián et al. 2005, Schwichtenberg & Doering 2008*]; and instead of psychiatrists or psychotherapists, first they visit dentist and insist on the somatic origin of their symptoms [*Ross et al. 1953, Fábián et al. 2005*]. Therefore, a simple referral to psychiatrist and/or psychotherapist would not solve PDI related problems in most cases. Consequently, an initial psychosomatic therapy is needed prior to definitive therapy, which is a scope of dental profession's duty [*Moulton et al. 1957, Pomp 1974*]. However, if the dentist is to manage PDI in a responsible way, competent clinical and psychological skills are also needed [*Figgener 1996*]. No wonder that, the need of a sufficient number of dentist undertaking the double role of mental therapist and dentist was indicated more than forty years ago [*Schweitzer 1964*].

The most important goals of initial psychosomatic therapy are avoidance of further useless invasive dental treatment [*Brodine & Hartshorn 2004, Sarlani et al. 2005, Reewes & Merrill 2007, Baad-Hansen 2008*] as well as obtaining decrease (recovery) of symptoms and motivation of patients to participate in a definitive psychosomatic therapy (which is the highest level care of psychogenic denture intolerance patients). Gradual escalation of therapy and avoidance of irreversible forms of treatment are "cornerstones" of the initial psychosomatic therapy [*Laskin & Block 1986*]; which utilizes several placebo and/or palliative methods (i.e. physiotherapies, medication, medicinal herb therapy, diet therapy, CAM therapy etc.) combined with supportive communication techniques. Administration of any mind-body therapies as "basic therapeutics" for psychosomatic disorders [*Iversen 1989, Binder & Bider 1989, Krause 1994*] is also an important goal of initial therapy. In contrast to initial therapy, definitive psychosomatic therapy should be carried out by *specialized dental professionals* as members of a specialized *psychosomatic team* including *experienced dentists and other medical and psychotherapeutical professionals*. Definitive psychosomatic therapy should be offered for patients being refractory to the initial psychosomatic therapy, and for patients responding to it but without a stable treatment outcome in a long run (i.e. patients with frequent relapses). Fundamentals of the complex processes of both initial and definitive psychosomatic therapies of PDI will be discussed more detailed in *Chapter 6*.

Medicinal herb and diet therapy are important supplemental modalities of psychosomatic dental therapy. Maintenance of a proper nutritional status and proper use of medicinal herbs seems to be highly important to maintain oral health and to prevent several oral manifestations [*Touger-Decker 1998, 2003, Touger-Decker et al. 2007*]. Proper alterations of patients' diet and administration of medicinal herbs may also be used for therapeutic purposes efficiently. However, to avoid potential health hazards, great care should be taken especially in the case of patients with severe systemic diseases, during pregnancy or lactation. Similarly, great care should be taken if long run administration of medicinal herbs and/or long run modification of the patient's diet that incorporates patient's total health needs are needed [*Palmer 2003, Touger-Decker 2003, Touger-Decker et al. 2007, Zhang et al. 2008*]. In such cases consultation with (or referral to) a registered dietitian and/or internist and/or family doctor is highly recommended before starting diet therapy or medicinal herb therapy. The most important aspects of medicinal herb and diet therapy are discussed more detailed in *Chapter 7*.

Complementary and alternative medicine (CAM) denotes a wide range of variable therapies, including also treatments with established benefits and few if any side effects [*Wahner-Roedler et al. 2005, Fábián in press*]. CAM therapies emphasize self-care, which can lead to advantageously decreased load of the much more expensive health care system [*Tindle et al. 2005*]. No wonder that, complementary and alternative medicine is increasingly accepted and frequently utilized for children [*Sanders et al. 2003; Losier et al. 2005; Wall 2005*] and adults also in such highly developed countries like the United States [*Cuellar et al. 2003; Barnes et al. 2004; Honda & Jacobson 2005, Tindle et al. 2005*], several countries of the European Union [*Langmead et al. 2002; Menniti-Ippolito et al. 2002; Hanssen et al. 2005, Walach 2006*], Canada [*Losier et al. 2005*] and Australia [*MacLennan et al. 1996*].

More than the half (roughly 54% - 62%) of normal adult population uses any CAM method [*Honda & Jacobson 2005; Goldstein et al. 2005; Barnes et al. 2004*]. Roughly one third (ca. 20% - 35%) of CAM methods belongs to mind-body type CAM therapies [*Barnes et al. 2004; Honda & Jacobson 2005; Upchurch & Chyu 2005; Goldstein et al. 2005*] like Tai-Chi therapy, Qigong therapy, breathing exercises, yoga therapy and some similar therapies. This proportion is at least doubled when prayer is also included [*Barnes et al. 2004, Honda & Jacobson 2005, Wahner-Roedler et al. 2005, Tindle et al. 2005*]. The rest proportion of CAM therapies include several other approaches like acupuncture, sleep deprivation (vigil), fasting therapy, light therapy and several other therapies. An overview of complementary and alternative medicine is presented in *Chapter 8.*

REFERENCES

[1] Baad-Hansen, L. Atypical odontalgia - pathophysiology and clinical management. *J Oral Rehabil*, 2008 35, 1-11.

[2] Barnes, PM; Powell-Griner, E; McFann, K; Nahin, RL. *Complementary and alternative medicine use among adults: United States, 2002. Advance data from vital and health statistics; no 343.* Hyattsville, Maryland: National Center for Health Statistics; 2004. 1-20.

[3] Barsby, MJ. The use of hypnosis in the management of "gagging" and intolerance to dentures. *Br Dent J*, 1994 176, 97-102.

[4] Bensing, J. Bridging the gap. The separate worlds of evidence-based medicine and patient-centered medicine. *Patient Education Counseling*, 2000 39, 17-25.

[5] Binder, H. & Binder, K. *Autogenes Training, Basispsychotherapeutikum.* Köln: Deutscher Ärzteverlag; 1989.

[6] Brodine, AL. & Hartshorn, MA. Recognition and management of somatoform disorders. *J Prosthet Dent*, 2004 91, 268-273.

[7] Cuellar, N; Aycock, T; Cahill, B; Ford, J. Complementary and alternative medicine (CAM) use by African American (AA) and Caucasian American (CA) older adults in a rural setting: a descriptive comparative study. *BMC Compl Altern Med*, 2003 3, 8.

[8] Demmel, H-J. & Lamprecht, F. Zahnheilkunde. In: von Uexküll T, editor. *Psychosomatische Medizin.* München, Wien, Baltimore: Urban & Schwarzenberg; 1996; 1125-1130.

[9] Derra, C. Psychosomatische Diagnostik und Therapie des atypischen Gesichtsschmerzes. *ZWR*, 2002 111, 485-490.

[10] Doering, S. & Wolowski, A. Psychosomatik als interdisciplinäres Fach. *Zahnärztl Nachr Sachsen-Anhalt*, 2007 12, 7.

[11] Dworkin, SF. & Sherman J. Chronic orofacial pain: biobehavioral perspectives. In: Mostofsky DI, Forgione AG, Giddon, DB. *Behavioral dentistry.* Ames (Iowa): Blackwell Munksgaard; 2006; 99-113.

[12] Engel, G. The need for a new medical model: a challenge for biomedicine. *Science*, 1977 196, 129-136.

[13] Fábián, TK. *Mind-body connections. Pathways of psychosomatic coupling under meditation and other altered states of consciousness.* New York: Nova Science Publishers; in press.

[14] Fábián, TK & Fábián, G. Dental stress. In: Fink G, editor in chef. *Encyclopedia of Stress. Vol. 1.* San Diego: Academic Press; 2000; 657-659.

[15] Fábián, TK. & Fejérdy, P. Denture intolerance [Fogpótlás intolerancia]. In: Fábián TK, Vértes G editors. *Psychosomatic dentistry* [*Fogorvosi pszichoszomatika*]. Budapest: Medicina; 2007; 127-146.

[16] Fábián, TK; Mierzwińska-Nastalska, E; Fejérdy P. Photo-acoustic stimulation. A suitable method in the treatment of psychogenic denture intolerance. *Protet Stomatol,* 2006 56, 335-340.

[17] Fábián, TK; Krause, WR; Krause, M; Fejérdy, P. Photo-acoustic stimulation and hypnotherapy in the treatment of oral psychosomatic disorders. *Hypnos,* 2005 32, 198-202.

[18] Fábián, TK; Fábián, G; Fejérdy, P. Dental Stress. In: Fink G, editor in chef. *Encyclopedia of Stress. 2-nd enlarged edition, Vol. 1.* Oxford: Academic Press; 2007; 733-736.

[19] Fejérdy, P. & Orosz, M. Personality of the dentist and patient-assistant-dentist interrelationships [A fogorvos személyisége, a beteg-asszisztens-fogorvos kapcsolatrendszer] In: Vértes G. Fábián TK. (Eds.) *Psychosomatic dentistry [Fogorvosi Pszichoszomatika]* Budapest: Medicina; 2007; 22-31.

[20] Fejérdy, P; Fábián, TK; Krause, WR. Mentalhygienische Aufgaben von Krankenschwestern in der Zahnmedizin. Kommunikation mit den Patienten und dem Zahnarzt. *Deutsche Z Zahnärztl Hypn,* 2004 3, 32-34.

[21] Figgener, L. Non-acceptance of prosthetic appliances at the focus of forensic consequences. *J Forensic Odontostomatol,* 1996 14, 28-29.

[22] Freeman, R. The determinants of dental health attitudes and behaviors. *Brit Dent J,* 1999 187, 15-18.

[23] Goldstein, MS; Brown, ER; Ballard-Barbash, R; Morgenstern, H; Bastani, R; Lee, J; Gatto, N; Ambs, A. The use of complementary and alternative medicine among California adults with and without cancer. *eCAM,* 2005 2, 557-565.

[24] Green, CS. & Laskin, DM. Temporomandibular disorders: Moving from a dentally based to a medically based model. *J Dent Res,* 2000 79, 1736-1739.

[25] Hanssen, B, Grimsgaard, S; Lauso, L; Fonnebo, V; Falkenberg, T; Rasmussen, NK. Use of complementary and alternative medicine in the Scandinavian countries. *Scand J Prim Health Care,* 2005 23, 57-62.

[26] Honda, K. & Jacobson, JS. Use of complementary and alternative medicine among United States adults: the influences of personality, coping strategies, and social support. *Preventive Medicine,* 2005 40, 46-53.

[27] Iversen, G. Geleitwort. In: Binder, H; Binder, K. *Autogenes Training, Basispsychotherapeutikum.* Köln: Deutscher Ärzteverlag; 1989.

[28] Krause, WR. Hypnose und Autogenes Training (Selbsthypnose) in der Rehabilitation. Ergänzung in: Schultz, JH. *Hypnose-Technik. Praktische Anleitung zum Hypnotisieren für Ärzte.* 9. Auflage - bearbeitet und ergänzt von G. Iversen und W.-R. Krause. Stuttgart - Jena - New York: Gustav Fischer Verlag; 1994. 71-79.

[29] Langmead, L; Chitnis, M; Rampton, DS. Use of complementary therapies by patients with IBD may indicate psychosocial distress. *Inflam Bowel Dis*, 2002 8, 174-179.

[30] Laskin, DM. & Block, S. Diagnosis and treatment of myofacial pain-dysfunction (MPD) syndrome. *J Prosthet Dent*, 1986 56, 75-84.

[31] Losier, A; Taylor, B; Fernandez, CV. Use of alternative therapies by patients presenting to a pediatric emergency department. *J Emergency Med*, 2005 28, 267-271.

[32] MacLennan, AH; Wilson, DH; Taylor, AW. Prevalence and cost of alternative medicine in Australia. *Lancet*, 1996 347, 569-573.

[33] Marxkors, R. & Müller-Fahlbusch, H. Zur Diagnose psychosomatischer Störungen in der zahnärztlich-prothetischen Praxis. *Dtsch Zahnärztl Z*. 1981 36, 787-790.

[34] Menniti-Ippolito, F; Gargiulo, L; Bologna, E; Forcella, E; Raschetti, R. Use of unconventional medicine in Italy: a nation-wide survey. *Eur J Clin Pharmacol*, 2002 58, 61-64.

[35] Moulton, R; Ewen, S; Thieman, W. Emotional factors in periodontal disease. *Oral Surg Oral Med Oral Pathol*, 1957 5, 833-860.

[36] Müller-Fahlbusch, H. & Marxkors, R. *Zahnärztliche Psychagogik. Vom Umgang mit dem Patienten.* München, Wien: Carl Hanser Verlag; 1981.

[37] Müller-Fahlbusch, H. & Sone, K. Präprotetische Psychagogik. *Dtsch Zahnärztl Z*, 1982 37, 703-707.

[38] Newton, AV. The psychosomatic component in prosthodontics. *J Prosthet Dent*, 1984 52, 871-874.

[39] Pertes, RA. Differential diagnosis of orofacial pain. *Mt Sinai J Med*, 1998 65, 348-354.

[40] Piko, BF. & Kopp, MS. Paradigm shifts in medical and dental education: behavioral sciences and behavioral medicine. *Eur J Oral Sci*, 2004 8 (Suppl. 4.), 25-31.

[41] Palmer, CA. Gerodontic nutrition and dietary counseling for prosthodontic patients. *Dent Clin North Am*, 2003 47, 355-371.

[42] Pomp, AM. Psychotherapy for the myofascial pain-dysfunction syndrome: a study of factors coinciding with symptom remission. *JADA*, 1974 89, 629-632.

[43] Reeves 2nd, JL. & Merrill, RL. Diagnostic and treatment challenges in occlusal dysesthesia. *J Calif Dent Assoc*, 2007 35, 198-207.

[44] Ross, GL; Bentley, HJ; Greene Jr., GW. The psychosomatic concept in dentistry. *Psychosom Med*, 1953 15, 168-173.

[45] Sanders, H; Davis, MF; Duncan, B; Meaney, FJ; Haynes, J; Barton, LL. Use of complementary and alternative medical therapies among children with special health care needs in Southern Arizona. *Pediatrics*, 2003 111, 584-587.

[46] Sarlani, E; Balciunas, BA; Grace, EG. Orofacial pain - Part II. Assessment and management of vascular, neurovascular, idiopathic, secondary, and psychogenic causes. *AACN Clin Issues*, 2005 16, 347-358.

[47] Schweitzer, JM. *Oral rehabilitation problem cases. Treatment and evaluation. Vol. 2.* Saint Louis: C.V. Mosby Company; 1964; 611-625.

[48] Schwichtenberg, J. & Doering, S. Success of referral in a psychosomatic-psychotherapeutic outpatient unit of a dental school. *Z Psychosom Med Psychother*, 2008 54, 285-292.

[49] Sugawara, N; Shiozawa, I; Masuda, T; Takei, H; Tsuruta, J; Ogura, N; Hasegawa, S. A survey on condition of outpatients at prosthodontics II, University Hospital, Faculty of

Dentistry, Tokyo Medical and Dental University. *Kokubyo Gakkai Zasshi*, 1998 65, 251-259.

[50] Swoope, CC. Predicting denture success. *J Prosthet Dent*, 1973 30, 860-865.

[51] Tindle, HA; Wolsko, P; Davis, RB; Eisenberg, DM; Phillips, RS; McCarthy, EP. Factors associated with the use of mind body therapies among United States adults with musculoskeletal pain. *Compl Ther Med*, 2005 13, 155-164.

[52] Touger-Decker, R. Oral manifestations of nutrient deficiencies. *Mt Sinai J Med*, 1998 65, 355-361.

[53] Touger-Decker, R. Clinical and laboratory assessment of nutrition status in dental practice. *Dent Clin North Am*, 2003 47, 259-278.

[54] Touger-Decker, R; Mobley, CC; & American Dietetic Association; Position of the American Dietetic Association: oral health and nutrition. *J Am Diet Assoc*, 2007 107, 1418-1428.

[55] Upchurch, DM. & Chyu, L. Use of complementary and alternative medicine among American women. *Women's Health Issues*, 2005 15, 5-13.

[56] Wahner-Roedler, DL; Elkin, PL; Vincent, A; Thompson, JM; Oh, TH; Loehrer, LL; Mandrekar, JN; Bauer, BA. Use of complementary and alternative medical therapies by patients referred to a fibromyalgia treatment program at a tertiary care center. *Mayo Clin Proc*, 2005 80, 55-60.

[57] Walach, H. Verfahren der Komplementärmedizin. Beispiel: Heilung durch Gebet und Geistiges Heilen. *Bundesgesundheitsbl gesundheitsforsch Gesundheitschutz*, 2006 8, 788-795.

[58] Wall, RB. Tai Chi and Mindfulness-Based Stress Reduction in a Boston public middle school. *J Pediatr Health Care*, 2005 19, 230-237.

[59] Wolowski, A. Orale Implantologie bei Patienten mit orofazialer Somatisierungsstörung. *Stomatologie*, 2000 97, 11-16.

[60] Zhang, AL; Story, DF; Lin, V; Vitetta, L; Xue, CC. A population survey on the use of 24 common medicinal herbs in Australia. *Pharmacoepidemiol Drug Saf*, 2008 17, 1006-1013.

Chapter 2

CONCEPT AND BACKGROUND OF PSYCHOGENIC DENTURE INTOLERANCE

ABSTRACT

In general, roughly 10 percent of the dental patients may be counted as a *risk patient* for any psychosomatic manifestations, from which more than a third (roughly 3-4 % of all patients with dentures) suffer from psychogenic denture intolerance. This is a not too large but still significant proportion, and the incidence may increase. Since even two or three of such patients may unbalance dentist's entire schedule and can occupy a large percentage of the dentist's time; the importance of psychogenic denture intolerance should not be underestimated, but considered as a rather important and difficult problem of dentistry. Although early complete denture related studies sometimes missed the point that psychogenic denture intolerance may develop in relation to other kind of dentures as well; later on psychogenic problems related to other kinds of dentures were also analyzed, and lastly a "holistic view" of psychogenic denture intolerance emerged. In this approach, denture intolerance is recognized as a member of the "large family" of orofacial psychosomatic manifestations; and may be defined as *patient's refusal accepting or wearing* truly prepared (standard, properly made) *fixed* and/or *removable denture*(s) because of appearing *any kind of psychogenic* symptom(s) in relation to the *denture* or to the *treatment procedure*. An abbreviation derived from the first letters of *p*sychogenic *d*enture *i*ntolerance (namely "PDI") may also be introduced.

2.1. INTRODUCTION

In general, roughly 10 percent of the dental patients may be counted as a *risk patient* for any psychosomatic manifestations [*Doering & Wolowski 2007*], from which more than a third (roughly 3-4 % of all dental patients) suffer from psychogenic denture intolerance [*Fábián & Fejérdy 2007*]. This is a not too large but still significant proportion, and the incidence may increase [*Sugawara et al. 1998, Fábián & Fejérdy 2007*]. Since even two or three of such patients may unbalance dentist's entire schedule [*Schweitzer 1964*] and can occupy a large percentage of the dentist's time [*Swoope 1973*]; the importance of psychogenic denture intolerance should not be underestimated, but considered as a rather important and difficult problem of dentistry. The problem of psychogenic denture intolerance stood in the limelight of scientific interest in the second half of the last century. Although early complete denture related studies sometimes missed the point that psychogenic denture intolerance may develop in relation to other kind of dentures as well; later on, psychogenic problems related to other kinds of dentures (i.e. removable partial dentures and/or fixed dentures) were also analyzed, and lastly a "holistic view" of psychogenic denture intolerance emerged. In this approach, denture intolerance is recognized as a member of the "large family" of orofacial psychosomatic manifestations [*Ross et al. 1953, Schweitzer 1964, Marxkors & Müller-Fahlbusch 1981, Müller-Fahlbusch & Marxkors 1981, Müller-Fahlbusch & Sone 1982, Newton 1984, Demmel & Lamprecht 1996, Wolowski 2000*].

2.2. CONCEPT OF PSYCHOGENIC DENTURE INTOLERANCE

2.2.1. Emergence of the Concept

The problem of psychogenic denture intolerance stood in the limelight of scientific interest because of comparatively frequent unsuccess during making complete dentures (full dentures). Although complete denture related studies sometimes missed the point that psychogenic denture intolerance may develop in relation to other kind of dentures as well (i.e. partial removable and/or fixed dentures); huge knowledge of the psychological and psychopathological mechanisms behind psychogenic denture intolerance were collected based on this approach. Importance of patient's personality structure [*Seifert et al. 1962, Ismail et al. 1974, Levin & Landesman 1976, Drost 1978/a,b, Reeve et al. 1984*] and affective state [*Golebiewska et al. 1998*] as well as patient's level of psychosocial stress [*Swoope 1973*] level of anxiety [*Swoope 1973*] and level of fear of death [*Dolder 1956, Kranz 1956*] were recognized. Similarly, the importance of various unconscious psychological processes [*Dolder 1956, Kranz 1956, Levin & Landesman 1976, Drost 1978/a,b*] and several mental disorders [*Levin & Landesman 1976, Drost 1978/a,b*] were documented. Further, significance of dentist's personality [*Langer et al. 1961, Seifert et al. 1962, Hirsch et al. 1973*] and communication skills [*Guckes et al. 1978, Reeve et al. 1984*] and quality of patient management [*Seifert et al. 1962, Hirsch et al. 1972, Guckes et al. 1978, Reeve et al. 1984*] were acknowledged. The importance of several transference and counter-transference processes [*Drost 1978/a,b*] were also recognized based on such studies.

Similarly, patient's persistence and motivation [*Michman & Langer 1975*] as well as patient's expectations [*Levin & Landesman 1976*] and emotional involvement in the development of a symptom [*Holland-Moritz 1980*] were documented. The importance of socio-cultural factors [*Lowental & Tau 1980, Tau & Lowental 1980*], self-image [*Silverman et al. 1976, Tau & Lowental 1980*], body-image [*Kranz 1956, Ament & Ament 1970, Swoope 1973, Silverman et al. 1976*] and gender differences [*Massler 1951, Kotkin 1985*] were also recognized. The significant influence of menopausal processes [*Niedermeier et al. 1979*] and the importance of quantitative and qualitative parameters of saliva secretion [*Niedermeier 1991*] were also recognized. The significance of neuromuscular coordination and adaptation [*Michman & Langer 1975, Landt 1978*], multifold sensory functions of mouth and teeth

[*Balters 1956/a,b*], several masticatory learning processes [*Michman & Langer 1975*] and localization of the denture (i.e. upper or lower jaw) [*Seifert et al. 1962*] was also acknowledged. Finally, the important correlation between the satisfaction with dentures and the patient's ability to adjust to general health [*Emerson & Giddon 1955*] as well as the importance of written documentation (including the mutual agreement of objectives before treatment is begun) [*Swoope 1972*] was also documented based on complete denture related studies primarily.

On the base of premised findings (and collaterally), psychogenic problems related to other kinds of dentures (i.e. removable partial dentures and/or fixed dentures) were also analyzed, and lastly a "holistic view" of psychogenic denture intolerance emerged. In this approach, denture intolerance is recognized as a member of the "large family" of orofacial psychosomatic manifestations [*Ross et al. 1953, Schweitzer 1964, Marxkors & Müller-Fahlbusch 1981, Müller-Fahlbusch & Marxkors 1981, Müller-Fahlbusch & Sone 1982, Newton 1984, Demmel & Lamprecht 1996, Wolowski 2000*]. Studies based on this concept investigate both peculiarities and general aspects of denture related psychogenic symptoms from the viewpoint of orofacial psychosomatics as a whole and more general problem [*Schweitzer 1964, Marxkors & Müller-Fahlbusch 1981, Müller-Fahlbusch & Marxkors 1981, Müller-Fahlbusch & Sone 1982, Demmel & Lamprecht 1996, Wolowski 2000*].

Major role of provocative life events like traumas and object loss and the consequent appearance of depression was primarily documented based on this "holistic" approach [*Müller-Fahlbusch 1972, 1975, 1976, Hach et al. 1978, Holland-Moritz 1979, Müller-Fahlbusch & Marxkors 1981, Müller-Fahlbusch & Sone 1982, Fassbind 1985, Kaán et al. 2004, Gáspár et al. 2002*]. Accordingly, the significance of traumatizing dental events (frequently causing traumas and object loss) and their role as a significant provocative life event was also acknowledged [*Schweitzer 1964, Miller 1970, Marxkors 1975, Müller-Fahlbusch & Marxkors 1981, Müller-Fahlbusch & Sone 1982, Kaán et al. 2004*]. The importance of learning processes (including classic/operant conditioning or model learning) [*Ross et al. 1953, Newton 1984*] was emphasized as well. The meaning of symptom chronification processes induced by repeated unsuccessful somatic dental treatments [*Müller-Fahlbusch 1975, Wolowski 2000, Fábián et al. 2004, Fábián & Fejérdy 2007*] as well as the significance of primary and secondary gain from illness [*Ross et al. 1953*] were also recognized mainly on the base of this approach.

Similarly, importance of the rather complex patient-nurse-dentist interrelationships [*Miller 1970, Fábián & Fábián 2000, Fejérdy et al. 2004, Fejérdy & Orosz 2007, Fábián et al. 2007*], meaning of the dental team's mental health [*Gerbert et al 1992, Fejérdy et al. 2004, Tóth & Fábián 2006, Fábián 2007*], as well as the significance of proper timing of the prosthodontic treatment [*Müller-Fahlbusch 1992*] were documented. Meaning of the impact of oral health on quality of life [*Giddon & Hittelman 1980, Leao & Sheiham 1996, McGrath & Bedi 1998, 1999, Watanabe 1998*], patient's oral health behavior [*Weinstein et al. 1979, Kiyak 1996, MacEntee 1996*] and patient's oral health-related beliefs [*MacEntee 1996, McGuire et al. 2007*] were recognized as well. The importance of social [*Nakaminami et al. 1989*], existential [*Graham 2005, Fábián et al. 2006*] and spiritual/religious [*Fábián et al. 2005, Fábián 2007/a*] aspects of psychogenic denture intolerance were also emphasized based on the latter "holistic" approach primarily.

2.2.2. Definition of Psychogenic Denture Intolerance (PDI)

Considering above described emergence of its concept no wonder if yet there is currently no consensus on the etiology and pathogenesis of psychogenic denture intolerance. Similarly, there is neither a prevalent definition nor a current abbreviation for convenient use in the scientific literature of psychogenic denture intolerance. Thus, a consensus definition of psychogenic denture intolerance is still keeping us waiting. Therefore, psychogenic denture intolerance will be defined in the present work as follows: *Patient's refusal accepting or wearing* truly prepared (standard, properly made) *fixed* and/or *removable denture*(s) because of appearing *any kind of psychogenic* symptom(s) in relation to the *denture* or to the *treatment procedure* [*Fábián & Fábián 2000, Fábián et al. 2004, 2007*]. Further, an abbreviation derived from the first letters of *p*sychogenic *d*enture *i*ntolerance (namely "PDI") will also be used in the text.

2.3. IMPORTANCE OF PSYCHOGENIC DENTURE INTOLERANCE

2.3.1. Frequency of Occurrence of PDI

In general, roughly 10 percent of the dental patients may be counted as a *risk patient* for any psychosomatic manifestations [*Doering & Wolowski 2007*]. In the case of complete denture patients, roughly 10-15 % is *strongly* unsatisfied with the denture [*Ruskin & Leeds 1959, Langer et al. 1961, Carlsson et al. 1967, Bergman & Carlsson 1972, Sauer 1975, Smith 1976, Brunner & Aeschbacher 1981, Berg 1993*]. From premised strongly unsatisfied patients about every second or third case (roughly 5 % of all complete denture wearers) may be considered of primarily psychogenic origin [*Schröder 1977*]. Similarly, in case of removable partial dentures (RPDs), roughly 6-10 % of patients are *strongly* unsatisfied [*Hicklin & Brunner 1972, Brunner 1977, Schwalm et al. 1977*], from which at least every second (at least 3-5 % of all RPD wearers) are unsatisfied because of psychogenic origin [*Hicklin & Brunner 1972, Körber et al. 1975*]. In case of clasp-retained RPDs premised incidence of dissatisfaction even may be roughly doubled [*Wagner & Kern 2000, Mazurat & Mazurat 2003/a*]. Although patients are usually more satisfied with fixed dentures comparing to other ones (i.e. complete and partial removable dentures), the percentage of *strongly* unsatisfied patients is likely to be relatively high (roughly 6-10 %) also in this group [*Goodacre et al. 2003/a,b*]. From strongly unsatisfied patients roughly one fourth of the cases (about 2-3 % of fixed denture wearers) are of psychogenic origin [*Authors unpublished data*]. Based on above data it may be concluded that, a not too large but still significant proportion (at least 3-4 % [*Fábián & Fejérdy 2007*]) of denture wearers suffer from PDI, and the incidence may increase [*Sugawara et al. 1998, Fábián & Fejérdy 2007*]. Since even two or three of such patients may unbalance dentist's entire schedule [*Schweitzer 1964*] and can occupy a large percentage of the dentist's time [*Swoope 1973*]; the importance of this "not too large proportion" of PDI patients should not be underestimated, but should be considered as a rather important and difficult problem of dentistry.

2.3.2. Consequences of Denture Intolerance

The most important *primary consequence* of psychogenic denture intolerance is the *unsuccessful* repetition(s) of prosthodontic treatment and/or carrying out other invasive somatic intervention [*Ross et al. 1953, Schweitzer 1964, Müller-Fahlbusch 1976, Fábián 1999*] because of misunderstanding of symptoms and consequent misdiagnosis of the disorder [*Brodine & Hartshorn 2004*]. Premised unsuccessful treatments frequently lead to *secondary consequences* such as: (1) moderate or excessive loss of teeth and other oral tissues [*Ross et al. 1953, Schweitzer 1964, Müller-Fahlbusch 1976, Fábián 1999*]; (2) chronification and/or aggravation of the oral (orofacial) symptoms [*Ross et al. 1953, Müller-Fahlbusch 1975, Harris et al. 1993, Wolowski 1999, Fábián 1999*]; (3) chronification and/or aggravation of the psychiatric condition behind the symptoms [*Ross et al. 1953, Schweitzer 1964, Müller-Fahlbusch 1975*]; (4) initiation of a "new" psychiatric condition (i.e. depressive episode, somatoform disorder, psychotic episode etc.) [*Schweitzer 1964, Müller-Fahlbusch 1972, Fábián 1999*]; (5) initiation of a "new" psychosomatic disorder of a new target organ [*Ross et al. 1953*] either with [*Ross et al. 1953*] or without disappearance of the already existing oral psychogenic symptoms. There are also *tertiary consequences,* which may include: (1) spending of rather long time for treatment of such cases with the overload of both patient and dentist [*Ross et al. 1953, Schweitzer 1964; Harris et al. 1993, Brodine & Hartshorn 2004*]; (2) long-run disturbances of patient's relationships to any dentist [*Schweitzer 1964, Fábián 1999*]; (3) highly increased expenses because of the repeated treatments and possible legal procedures [*Harris et al. 1993, Curley 1997*]; (4) consequences of all premised elements on the general health and quality of life of patient [*Ross et al. 1953, Olsen-Noll & Bosworth 1989*] and dentist.

2.4. PSYCHOLOGICAL PECULIARITIES OF MOUTH AND TEETH

The orofacial region is an area of human privacy of special personality relevance with overproportional cortical representation, which appears to be particularly predisposed for a large number of different functional and somatoform psychosomatic disorders [*Kreyer 2000*]. There are several deep-seated psychological reasons for this sensitivity. The oral psychogenic manifestations (including PDI) are based on the unique psychological and dept-psychological function of the mouth, and teeth during infancy (breasting), sexuality, aggressiveness and communication [*Fábián & Fábián 2000, Fábián et al. 2000, 2007*]. There is also a great importance of the symbolic values of the mouth, teeth, tongue, and face [*Fábián & Fábián 2000, Fábián et al. 2000, 2007*]. The mouth (including the teeth and tongue) also serves as a primary zone of interaction with the environment, and as such can have far-reaching emotional significance [*Ament & Ament 1970, Benson 2000*]. It is surely tremendously important already in the baby's life as an organ through which to receive nourishment, as an organ of pleasure, as an organ of contact with the mother, as an organ of testing, learning and understanding and as an organ of social signal [*Ament & Ament 1970*]. The mouth should be considered also as a highly charged erotogenic region already from the childhood [*Ament & Ament 1970, Benson 2000*]. The mouth (including the teeth and tongue) is also a source of contention, and when speech comes, the mouth becomes a seat of power in a new sense as well [*Ament & Ament 1970*].

Psychoemotional consequences of certain traumas like the experience of forced feeding by parents in the childhood, as well as the forced manipulation of the tongue blade by the physician, or a forced (or even painful) approach by the dentist (already in the early childhood) should also be considered [*Ament & Ament 1970*]. The early traumatizing experience of the infant related to losing somebody (the baby must be taken off the breast) and destroying something (intake of food with the use of the teeth) is strongly coupled to the oral region and the teeth too. (Premised coupling may be especially important during the so-called oral stage and oral-sadistic stage of the psychological development [*Fábián et al. 2000, Fábián et al. 2006*].) Loss of milk teeth (deciduous teeth) is usually the first loss of any part of the body and the first significant injury of body image [*Ament & Ament 1970*]. Next, wearing orthodontic appliances may lead to shame and body image disturbances. In many cases the dental treatment may also be traumatic for adults, and the dental experience may be perceived as an "assault" which recapitulates the old feelings (i.e. from the childhood) of helplessness, aggression, defenselessness etc. [*Ament & Ament 1970*]. Tooth loss may profoundly affect the psychosocial well-being of patients, even those who are apparently coping well with dentures [*Fiske et al. 1998, Allen & McMillan 2003*]. Complete edentulousness is a serious life event which can be perceived as more stressful than retirement [*Bergendal 1989, Trullson et al. 2002*], because tooth loss (especially edentulousness) also symbolizes the loss of living force, and evokes a symbolic meaning of growing old, evanescence and death [*Fábián & Fábián 2000, Fábián et al. 2000, 2006, 2007*].

The importance of dental appearance to overall appearance is also rated high [*Hassel et al. 2008*], and tooth loss can have tremendous patient impact and social implication [*Roumanas 2009*]. Therefore, significant alteration of the patient's self image may occur with an increasingly worsened dental status [*Fiske et al. 1998, Trullson et al. 2002, Allen & McMillan 2003*]; which may lead (in the absence of dental restorations and/or dentures) to a self-image can be labeled as "becoming a deviating person" [*Trullson et al. 2002*]. Bed dental status also may lead to feeling of guilt and shame [*Trullson et al. 2002*]. Notwithstanding that, removable dentures may significantly improve oral health-related quality of life [*Adam et al. 2007, Ellis et al. 2007*]; living and coping with removable dentures (especially with full dentures) may lead to a self-image can be labeled as "becoming an uncertain person" [*Trullson et al. 2002*]. (Premised self-image may appear because of the uncertainty and insecurity when having to cope with a removable denture.) In order to manage premised uncertainty and being in control, patient often develops avoiding strategies to ensure that no-one would notice his/her removable denture [*Trullson et al. 2002*]. Such patient frequently keeps the hand in front of the mouth when talking or laughing, and avoids social interactions, especially when eating. These avoiding strategies contribute to restricted social participation and a further change (worsening) of self-image [*Trullson et al. 2002*].

Besides premised psychological and psychosocial aspects (see above), certain neuro*biological* aspects of the orofacial region should also be considered. Importantly, those tissues, which are of mesodermic origin in most part of the body, are of *ecto*dermic (ectomesodermic) origin in the orofacial region indicating a strong coupling of orofacial and nervous structures. Accordingly, stem cells present in the human dental pulp has a tendency to differentiate into functionally active neurons under certain experimental circumstances

[*Király et al. 2009*]; which may be another indication of the above mentioned relatively strong coupling of several orofacial and nervous tissues. Further, innervation of the orofacial region is originated from the brain stem (instead of spinal cord); which may also be a base of a strong influence of psycho-emotional functions on the orofacial tissues and function.

Premised peculiarities may also be responsible for the finding that, facial and masticatory muscles are highly sensitive to psycho-emotional processes, reacting earlier, stronger and longer lasting with muscle spasm to psychoemotional stress comparing to other muscles of the body [*Heggendorn et al. 1979*]. It is also likely that, increased activity of facial and masticatory muscles have a special extraordinary role in the attenuation (elimination due to motor activity) of psychoemotional stress [*Sato et al. in press*]. A similar extraordinary role in the attenuation of psychoemotional stress due to autonomic activity (i.e. similar to that of shedding tears) may also be expected in relation with the psychoemotional stress induced alterations of saliva secretion [*Fábián 2007/b*]. In addition, mouth, teeth and tongue act as organs of sense of touch temperature and taste, leading to a reach representation of these organs in the central nervous system [*Fábián et al. 2007*]. Taking together all above data it is no wonder that, the orofacial region is affected by psychosomatic manifestations much more frequently comparing to most other parts of the body [*Böning 1990*].

2.5. BACKGROUND FACTORS OF DENTURE INTOLERANCE

2.5.1. Psychiatric Background

In general, orofacial psychosomatic patients usually display a lower level of psychopathology comparing to psychiatric patients [*Meldolesi et al. 2000, Ommerborn et al. 2008*]. Although there are certain differences between several orofacial manifestations [*Auerbach et al. 2001, Ommerbor et al. 2008*], the *most frequently* appearing psychiatric background of most orofacial psychosomatic disorders are similar. The psychiatric background frequently include increased level of depression [*Müller-Fahlbusch & Sone 1982, Böning 1990, Trikkas et al. 1996, Meldolesi et al. 2000, Israel & Scrivani 2000, Toyofuku & Kikuta 2006*], increased level of anxiety [*Kampe et al. 1997, Meldolesi et al. 2000, Israel & Scrivani 2000*] and increased level of neuroticism [*Pilling 1983, Trikkas et al. 1996, al Quran et al. 2001, Fenlon et al. 2007*]. Conversion phenomena [*Engel 1951, Baker et al. 1961, Lupton 1969, Pilling 1983, Böning 1990, Meldolesi et al. 2000*], somatoform disorder [*Schwartz et al. 1979, Egle 1985, Reeves & Merrill 2007*], hypochondriasis [*Baker et al. 1961, Pilling 1983, Böning 1990, Meldolesi et al. 2000*], dysmorphophobia [*Pilling 1983, Böning 1990*] and alexithimia [*Sipilä et al. 2001, Ahlberg et al. 2004*] also frequently appear. Importantly, in some cases orofacial symptoms of a patient may serve as a defense *against* psychiatric *decompensation* (i.e. outbreak of paranoia or other *not yet* manifest psychotic symptoms) [*Lesse 1956, Delaney 1976, Violon 1980, Marbach 1978, Kaban & Belfer 1981, Fábián 1999*]. In rare cases, *manifest* (already decompensated) severe psychopathologies (including paranoid ideation or other psychosis) are clearly recognizable as a background of orofacial symptoms [*Marbach 1978, Kaban & Belfer 1981, Pilling 1983, Ommerborn et al. 2008*].

2.5.2. Personality

The characteristics displayed by many orofacial psychosomatic patients are high level of perceived stress (increased stress and/or stress sensitivity) [*Schwartz et al. 1979, Israel & Scrivani 2000*], dependence on family, friends and doctors [*Moulton et al. 1957, Lupton 1969, Pomp 1974, Israel & Scrivani 2000*], loss of self-esteem [*Israel & Scrivani 2000*], apathy [*Israel & Scrivani 2000*], and withdrawal behavior [*Israel & Scrivani 2000*]. Increased level of aggression [*Graber 1971, Frei & Graber 1976, Fallschüssel 1983*] anger [*Lupton 1969, Israel & Scrivani 2000*] and hostility [*Trikkas et al. 1996, Israel & Scrivani 2000*] (especially their introverted forms [*Fallschüssel 1983, Trikkas et al. 1996*]) also rather frequently appear. High degree of sense of responsibility may also be a cause in certain cases especially of symptoms of muscle dysfunction origin [*Serra-Negra et al. in press*]. Masochism and self-punishment [*Engel 1951, Lupton 1969, Violon 1980, Wolowski 2002*] is also not rare in the case of PDI patients. A marked tendency towards pharmacological drug tolerance and dependence also may appear [*Israel & Scrivani 2000*]. Low level of the sense of coherence (SOC) may also increase the frequency of occurrence of PDI symptoms [*Savolainen et al. 2005*]. However, even if there is a clear association between personality and dissatisfaction with dentures [*Klages et al. 2005*], it should not be assumed that, PDI is a deficiency of personality [*Salter et al. 1983, Marbach 1992, Dahlström 1993, Fiske et al. 1998, Allen & McMillan 2003*]. Moreover, in certain cases weaknesses of PDI patients' personality may also be a consequence (rather than a cause) of the appearing unpleasant or torturing symptoms [*McCall et al. 1961, Kaban & Belfer 1981, Salter et al. 1983, Marbach 1992, Dahlström 1993*]. Similarly, the psycho-emotional traumatism caused by tooth loss and consequent need of denture wearing may also lead to personality alterations [*Fiske et al. 1998, Allen & McMillan 2003*].

2.5.3. Gender

Most of the orofacial psychogenic symptoms are much more prevalent in women than in men. Gender difference is especially obvious in the case of temporomandibular disorders [*Lundeen et al. 1986, Sarlani et al. 2005/a, Ommerborn et al. 2008*] and other oral and orofacial pain symptoms [*Sarlani et al. 2005/a,b, Ommerborn et al. 2008*], as well as in the case of xerostomia [*Guggenheimer & Moore 2003*], irritative/allergic reactions to dental materials [*Garhammer et al. 2001, Vamnes et al. 2004, van Noort et al. 2004*] and denture induced inflammatory fibrous tissue hyperplasia [*Macedo-Firoozmand et al. 2005*]. Similarly, soft tissue parafunctions (such as buccal mucosa ridging and tongue indentation) [*Piquero et al. 1999*] more frequently occur in female than in male. Interestingly, presence of a preferred chewing side (which may lead to several disadvantageous consequences and symptoms [*Miyake et al. 2004, Diernberger et al. 2008*]) also occur more frequently in women [*Diernberger et al. 2008*]. Depending on symptom, female/male ratio can be roughly between 2:1 and 8:1 in these cases [*Laskin & Block 1986, Garhammer et al. 2001, Sarlani et al. 2005/a,b, Ommerborn et al. 2008*].

A gender difference is also likely to exist in relation with PDI, affecting more women than men [*Müller-Fahlbusch & Sone 1982, Wöstmann 1996*]. Denture related chewing difficulties [*Foerster et al. 1998, Pan et al. 2008*] and esthetic problems are likely to occur more frequently in women [*Baran et al. 2007, Pan et al. 2008*]. There is likely also a gender difference in the acceptance (or refusal) of tooth extraction as a treatment possibility [*Hunter & Arbona 1995*], and in the use of dentures [*Hunter & Arbona 1995*]. General satisfaction is also likely to be lower in female than male [*Hassel et al. 2008, Pan et al. 2008*]. However, it should also be considered that, the appearance of a gender difference is likely to be depending on the type of denture [*Pan et al. 2008*]. Some data in the literature [*Baran et al. 2007, Pan et al. 2008*] as well as authors' experience may indicate that, PDI related gender differences are not as pronounced as in the case of other orofacial symptoms.

2.5.4. Age

It is rather difficult to interpret the possible influence of age on the incidence of PDI. *There are some symptoms, which may appear in relatively young patients, whereas others may appear in adults or in the elderly.* Bruxism frequently appear already in the childhood [*Ozaki et al. 1990, Widmalm et al. 1995, Glaros 2006, Serra-Negra et al. in press*]; and soft tissue parafunctions also appear relatively early, with the highest frequency of occurrence in the 20 to 29 years age group [*Piquero et al. 1999*]. TMD and related symptoms appear somewhat later, but still relatively early with a maximum frequency of occurrence in the 20 to 40 years age group [*Laskin & Block 1986, Lundeen et al. 1986*]. Irritative/allergic reactions to dental materials most frequently appear in the age group of 40 to 49 years [*Lygre et al. 2003, Vamnes et al. 2004*]. Presence of a preferred chewing side (with several disadvantageous consequences [*Diernberger et al. 2008*]) occurs most frequently in the age group of 40 to 69 years [*Diernberger et al. 2008*]. Frequency of occurrence of most other types of denture related psychological symptoms are likely to increase with age [*Wöstmann 1996, Ringland et al. 2004, Ommerborn et al. 2008*] with a maximum at the 50 to 60 years age group [*Wöstmann 1996*].

There are likely to be *six major age dependent factors* behind the relatively late appearance of most PDI symptoms (comparing to parafunction and TMD) as follows: (1) there is a clear association between age and the irreversible complications during prosthetic rehabilitation [*De Backer et al. 2007*]; (2) perceived oral health rating worsens gradually with increase of number of compromised and missing teeth [*Cunha-Cruz et al. 2007*] (thus also with age); (3) frequency of occurrence of denture discomfort increases gradually with increase of the number of missing teeth [*Cunha-Cruz et al. 2007*] (thus also with age); (4) frequency of appearance of uneasiness, nervousness, self-consciousness during social gathering increases gradually with increase of the number of missing teeth [*Cunha-Cruz et al. 2007*] (thus also with age); (5) an increase of the incidence of PDI at the age of menopause (in women) and also at the age of pensioning (in both genders) is also very likely to occur [*Friedlander 2002, Frutos et al. 2002, Fábián & Fejérdy 2007*]; (6) there is a noticeable rise in the number of depressions and other abnormal reactions of organic origin in the older age groups [*Müller-Fahlbusch 1983*].

On the other hand, denture satisfaction [*Müller et al. 1994*] and complaint intensity on the initial visit [*Lowenthal & Tau 1980*] do not necessarily increase but may even decrease with age [*Müller et al. 1994, Lowenthal & Tau 1980*]. Farther, there is no simple linear association between *common* oral health-related quality of life and the number of missing teeth [*Cunha-Cruz et al. 2007*]. Common oral health-related quality of life worsen with increase of the number of missing teeth *only up to a maximum of 8 - 11 missing teeth*; but thereafter it *improves* with farther increase of number of missing teeth [*Cunha-Cruz et al. 2007*]. Similarly, frequency of occurrence of irritative/allergic mucosal reactions increases with age in adults, with a maximum at the 50 to 60 years age group; however, thereafter the incidence significantly decreases in higher age groups [*Garhammer et al. 2001*]. Thus, *several significant PDI related parameters* including complaint intensity on the initial visit and common oral health-related quality of life as well as the frequency of occurrence of mucosal irritative/allergic reactions *is not necessarily worsen with age, moreover it may even improve in the elderly* [*Lowenthal & Tau 1980, Garhammer et al. 2001, Cunha-Cruz et al. 2007*].

2.5.5. Social- and General Health Factors

In an image-conscious society, dentures restore a sense of normalcy and allow the patient the ability to interact with others [*Roumanas 2009*]. No wonder that, majority of patients in such societies are primarily focused on *social meaning of the mouth* (rather than physical function of teeth) when defining subjective need for replacement of missing teeth [*Graham et al. 2006*]. Besides influencing the *subjective* need for tooth replacement [*Graham et al. 2006, Müller et al. 2007*], social factors significantly influence the acceptance (or refusal) of tooth extraction as a dental treatment possibility [*Müller et al. 2007*]. Similarly, social factors significantly influence patients' preference related to fixed versus removable dentures [*Zittmann et al. 2007*] and the level of perceived oral health [*Atchison & Gift 1997*]. *Ethnocultural* background is likely to be another important factor influencing social meaning of mouth and teeth [*Lowenthal & Tau 1980, Payne & Locker 1994, Strauss 1996, Kawamura et al. 2005*]. In contrast, there is no clear evidence in relation with the *socioeconomic status*. Subjects of higher socioeconomic status may be more likely to accept dentures [*Allen & McMillan 2003, Ringland et al. 2004*], however not necessarily the socioeconomic status itself, but the high self-image [*Silvermann et al. 1976*] and premised social meaning of the mouth (and teeth) are likely to be the primary factors in this case. *Perceived general health* [*Emerson & Giddon 1955, Moroi et al. 1999*] and *mental well-being* [*Moroi et al. 1999*] also significantly improve general denture satisfaction, especially because level of perceived *general health status* significantly influences and positively correlates with the level of perceived oral health [*Atchison & Gift 1997, Tickle et al. 1997*]. Being unable to travel alone may also increase the frequency of appearance of tooth-, mouth- or denture related problems [*Ringland et al. 2004*].

2.6. CONCLUSION

In summary, even though prosthesis is fabricated conscientiously and properly, there is no assurance that the patient will be comfortable while wearing it or satisfied with the therapy [*Mazurat & Mazurat 2003/b*]. A normative evaluation by a dentist and a subjective evaluation by the patient related to the denture or to the dental treatment may be rather different [*Lechner & Roessler 2001*]. The factors not related to operative/technological dental skills that contribute to the success of denture wearing are becoming more and more important [*Ma et al. 2008*].

REFERENCES

[1]   Adam, RZ; Geerts, GA; Lalloo, R. The impact of new complete dentures on oral health-related quality of life. *SADJ*, 2007 62, 264-268.

[2]   Ahlberg, J; Nikkilä, H; Könönen, M; Partinen, M; Lindholm, H; Sarna, S; Savolainen, A. Associations of perceived pain and painless TMD-related symptoms with alexithymia and depressive mood in media personnel with or without irregular shift work. *Acta Odontol Scand*, 2004 62, 119-123.

[3]   Al Quran, F; Clifford, T; Cooper, C; Lamey, PJ. Influence of psychological factors on the acceptance of complete dentures. *Gerodontology*, 2001 18, 35-40.

[4]   Allen, PF. & McMillan, AS. A review of the functional and psychosocial outcomes of edentulousness treated with complete replacement dentures. *J Can Dent Assoc*, 2003 69, 662.

[5]   Ament, P. & Ament, A. Body image in dentistry. *J Prosthet Dent*, 1970 24, 362-366.

[6]   Atchison, KA. & Gift, HC. Perceived oral health in a diverse sample. *Adv Dent Res*, 1997 11, 272-280.

[7]   Baker, EG; Crook, GH; Schwabacher, ED. Personality correlates of periodontal disease. *J Dent Res*, 1961 40, 396-403.

[8]   Balters, W. Die Bedeutung von Zahnverlust und Zahnersatz für den Patienten - von der Psychologie her gesehen. *Dtsch Zahnärztl Z*, 1956/a 11, 112-120.

[9]   Balters, W. Die Bedeutung von Zahnverlust und Zahnersatz für den Patienten - von der Psychologie her gesehen. (Fortsetzung). *Dtsch Zahnärztl Z*, 1956/b 11, 465-468.

[10]   Baran, I; Ergün, G; Semiz, M. Socio-demographic and economic factors affecting the acceptance of removable dentures. *Eur J Dent*, 2007 2, 104-110.

[11]   Benson, PE. Suggestion can help. *Ann R Australas Coll Dent Surg*, 2000 15, 284-285.

[12]   Berg, E. Acceptance of full dentures. *Int Dent J*, 1993 43, 299-306.

[13]   Bergendal, B. The relative importance of tooth loss and denture wearing in Swedish adults. *Community Dent Health*, 1989 6, 103-111.

[14]   Bergman, B. & Carlsson, GE. Review of 54 complete denture wearers. Patients' opinions 1 year after treatment. *Acta Odont Scand*, 1972 30, 399-414.

[15]   Böning, J. Psychosomatic and psychopathological aspects in dental-orofacial medicine with special reference to old age. *Z Gerontol*, 1990 23, 318-321.

[16]   Brodine, AH. & Hartshorn, MA. Recognition and management of somatoform disorders. *J Prosthet Dent*, 2004 91, 268-273.

[17]   Brunner, T. Spätresultate mit hybriden Prothesen unterschiedlicher Konstruktion. *Schweiz Mschr Zahnheilk*, 1977 87, 1135-1137.

[18]   Brunner, T. & Aeschbacher, A. Nachkontrolle von Totalprothesen aus der Zürcher Volkszahnklinik - I. Ergebnisse einer Patientenbefragung nach mehr als 10jähriger Tragezeit. *Schweiz Mschr Zahnheilk*, 1981 91, 87-105.

[19]   Carlsson, GE; Otterland, A; Wennström, A. Patient factors in appreciation of complete dentures. *J Prosthet Dent*, 1967 17, 322-328.

[20]   Cunha-Cruz, J; Hujoel, PP; Kressin, NR. Oral health-related quality of life of periodontal patients. *J Periodont Res*, 2007 42, 169-176.

[21]   Curley, AW. Malpractice - The dentist's perspective. *J Am Coll Dent*, 1997 64, 21-24.

[22]   Dahlström, L. Psychometrics in temporomandibular disorders. An overview. *Acta Odontol Scand*, 1993 51, 339-352.

[23]   De Backer, H; Van Maele, G; De Moor, N; Van der Berghe, L. The influence of gender and age on fixed prosthetic restoration longevity: an up to 18- to 20-year follow-up in an undergraduate clinic. *Int J Prosthodont*, 2007 20, 579-586.

[24]   Delaney, JF. Atypical facial pain as a defense against psychosis. *Am J Psychiat*, 1976 133, 1151-1154.

[25]   Demmel, H-J. & Lamprecht, F. Zahnheilkunde. In: von Uexküll T, editor. *Psychosomatische Medizin*. München, Wien, Baltimore: Urban & Schwarzenberg; 1996; 1125-1130.

[26]   Diernberger, S; Bernhardt, O; Schwahn, C; Kordass, B. Self-reported chewing side preference and its association with occlusal, temporomandibular and prosthodontic factors: results from the population-based study of health in Pomerania (SHIP-0). *J Oral Rehabil*, 2008 35, 613-620.

[27]   Doering, S. & Wolowski, A. Psychosomatik als interdisciplinäres Fach. *Zahnärztl Nachr Sachsen-Anhalt*, 2007 12, 7.

[28]   Dolder, E. Zur Psychologie des Zahn-Verlustes und des Zahn-Ersatzes. *Dtsch Zahnärztl Z*, 1956 11, 469-477.

[29]   Drost, R. Sogenannte prothesenunverträglichkeit (oder: Die nichtacceptierte Prothese). Psychosomatische Aspekte - I. Teil -. *ZWR*, 1978 87, 848-852.

[30]   Drost, R. Sogenannte prothesenunverträglichkeit (oder: Die nichtacceptierte Prothese). Psychosomatische Aspekte - II. Teil -. *ZWR*, 1978 87, 907-913.

[31]   Egle, UT. Auf der Suche nach den Wurzeln psychogen bedingter Mund-Krankheiten. *Zahnärztliche Mitteilungen*, 1985 75, 2413-2420.

[32]   Ellis, JS; Pelekis, ND; Thomason, JM. Conventional rehabilitation of edentulous patients: the impact on oral health-related quality of life and patient satisfaction. *J Prosthodont*, 2007 16, 37-42.

[33]   Emerson, WA. & Giddon, DR. Psychologic factors in adjustment to full denture prothesis. *J Dent Res*, 1955 34, 683-684.

[34]   Engel, GL. Primary atypical facial neuralgia: hysterical conversion symptom. *Psychosom Med*, 1951 13, 375-396.

[35]   Fallschüssel, GKH. Persönlichkeitsprofil und Persönlichkeitsentwicklung von Patienten mit Funktionsstörungen im Kausystem. *Deutsch Zahnärztl Z*, 1983 38, 670- 674.

[36]   Fábián, TK. Treatment possibilities of denture intolerance. Use of photo-acoustic stimulation and hypnotherapy in a difficult clinical case. [Adalékok a protézis

intolerancia gyógyításához. Fény-hang kezeléssel kombinált hipnoterápia alkalmazásának szokatlan módja egy eset kapcsán.] *Hipno Info*, 1999 38, 81-88.

[37] Fábián, TK. Mental health and pastoral counseling [Mentálhigiéné és lelkigondozás]. In: Fábián TK, Vértes G. editors. *Psychosomatic dentistry [Fogorvosi pszichoszomatika]*. Budapest: Medicina; 2007/a; 158-168.

[38] Fábián, TK. Psychosomatics of salivation problems [A nyálszekréciós zavarok pszichoszomatikája]. In: Fábián TK, Vértes G editors. *Psychosomatic dentistry [Fogorvosi pszichoszomatika]*. Budapest: Medicina; 2007/b; 121-126.

[39] Fábián, TK. & Fábián, G. Dental stress. In: Fink G, editor in chef. *Encyclopedia of Stress. Vol. 1*. San Diego: Academic Press; 2000; 657-659.

[40] Fábián, TK. & Fejérdy, P. Denture intolerance [Fogpótlás intolerancia]. In: Fábián TK, Vértes G editors. *Psychosomatic dentistry [Fogorvosi pszichoszomatika]*. Budapest: Medicina; 2007; 127-146.

[41] Fábián, TK; Vértes, G; Tóth, Zs. Some depth-psychological aspects of the psychogenic symptoms of the orofacial tissues. *Fogorv Szle*, 2000 93, 262-267.

[42] Fábián, TK; Kovács, Sz; Müller, O; Fábián, G; Marten, A; Fejérdy, P. Some aspects of existential psychotherapy in dentistry. *Fogorv Szle*, 2006 99, 246.

[43] Fábián, TK; Kaán, B; Fejérdy, L; Tóth, Zs; Fejérdy, P. Effectiveness of psychotherapy in the treatment of denture intolerance. Evaluation of 25 cases. *Fogorv Szle*, 2004 97, 163-168.

[44] Fábián, TK; Vértes, G; Fejérdy, P. Pastoral psychology, spiritual counseling in dentistry. Review of the literature. *Fogorv Szle*, 2005 98, 37-42.

[45] Fábián, TK; Kovács, Sz; Müller, O; Fábián, G; Marten, A; Fejérdy, P. Some aspects of existential psychotherapy in dentistry. *Fogorv Szle*, 2006 99, 246.

[46] Fábián, TK; Fábián, G; Fejérdy, P. Dental Stress. In: Fink G, editor in chef. *Encyclopedia of Stress. 2-nd enlarged edition, Vol. 1*. Oxford: Academic Press; 2007; 733-736.

[47] Fassbind, O. Psychogene Prothesenunverträglichkeit: Therapiemöglichkeiten. *Schweiz Mschr Zahnmed*, 1985 95, 595-598.

[48] Fejérdy, P; Fábián, TK; Krause, W-R. Mentalhygienische Aufgaben von Krankenschwestern in der Zahnmedizin. Kommunikation mit den Patienten und dem Zahnarzt. *Dtsch Z Zahnärztl Hypn*. 2004 4; 32-34.

[49] Fejérdy, P. & Orosz, M. Dentist's personality, patient-nurse-dentist interrelationships [A fogorvos személyisége, a beteg-asszisztens-fogorvos kapcsolatrendszer]. In: Fábián TK, Vértes G editors. *Psychosomatic dentistry [Fogorvosi pszichoszomatika]*. Budapest: Medicina; 2007; 22-31.

[50] Fenlon, MR; Sherriff, M; Newton, JT. The influence of personality on patients' satisfaction with existing and new complete dentures. *J Dentistry*, 2007 35, 744-748.

[51] Fiske, J; Davis, DM; Frances, C; Gelbier, S. The emotional effects of tooth loss in edentulous people. *Brit Dent J*, 1998 184, 90-93.

[52] Foerster, U; Gilbert, GH; Duncan, RP. Oral functional limitation among dentate adults. *J Public Health Dent*, 1998 58, 202-209.

[53] Frei, P. & Graber, G. Der Kaumuskelsynchronisator (KMS). Gesteuerte funktionelle Therapie der Myoarthropathien. des Kiefergelenkes. *Schweiz Monatsch Zahnheilk (SMfZ/RMSO)*, 1976 86, 1195-1206.

[54] Friedlander, AH. The physiology, medical management and oral implications of menopause. *JADA*, 2002 133, 73-81.

[55] Frutos, R; Rodríguez, S; Miralles, L; Machuca, G. Oral manifestations and dental treatment in menopause. *Med Oral*, 2002 7, 26-35.

[56] Garhammer, P; Schmalz, G; Hiller, KA; Reitinger, T; Stolz, W. Patients with local adverse effects from dental alloys: frequency, complaints, symptoms, allergy. *Clin Oral Invest*, 2001 5, 240-249.

[57] Gáspár, J; Fejérdy, L; Fábián, TK. Psychic aspects of the overactive gag reflex (gagging) in connection with a clinical case. *Fogorv Szle*, 2002 95, 199-267.

[58] Gerbert, B; Bernzweig, J; Bleecker, T; Bader, J; Miyasaki, C. How dentists see themselves, their profession, the public. *JADA*, 1992 123, 72-78.

[59] Giddon, DB. & Hittelman, E. Psychologic aspects of prosthodontic treatment for geriatric patients. *J Prosthet Dent*, 1980 43, 374-379.

[60] Glaros, AG. Bruxism. In: Mostofsky DI, Forgione AG, Giddon, DB editors. *Behavioral dentistry*. Ames (Iowa): Blackwell Munksgaard; 2006; 127-137.

[61] Golebiewska, M; Sierpińska, T; Namiot, D; Likeman, PR. Affective state and acceptance of dentures in elderly patients. *Gerodontology*, 1998 15, 87-92.

[62] Goodacre, CJ; Bernal, G; Rungcharassaeng, K; Kan, YKK. Clinical complications in fixed prosthodontics. *J Prosthet Dent*, 2003/a 90, 31-41.

[63] Goodacre, CJ; Bernal, G; Rungcharassaeng, K; Kan, YKK. Clinical complications with implant and implant prostheses. *J Prosthet Dent*, 2003/b 90, 121-132.

[64] Graber, G. Psychisch motivierte Parafunktionen auf Grund von Aggressionen und Myoarthropathien des Kauorgans. *Schweiz Monatsch Zahnheilk (SMfZ/RMSO)*, 1971 81, 713-718.

[65] Graham, G. Two case-histories of ladies who were unable to wear their dentures without feeling sick and retching. *Hypnos*, 2005 32, 210-212.

[66] Graham, R; Mihaylov, S; Jepson, N; Allen, PF; Bond, S. Determining "need" for a removable partial denture: a qualitative study of factors that influence dentist provision and patient use. *Brit Dent J*, 2006 200, 155-158,

[67] Guckes, AD; Smith, DE; Swoope, CC. Counseling and related factors influencing satisfaction with dentures. *J Prosthet Dent*, 1978 39, 259-267.

[68] Guggenheimer, J. & Moore, PA. Xerostomia. Etiology, recognition and treatment. *JADA*, 2003 134, 61-69.

[69] Hach, B; Lehrl, S; Niedermeier, W. Psychopathological and psychopathometric findings in patients with dental prosthesis intolerance. *Dtsch Zahnärztl Z*, 1978 33, 238-244.

[70] Harris, M; Feinmann, C; Wise, M; Treasure, F. Temporomandibular joint and orofacial pain: clinical and medicolegal management problems. *Brit Dent J*, 1993 174, 129-136.

[71] Hassel, AJ; Wegener, I; Rolko, C; Nitschke, I. Self-rating of satisfaction with dental appearance in an elderly German population. *Int Dent J*, 2008 58, 98-102.

[72] Heggendorn, H; Voght, HP; Graber, G. Experimentelle Untersuchungen über die orale Hyperaktivität bei psychischer belastung, im besonderen bei Aggression. *Schweiz Mschr Zahnheilk*, 1979 89, 1148-1161.

[73] Hicklin, B. & Brunner, Th. Ergebnisse einer Nachkontrolle von doppelseitigen Freiendprothesen im Unterkiefer aus der Kantonalen Volkszahnklinik Zürich. *Schweiz Mschr Zahnheilk*, 1972 82, 735-762.

[74] Hirsch, B; Levin, B; Tiber, N. Effects of patient involvement and esthetic preference on denture acceptance. *J Prosthet Dent*, 1972 28, 127-132.

[75] Hirsch, B; Levin, B; Tiber, N. Effects of dentist authoritarianism on patient evaluation of dentures. *J Prosthet Dent*, 1973 30, 745-748.

[76] Holland-Moritz, R. Systematische Befunderhebung bei Zahnersatzunverträglichkeit. *Dtsch Zahnärztl Z*, 1979 34, 786-788.

[77] Holland-Moritz, R. Zahnersatzunverträglichkeit und Schleimhautbrennen. *Dtsch Zahnärztl Z*. 1980 35, 948-952.

[78] Hunter, JM. & Arbona, SI. The tooth as a marker of developing world quality of life: a field study in Guatemala. *Soc Sci Med*, 1995 41, 1217-1240.

[79] Ismail, Y; Zullo, T; Kruper, D. The use of the psychological screening inventory as a predictor of problem denture patients. *J Dent Res*, 1974 54 (spec. issue. A), L128.

[80] Israel, HA. & Scrivani, SJ. The interdisciplinary approach to oral, facial and head pain. *JADA*, 2000 131, 919-926.

[81] Kaán, B; Tóth, Zs; Fábián, TK. The role of sexual trauma as a cause of orofacial symptoms. Case report. *Fogorv Szle*, 2004 97, 37-40.

[82] Kaban, LB. & Belfer, ML. Temporomandibular joint dysfunction: an occasional manifestation of serious psychopathology. *J Oral Surg*, 1981 39, 742-746.

[83] Kampe, T; Edman, G; Bader, G; Tagdae, T; Karlsson, S. Personality traits in a group of subjects with long-standing bruxing behavior. *J Oral Rehabil*, 1997 24, 588-593.

[84] Kawamura, M; Wright, FA; Declerck, D; Freire, MC; Hu, DY; Honkala, E; Lévy, G; Kalwitzki, M; Polychronopoulou, A; Yip, HK; Kinirons, MJ; Eli, I; Petti, S; Komabayashi, T; Kim, KJ; Razak, AA; Srisilapanan, P; Kwan, SY. An exploratory study on cultural variations in oral health attitudes, behavior and values of freshman (first-year) dental students. *Int Dent J*, 2005 55, 205-211.

[85] Kreyer, G. Psychosomatics of the orofacial system. *Wien Med Wochenschr*, 2000 150, 213-216.

[86] Király, M; Porcsalmy, B; Pataki, A; Kádár, K; Jelitai, M; Molnár, B; Hermann, P; Gera, I; Grimm, WD; Ganss, B; Zsembery, A; Varga, G. Simultaneous PKC and cAMP activation induces differentiation of human dental pulp stem cells into functionally active neurons. *Neurochem Int*, 2009 55, 323-332.

[87] Kiyak, HA. Measuring psychosocial variables that predict older persons' oral health behavior. *Gerodontology*, 1996 13, 69-75.

[88] Klages, U; Esch, M; Wehrbein, H. Oral health impact in patients wearing removable prostheses: relations to somatization, pain sensitivity, and body consciousness. *Int J Prosthodont*, 2005 18, 106-111.

[89] Kotkin, H. Diagnostic significance of denture complaints. *J Prosthet Dent*, 1985 53, 73-77.

[90] Körber, E; Lehman, K; Pangidis, C. Kontrolluntersuchungen an parodontal und parodontal-gingival getragenen Prothesen. *Dtsch Zahnärztl Z*. 1975 30, 77.

[91] Kranz, H. Zahnverlust und Zahnersatz als psychologisches Problem. *Dtsch Zahnärztl Z*, 1956 11, 105-112.

[92] Landt, H. Adaptationsprobleme bei der oralen prothetischen Rehabilitation des alternden Menschen. In: Körber E, editor. *Die zahnärztlich-protetische Versorgung des älternden Menschen*. München, Wien: Carl Hanser Verlag; 1978; 69-92.

[93] Langer, A; Michman, J; Seifert, I. Factors influencing satisfaction with complete dentures in geriatric patients. *J Prosthet Dent*, 1961 11, 1019-1031.

[94] Laskin, DM. & Block, S. Diagnosis and treatment of myofacial pain-dysfunction (MPD) syndrome. *J Prosthet Dent*, 1986 56, 75-84.

[95] Leao, A. & Sheiham, A. The development of a socio-dental measure of dental impacts on daily living. *Community Dent Health*, 1996 13, 22-26.

[96] Lechner, SK. & Roessler, D. Strategies for complete denture success: beyond technical excellence. *Compend Contin Educ Dent*, 2001 22, 553-559.

[97] Lesse, S. Atypical facial pain syndromes of psychogenic origin. Complications of their misdiagnosis. *J Nerv Ment Dis*, 1956 124, 346- 351.

[98] Levin, B. & Landesman, HM. A practical questionnaire for predicting denture success or failure. *J Prosthet Dent*, 1976 35, 124-130.

[99] Lowenthal, U. & Tau, S. Effects of ethnic origin, age, and bereavement on complete denture patients. *J Prosthet Dent*, 1980 44, 133-136.

[100] Lundeen, TF; Levitt, SR; McKinney, MW. Discriminative ability of the TMJ scale: age and gender differences. *J Prosthet Dent*, 1986 56, 84-92.

[101] Lupton, DE. Psychological aspects of temporomandibular joint dysfunction. *JADA*, 1969 79, 131-136.

[102] Lygre, GB; Gjerdet, NR; Grønningsæter, AG; Björkman, L. Reporting on adverse reactions to dental materials - intraoral observations at a clinical follow-up. *Community Dent Oral Epidemiol*, 2003 31, 200-206.

[103] Ma, H; Sun, HQ, Ji, P. How to deal with esthetically overcritical patients who need complete dentures: A case report. *J Contemp Dent Pract*, 2008 9, 22-27.

[104] Macedo Firoozmand, L; Dias Almeida, J; Guimarães Cabral, LA. Study of denture-induced fibrous hyperplasia cases diagnosed from 1979 to 2001. *Quintessence Int*, 2005 36, 825-829.

[105] MacEntee, MI. Measuring the impact of oral health in old age: a qualitative reaction to some quantitative views. *Gerodontology*, 1996 13, 76-81.

[106] Marbach, JJ. Phantom bite syndrome. *Am J Psychiatry*, 1978 135, 476-479.

[107] Marbach, JJ. The "temporomandibular pain dysfunction syndrome" personality: fact or fiction? *J Oral rehabil*, 1992 19, 545-560.

[108] Marxkors, R. Psychische Konditionierung. *ZWR*, 1975 84, 461-462.

[109] Marxkors, R. & Müller-Fahlbusch, H. Zur Diagnose psychosomatischer Störungen in der zahnärztlich-prothetischen Praxis. *Dtsch Zahnärztl Z.* 1981 36, 787-790.

[110] Massler, M. Oral manifestations during the female climacteric (the postmenopausa syndrome). *Oral Surg Oral Med Oral Pathol*, 1951 4, 1234-1243.

[111] Mazurat, NM. & Mazurat, RD. Discuss before fabricating: Communicating the realities of partial denture therapy. Part I: Patient expectations. *J Can Dent Assoc*, 2003/a 69, 90-94.

[112] Mazurat, NM. & Mazurat, RD. Discuss before fabricating: Communicating the realities of partial denture therapy. Part II: Clinical outcomes. *J Can Dent Assoc*, 2003/b 69, 90-94.

[113] McCall, CM; Szmyd, L; Ritter, RM. Personality characteristics in patients with temporomandibular joint symptoms. *JADA*, 1961 62, 694-698.

[114] McGrath, C. & Bedi, R. A study of the impact of oral health on the quality of life of older people in the UK - findings from a national survey. *Gerodontology*, 1998 15, 93-98.

[115] McGrath, C. & Bedi, R. The importance of oral health to older people's quality of life. *Gerodontology*, 1999 16, 59-63.

[116] McGuire, L; Millar, K; Lindsay, S. A treatment trial of an information package to help patients accept new dentures. *Behav Res Ther*, 2007 45, 1941-1948.

[117] Meldolesi, GN; Picardi, A; Accivile, E; Toraldo di Francia, R; Biondi, M. Personality and psychopathology in patients with temporomandibular joint pain-dysfunction syndrome. *Psychother Psychosom*, 2000 69, 322-328.

[118] Michman, J. & Langer, A. Postinsertion changes in complete dentures. *J Prosthet Dent*, 1975 34, 125-134.

[119] Miller, AA. Psychological Considerations in Dentistry, *JADA*, 1970 81, 941-947.

[120] Miyake, R; Ohkubo, R; Takehara, J; Morita, M. Oral parafunctions and association with symptoms of temporomandibular disorders in Japanese university students. *J Oral Rehabil*, 2004 31, 518-523.

[121] Moroi, HH; Okimoto, K; Terada, Y. The effect of an oral prosthesis on the quality of life for head and neck cancer patients. *J Oral Rehabil*, 1999 26, 265-273.

[122] Moulton, R; Ewen, S; Thieman, W. Emotional factors in periodontal disease. *Oral Surg Oral Med Oral Pathol*, 1957 5, 833-860.

[123] Müller, F; Wahl, G; Fuhr, K. Age-related satisfaction with complete dentures, desire for improvement and attitudes to implant treatment. *Gerodontology*, 1994 11, 7-12.

[124] Müller, F; Naharro, M; Carlsson, GE. What are the prevalence and incidence of tooth loss in the adult and elderly population in Europe? *Clin Oral Implants Res*, 2007 18 (suppl. 3), 2-14.

[125] Müller-Fahlbusch, H. Über situative Provokation endogener depressiver Phase. *Med Welt*, 1972 23, 919.

[126] Müller-Fahlbusch, H. Nervenärztliche Befunde bei Prothesenunverträglichkeits-erscheinungen *ZWR*, 1975 84, 574-578.

[127] Müller-Fahlbusch, H. Nervenärztliche Aspekte der Prothesenunverträglichkeit. *Dtsch Zahnärztl Z*, 1976 31, 13-17.

[128] Müller-Fahlbusch, H. Psychosomatic aspects of stomatology in the aged. *Z Gerontol*, 1983 16, 66-69.

[129] Müller-Fahlbusch, H. Therapie nach erkannter psychosomatischer Störung. *Dtsch Zahnärztl Z*, 1992 47, 157-161.

[130] Müller-Fahlbusch, H. & Marxkors, R. *Zahnärztliche Psychagogik. Vom Umgang mit dem Patienten*. München, Wien: Carl Hanser Verlag; 1981.

[131] Müller-Fahlbusch, H. & Sone, K. Präprotetische Psychagogik. *Dtsch Zahnärztl Z*, 1982 37, 703-707.

[132] Nakaminami, T; Omae, T; Akanishi, M; Maruyama, T. Psychosomatic aspects of the patients with stomatognathic dysfunction. 2. *Nihon Hotetsu Shika Gakkai Zasshi*, 1989 33, 395-400.

[133] Newton, AV. The psychosomatic component in prosthodontics. *J Prosthet Dent*, 1984 52, 871-874.

[134] Niedermeier, W. Physiology and pathophysiology of the minor salivary glands. *Dtsch Z Mund Kiefer Gesichtschir*, 1991 15, 6-15.

[135] Niedermeier, W; Becker, H, Christ, F; Habermann, PG. Effect of menopausal syndromes on symptoms of denture intolerance. *Schweiz Mschr Zahnheilk*, 1979 89, 1011-1018.

[136] Olsen-Noll, CG; Bosworth, MF. Anorexia and weight loss in the elderly. Causes range from loose dentures to debilitating illness. *Postgrad Med*, 1989 85, 140-144.

[137] Ommerborn, MA; Hugger, A; Kruse, J; Handschel, JGK; Depprich, RA; Stüttgen, U; Zimmer, S; Raab, WHM. The extent of the psychological impairment of prosthodontic outpatients at a German University Hospital. *BMC Head & Face Med*, 2008 4, 23.

[138] Ozaki, M; Ishii, K; Ozaky, Y; Hayashida, H; Motokawa, W. Psychosomatic study on the relation between oral habits and personality characteristics of the children in a mountain village. *Shoni Shikagaku Zassi*, 1990 28, 699-709.

[139] Pan, S; Awad, M; Thomason, JM; Dufresne, E; Kobayashi, T; Kimoto, S; Wollin, SD; Feine, JS. Sex differences in denture satisfaction. *J Dentistry*, 2008 36, 301-308.

[140] Payne, BJ. & Locker, D. Preventive oral health behaviors in a multi-cultural population: the North York Oral Health Promotion Survey. *J Can Dent Assoc*, 1994 60, 129-130.

[141] Pilling, LF. Psychiatric aspects of diagnosis and treatment. In: Laney WR, Gibilisco JA editors *Diagnosis and treatment in prosthodontics*. Philadelphia: Lea & Febiger; 1983; 129-140.

[142] Piquero, K; Ando, T; Sakurai, K. Buccal mucosa ridging and tongue indentation: incidence and associated factors. *Bull Tokyo Dent Coll*, 1999 40, 71-78.

[143] Pomp, AM. Psychotherapy for the myofascial pain-dysfunction syndrome: a study of factors coinciding with symptom remission. *JADA*, 1974 89, 629-632.

[144] Reeve, PE; Watson, CJ; Stafford, GD. The role of personality in the management of complete denture patients. *Brit Dent J*, 1984 156, 356-362.

[145] Reeves 2nd, JL. & Merrill, RL. Diagnostic and treatment challenges in occlusal dysesthesia. *J Calif Dent Assoc*, 2007 35, 198-207.

[146] Ringland, C; Taylor, L; Bell, J; Lim, K. Demographic and socio-economic factors associated with dental health among older people in NSW. *Aust N Z J Public Health*, 2004 28, 53-61.

[147] Ross, GL; Bentley, HJ; Greene Jr., GW. The psychosomatic concept in dentistry. *Psychosom Med*, 1953 15, 168-173.

[148] Roumanas, ED. The social solution - denture esthetics, phonetics, and function. *J Prosthodont*, 2009 18, 112-115.

[149] Ruskin, IR. & Leeds, MH. Dentistry for the elderly. *JADA*, 1959 59, 1248-1250.

[150] Salter, M; Brooke, RI; Merskey, H; Fichter, GF; Kapusianyk, DH. Is the temporomandibular pain and dysfunction syndrome a disorder of the mind? *Pain*, 1983 17, 151-166.

[151] Sarlani, E; Balciunas, BA; Grace, EG. Orofacial pain - Part I. Assessment and management of musculoskeletal and neuropathic causes. *AACN Clin Issues*, 2005/a 16, 333-346.

[152] Sarlani, E; Balciunas, BA; Grace, EG. Orofacial pain - Part II. Assessment and management of vascular, neurovascular, idiopathic, secondary, and psychogenic causes. *AACN Clin Issues*, 2005/b 16, 347-358.

[153] Sato, C; Sato, S; Takashina, H; Ishii, H; Onozuka, M; Sasaguri, K. Bruxism affects stress responses in stressed rats. *Clin Oral Invest*, in press. DOI: 10.1007/s00784-009-0280-6

[154] Sauer, G. Beurteilung und Traggewohnheiten von totalem Zahnersatz - Ergebnisse einer Patientenbefragung. *Dtsch zahnärztl Z*, 1975 30, 702-705.

[155] Savolainen, J; Suominen-Taipale, AL; Hausen, H; Harju, P; Uutela, A; Martelin, T; Knuuttila, M. Sense of coherence as a determinant of the oral healt-related quality of life: a national study of Finnish adults. *Eur J Oral Sci*, 2005 113, 121-127.

[156] Schröder, D. Nachuntersuchungsbefunde bei Vollprothesenträgern. *Dtsch Zahnärztl Z*, 1977 32, 976-980.

[157] Schwalm, CA; Smith, DE; Erickson, JD. A clinical study of patients 1 to 2 years after placement of removable partial dentures. *J Prosthet Dent*, 1977 38, 380-391.

[158] Schwartz, RA; Green, C; Laskin, DM. Personality characteristics of patients with myofascial pain-dysfunction (MPD) syndrome unresponsive to conventional therapy. *J Dent Res*, 1979 58, 1435-1439.

[159] Schweitzer, JM. *Oral rehabilitation problem cases. Treatment and evaluation. Vol. 2.* Saint Louis: C.V. Mosby Company; 1964; 611-625.

[160] Seifert, I; Langer, A; Michmann, J. Evaluation of psychologic factors in geriatric denture patiens. *J Prosthet Dent*, 1962 12, 516-523.

[161] Serra-Negra, JM; Ramos-Jorge, ML; Flores-Mendoza, CE; Paiva, SM; Pordeus, IA. Influence of psychosocial factors on the development of sleep bruxism among children. *Int J Paediatr Dent*, in press.

[162] Silverman, S; Silverman, SI; Silverman, B; Garfinkel, L. Self-image and its relation to denture acceptance. *J Prosthet Dent*, 1976 35, 131-141.

[163] Sipilä, K; Veijola, J; Jokelainen, J; Järvelin, MR; Oikarinen, KS; Raustia, AM; Joukamaa, M. Association of symptoms of TMD and orofacial pain with alexithymia: an epidemiological study of the Northern Finland 1966 Birth Cohort. *Cranio*, 2001 19, 246-251.

[164] Smith, M. Measurement of personality traits and their relation to patient satisfaction with complete dentures. *J Prosthet Dent*, 1976 35, 492-503.

[165] Strauss, RP. Culture, dental professionals and oral health values in multicultural societies: measuring cultural factors in geriatric oral health research and education. *Gerodontology*, 1996 13, 82-89.

[166] Sugawara, N; Shiozawa, I; Masuda, T; Takei, H; Tsuruta, J; Ogura, N; Hasegawa, S. A survey on condition of outpatients at prosthodontics II, University Hospital, Faculty of Dentistry, Tokyo Medical and Dental University. *Kokubyo Gakkai Zasshi*, 1998 65, 251-259.

[167] Swoope, CC. Identification and management of emotional patients. *J Prosthet Dent*, 1972 27, 434-440.

[168] Swoope, CC. Predicting denture success. *J Prosthet Dent*, 1973 30, 860-865.

[169] Tau, S. & Lowental, U. Some personality determinants of denture preference. *J Prosthet Dent*, 1980 44, 10-12.

[170] Tickle, M; Craven, R; Worthington, HV. A comparison of the subjective oral health status of older adults from deprived and affluent communities. *Community Dent Oral Epidemiol*, 1997 25, 217-222.

[171] Tóth, Zs. & Fábián, TK. Relaxation techniques in dentistry. *Fogorv Szle*, 2006 99, 15-20.

[172] Toyofuku, A. & Kikuta, T. Treatment of phantom bite syndrome with milnacipran - a case series. *Neuropsych Dis Treatment*, 2006 2, 387-390.

[173] Trikkas, G; Nikolatou, O; Samara, C; Bazopoulou-Kyrkanidou, E; Rabavilas, AD; Christodoulou, GN. Glossodynia: personality characteristics and psychopathology. *Psychother Psychosom*, 1996 65, 163-168.

[174] Trulsson, U; Engstrand, P; Berggren, U; Nannmark, U; Brånemark, PI. Edentulousness and oral rehabilitation: experiences from the patients' perspective. *Eur J Oral Sci*, 2002 110, 417-424.

[175] Vamnes, JS; Lygre, GB; Grönningsæter, AG, Gjerdet, NR. Four years of clinical experience with an adverse reaction unit for dental biomaterials. *Community Dent Oral Epidemiol*, 2004 32, 150-157.

[176] van Noort, R; Gjerdet, NR; Schedle, A; Björkman, L. Berglund, A. An overview of the current status of national reporting systems for adverse reactions to dental materials. *J Dentistry*, 2004 32, 351-358.

[177] Violon, A. The onset of facial pain. A psychological study. *Psychother Psychosom*, 1980 34, 11-16.

[178] Wagner, B. & Kern, M. Clinical evaluation of removable partial dentures 10 years after insertion: success rates, hygienic problems, and technical failures. *Clin Oral Investig*, 2000 4, 74-80.

[179] Watanabe, I. Masticatory function and life style in aged. *Nippon Rogen Igakkai Zasshi*, 1998 35, 194-200.

[180] Weinstein, P; Milgrom, P; Ratener, P; Morrison, K. Patient dental values and their relationship to oral health status, dentist perceptions and quality of care. *Community Dent Oral Epidemiol*, 1979 7, 121-127.

[181] Widmalm, SE; Christiansen, RL; Gunn, SM. Oral parafunctions as temporomandibular disorder risk factors in children. *Cranio*, 1995 13, 242-246.

[182] Wolowski, A. Prohesenunverträglichkeit. *Zahnärztl Mitteilungen*, 1999 89, 1246-1250.

[183] Wolowski, A. Orale Implantologie bei Patienten mit orofazialer Somatisierungsstörung. *Stomatologie*, 2000 97, 11-16.

[184] Wolowski, A. Bruxismus und psychovegetative Spannungszustände. *Zahnärztl Mitteilungen*, 2002 92, 30-33.

[185] Wöstmann, B. Psychogene Zahnersatzunverträglichkeit. In: Sergl HG editor *Psychologie und Psychosomatik in der Zahnheilkunde*. München - Wien - Baltimore: Urban & Schwarzenberg; 1996; 187-213.

[186] Zitzmann, NU; Hagmann, E; Weiger, R. What is the prevalence of various types of prosthetic dental restorations in Europe? *Clin Oral Implant Res*, 2007 18 (Suppl. 3), 20-33.

Chapter 3

PATHOMECHANISMS AND CLINICAL MANIFESTATIONS

ABSTRACT

There are various symptoms of psychogenic denture intolerance including pain manifestations, neuromuscular symptoms, immune and inflammatory reactions as well as several other symptoms like cognitive-behavioral symptoms, salivation related problems, halithosis, alterations of taste sensation, alterations of speech, pseudoneurological symptoms etc. Premised symptoms can be triggered due to the preparation, insertion or wearing of fixed and/or removable dentures. Their pathomechanisms may include both somatic and psychogenic mechanisms. PDI related symptoms are usually multifactorial (multicausal), therefore both somatic and psychogenic pathways of pathomechanism should be considered carefully for both diagnosis and treatment. It is also highly important to recognize the "point of attack" at which psychogenic pathways join major somatic pathways of pathomechanisms. Especially, because somatic type treatment modalities (i.e. physiotherapy, medication therapy, diet- or medicinal herb therapy etc.) may be introduced most efficiently at that particular point of pathomechanism (and along) within the frame of multimodal therapies utilizing both somatic type and psychological approaches. Therefore, besides the most important clinical findings, fundamentals of the pathomechanisms including recognized psychogenic pathways as well as major somatic pathways will be introduced in this chapter.

3.1. INTRODUCTION

There are various symptoms of psychogenic denture intolerance including pain manifestations, neuromuscular symptoms, immune and inflammatory reactions as well as several other symptoms like cognitive-behavioral symptoms, salivation related problems, halithosis, alterations of taste sensation, alterations of speech, pseudoneurological symptoms etc. [*Fábián & Fábián 2000; Fábián et al. 2006, 2007/a*]. Premised symptoms can be triggered due to the preparation, insertion or wearing of fixed and/or removable dentures [*Fábián & Fábián 2000, Fábián et al. 2006, 2007/a*]. There are various pathways, which can lead to a denture induced appearance of such symptoms. Some of these pathways are primarily of somatic origin (including also preparative and/or technical causes), whereas others are primarily psychogenic. Pathways of somatic origin are more or less well characterized, whereas much less is known about the *concrete* pathomechanisms of most psychogenic manifestations. However, it is very likely that, pathways of psychogenic manifestations join major somatic pathways at a certain level of pathomechanism. Therefore, besides the most important clinical findings, fundamentals of the pathomechanisms including recognized psychogenic pathways as well as major somatic pathways will be introduced in this chapter.

3.2. PAIN MANIFESTATIONS

3.2.1. Concept and Features of Pain

Pain is an unpleasant sensory and emotional experience associated with actual or potential tissue damage, or described in terms of such damage [*Merskey 1979*]. Pain is a multifaceted and multilevel phenomenon including a specific sensation, a variable emotional state, an aspect of interoception and a specific behavioral motivation [*Carli 2009*]; all of which are strongly influenced by personality, cultural background, as well as social and economic factors [*Dworkin & Sherman 2006, Vanhaudenhuyse et al. 2009*]. Previous pain experiences [*Vanhaudenhuyse et al. 2009*], the significance of the organ involved [*Vanhaudenhuyse et al. 2009*], local pain threshold of tissues [*Ogawa et al. 2004*] as well as individual's current pain tolerance, mood (depression) and level of anxiety also influence pain experience significantly [*Dworkin & Sherman 2006*]. There are three major components of pain such as *psychogenic-*, *neuropathic-* and *nociceptive* pain components [*Burton 1969, Gerbershagen 1995, Baldry 2005*]. Importantly, pain of *vascular* and *muscular* origin also *belong to nociceptive pain*, because nociceptors of blood vessels or muscles (or other related tissues) are the primary sources of pain impulses in these cases [*Baldry 2005*] (see also *paragraphs 3.2.2., 3.2.10., 3.2.15.*) In some cases pain symptom is solely due to a single pain component; in other cases two or three components may be present concomitantly [*Burton 1969, Gerbershagen 1995, Baldry 2005*].

3.2.2. Major Pain Components

Psychogenic pain components are induced by the dysfunction of the mind [*Baldry 2005*], usually because of several psychiatric disorders including primarily somatoform disorders, depression or psychotic disorders. Psychogenic pain component usually belongs to the core of psychopathology and play an important role to maintain and keep the (pathological) balance of the personality and/or to prevent decompensation. Psychogenic pain component also plays an important role in patient's communication, may symbolically refer to the underlying psychological problem or may express patient's anger, disappointment or need for warmth and help. *Neuropathic pain component* is caused by an injury or damage of the central or peripheral nerval tissues [*Baldry 2005*]. In such cases the injury or structural damage cause a transient or permanent disruption of the pain sensory apparatus, so that a normal pattern of neural activity is no longer transmitted [*Fields 1987, Baldry 2005*]. Therefore, those cells whose peripheral pain related input has been cut increase their excitability (they are "searching" for inputs) to such an extent that, they begin to fire either spontaneously or to distant inappropriate inputs [*Melzack & Wall 1988, Baldry 2005*]. *Nociceptive pain component* develops because of the primary activation and/or sensitization of nociceptors in any tissues [*Baldry 2005*] including the facial skin, the oral mucosa, the bone, a muscle, a tendon, an articular capsule, a blood vessel, a lymph vessel, a viscera etc.. Nociceptive pain of the skin and oral mucosa is typically superficial and not radiating. Nociceptive pain of other origin is usually deep-seated, frequently radiating (referred pain), and concomitant autonomic phenomena frequently appear. Nociceptive pain also frequently triggers off several muscular responses.

3.2.3. Pain Related Nervous Structures

The *pain related nervous structures* that are of particular importance in the complex processes of oral and orofacial pain are: (1) *sensory receptors* including pain signaling *mechanosensitive nociceptors*, *thermosensitive nociceptors* and *polymodal nociceptors* as well as several other not pain-related receptors such as mechanoreceptors or thermal receptors; (2) their *associated afferent trigeminal nerve* fibers such as low conduction velocity *C-fibers* conducting impulses of mechanoreceptors, thermal receptors and *mechanosensitive- thermosensitive-* and *polymodal* nociceptors [*Zimmermann 2004, Baldry 2005*], and high conduction velocity *A-delta fibers* conducting impulses of mechanoreceptors, thermal receptors and *mechanosensitive nociceptors* [*Zimmermann 2004, Baldry 2005*]. The highest conduction velocity *A-beta fibers* conduct signals of sensitive mechanoreceptors, but not those of nociceptors [*Zimmermann 2004*]; (3) *brainstem* including the *nuclei of the trigeminal nerve*, and their connecting nervous paths (*interneurons*) towards the ascending and descending pain tracts as well as towards the reticular formation; (4) the *ascending pain tracts* which could be either those which conduct pain signals of spinal cord (i.e. spinoreticular tract, spinothalamic tract, and spinomesencephalic tract) [*Treede & Magerl 2003, Zimmermann 2004*], or could be other not yet recognized or clearly characterized ascending nervous paths conducting pain stimuli of trigeminal nerve; (5) *descending inhibitory* serotonergic-, endomorphinergic- and noradrenergic *tracts*; and the *local* ("segmental") *inhibitory interneurons* acting on the postsynaptic receptors of the ascending tracts [*Gebhardt et al. 1984, Fields & Basbaum 1994, Strasbaugh & Levine 2000*]; (6) *reticular formation* which is a dense net-like mass of neurons with overlapping and intertwining dendrites that ramifies throughout the brainstem [*Baldry 2005*]. It is responsible primarily for pain related changes of arousal level, attention as well as for pain related autonomic changes of breathing-, cardiac- and vascular function. Reticular formation also mediates descending inhibition of pain due to the descending inhibitory tracts [*Zimmermann 2004*]; (7) *thalamus* responsible for pain related affective, autonomic and hormonal changes due to the *medial thalamic nuclei* being interconnected with the *limbic* system and the *hypothalamic-pituitary-adrenocortical axis,* as well as for determination of quality and localization of pain due to the *lateral thalamic nuclei* being interconnected with the *somatosensory cortex*. Importantly, concomitant activation of both premised groups of thalamic nuclei is needed for the appearance of a real pain experience indicating a key position of thalamus in pain experience [*Peyron et al. 2000, Zimmermann 2004, Baldry 2005*]; (8) *other subcortical structures* including periaqueductal grey, locus ceruleus, and nuclei of the raphe which modulate pain impulses and mediate descending inhibition due to the descending inhibitory tracts (mentioned above) [*Gebhardt et al. 1984, Fields & Basbaum 1994, Strasbaugh & Levine 2000, Baldry 2005*]; (9) *somatosensory cortex* responsible for the integration of pain related sensory stimuli with other sensory inputs (i.e. visual, acoustic, tactile, mechanosensory, somatesthesic, kinesthesic, thermal, taste, smell); (10) *frontal cortex and limbic system* which are responsible for the highest integration resulting in pain experience, pain related cognitive and emotional activities, changes of mood, as well as initiation of pain related behavioral-, autonomic- and hormonal responses [*Zimmermann 2004, Baldry 2005*].

3.2.4. Concomitant Phenomena of Pain

There are also several *concomitant phenomena of pain* including hormonal-, autonomic nervous- and motor responses. *Hormonal changes* are primarily because of the activation of the *hypothalamic-pituitary-adrenocortical axis* (HPA axis) due to the *medial thalamic nuclei*, and consequent release of the major stress hormone cortisol. *Autonomic nervous changes* occur *either* due to the *reticular formation* resulting in a shift towards sympathetic activation and consequent changes of breathing-, cardiac- and vascular function, *or* due to *local* ("segmental") *autonomic brainstem reflexes* [*Zimmermann 2004*]. *Motoric responses* may occur either because of a pain related *general increase of muscle tone* induced by several higher brain centers of pain sensation (i.e. limbic system, thalamus, hypothalamus, reticular formation) or because of *local motor reflexes of brainstem origin*. Local motor reflexes include prompt protective muscle reflexes and reflex myospasm. *Protective muscle reflexes* (see also *paragraphs 3.3.3., 3.3.5., 3.3.6.*) are triggered by suddenly appearing nociceptive pain of the facial skin and oral mucosa, and result in pulling away the head (i.e. accidental facial injuries), or reflex jaw opening (i.e. accidental biting on tongue, lip or cheek). *Reflex myospasm* (see also *paragraph 3.3.3.*) may occur as a frequent concomitant phenomena of deep-seated pain of any tissues.

3.2.5. Local Radiation of Pain

Local radiation of pain leading to *local (near) referred pain* is also a frequent *concomitant phenomenon* of pain, especially when deep-seated pain appears (i.e. painful teeth radiating pain into other teeth or the ear). There are two basic theories of pain radiation, namely the theory of *convergence* and the theory of *facilitation* [*Ganong 1990*]. Both theories hypothesize that, the number of peripheral sensory fibers are higher than the number of ascending sensory fibers; therefore, an only ascending fiber should conduct stimuli arriving from more than one afferent fiber [*Ganong 1990*]. *Convergence theory* hypothesizes that, conducing stimuli of more than one afferent fibers *via* an only ascending fiber may lead to mislocalization of conducted impulses resulting in pain (or other sensory) radiation phenomena [*Ganong 1990*]. *Theory of facilitation* hypothesizes that *sub*liminal impulses arriving from more than one afferent fibers to an only ascending fiber may increase the excitability of this ascending fibers to such an extent that it begin to fire in an inappropriate manner, which may lead to misdetermination of impulse quality. Consequently, higher brain centers may recognize non-painful sensory stimuli as if they were nociceptive pain stimuli [*Ganong 1990*]. Although both convergence- and facilitation theories are important, *both theories have some weaknesses* and none of them explains the appearance of referred pain thoroughly. (Please consider that: following the convergence theory, administration of local anesthesia into a referred pain area should not have any effect on the referred pain at issue; however, such a treatment clearly can lead to improvement in some cases. Similarly, following the facilitation theory, administration of local anesthesia into a referred pain area should have an analgesic effect in all the cases; however, such a treatment lead to improvement in some (but far not all) of the cases only.)

3.2.6. Distant Radiation of Pain

Distant radiation of pain may also occur, according to the location of *dermatomes* which are *skin* areas having sensory innervations from the same central nervous segment. Visceral pain is frequently radiated into the dermatome of that central nervous segment, which the visceral organ itself belongs to [*Gerbershagen 1995*]. This phenomenon is referred to as "*rule of dermatome*" which (at least partly) may also be explained utilizing the theories of *convergence* or *facilitation* (as described above). Importantly, radiating visceral pain usually *does not cover the whole dermatome* surface, but specific smaller areas of the dermatome, which are referred to as *Head-zones* [*Hansen & Schliack 1962, Gerbershagen 1995*]. Although the "classical" dermatomes typically belong to the spinal cord segments; brainstem is also considered as a "segment" of the central nervous system in this relation, and *skin innervations areas of the branches of trigeminal nerve are considered as dermatomes of the facial region* [*Gerbershagen 1995*]. There are also smaller facial skin areas located roughly concentric around the mouth called „*trigeminal projection fields*" [*Gerbershagen 1995*] which are considered as *facial Head zones*. Importantly, facial dermatomes or facial head zones may become targets of distant pain radiations (referred pain symptoms) originating from those visceral organs having their innervations from the brainstem (i.e. *via* the vagus nerve or glossopharyngeal nerve). Please note that, referred pain appearing in facial dermatomes (or facial Head zones) can be the presenting symptom of cardiac angina pectoris or myocardial infarction [*Sandler et al. 1995*] and on rare occasions of lung cancer [*Sarlani et al. 2005/b*].

3.2.7. Inflammation Related Pain

Inflammation related pain is another important phenomenon, which should also be considered in relation with orofacial pain symptoms. Pain sensitivity of nociceptors can be enhanced by numerous agents of immune/inflammatory processes (i.e. bradikinin, interleukins, prostaglandins, serotonin etc.) which phenomenon is referred to as *nociceptor sensitization* [*Zimmermann 2004*]. This process occurs in a few seconds or minutes, and triggers a release of *neuropeptides* (i.e. Substance-P, CGRP) from the afferent neuron. Since neuropeptides facilitate inflammatory processes, a *circulus vitiosus* appears and the sensitization of *very low sensitivity* "*silent nociceptors*" occurs [*Zimmermann 2004*]. Importantly, a release of neuropeptides also occurs at the *central endings* of the afferent fibers, and certain neuropeptides (especially Substance-P) may act as *synaptic transmitters* on the ascending pain fibers [*Zimmermann 2004, Baldry 2005*]. Therefore an intense stimulation of ascending pain tracts and pain related brain centers also occur [*Woolf 1983*], resulting in increased pain experience at the location of inflamed tissues.

3.2.8. Pain Chronification Processes

Pain chronification processes are also highly important in relation with orofacial pain. Whenever *increased activity* of pain related afferent fibers and other neurons of pain related centers appears, *profound intracellular changes* occur in few hours (but latest in few days). Premised profound changes are referred to as *activity dependent neuronal plasticity* which includes activation of immediate early genes and several transcription factors as well as altered synthesis of neurotransmitters, receptor precursors, or secondary messengers like kinases or phosphatases (etc.) [*Hunt et al. 1987, Besson 1999, Zimmermann 2004*]. Although premised changes are *reversible* at the beginning, they may become *irreversible* in the course of time (roughly in months). Whenever irreversible changes appeared, the pain sensation may become *independent* from the primary cause and may *become chronic,* because at this stage neurones may fire spontaneously in an irreversible manner. (Simply to say, the neurons "acquire the habit" of firing continuously.) Importantly, any neuron involved in pain related processes [*Zimmermann 2004*] may fire spontaneously at this stage, therefore the elimination of the primary cause, or a neurotomy of peripheral nerves (afferent fibers) not necessarily lead to the improvement of chronic pain.

3.2.9. Atypical Facial Pain

Atypical facial pain is an idiopathic symptom. It is a diagnosis of exclusion, after other conditions have been considered and eliminated. Although any area of the face can be involved, the most commonly affected areas are the maxillary region [*Sarlani et al. 2005/b*] and other non-muscular non-joint orofacial areas [*Köling 1998*]. It is characterized by continuous, daily pain (with or without intermittent episodes) that is described as dull and aching [*Köling 1998, Sarlani et al. 2005/b*]. The pain is usually deep and diffuse and does not interfere with sleep [*Sarlani et al. 2005/b*]. At onset, the pain may be confined to a limited area on one side of the face, while later it may spread to involve a larger area [*Sarlani et al. 2005/b*]. In latter case, larger pain areas usually do not respect any recognizable area of innervations or dermatome [*Sandler et al. 1995*]. Atypical facial pain may also appear in relation with PDI [*Fábián 1999, Fábián et al. 2006*]. Although atypical facial pain is considered as idiopathic [*Sarlani et al. 2005/a,b*], in PDI related cases the psychogenic origin of the manifestation is rather likely. Psychological distress, anxiety and depression are prevalent among atypical facial pain patients. A small subset of patients develops later a trigeminal neuralgia, in the course of the conditions, which cases can be referred to as *pretrigeminal neuralgia* that may precede the development of trigeminal neuralgia even by years [*Sarlani et al. 2005/a,b*].

3.2.10. Myofascial Pain

Myofascial pain is characterized by the presence of focal, exquisitely tender muscle areas called trigger points typically found in the taut muscle band and producing a characteristic pain referral pattern on palpation [*Sarlani et al. 2005/a*] (see also *paragraph 4.2.4.*). Besides trigger points, myofascial pain may also lead to the appearance of heterotopic orofacial pain [*Sieber et al. 2003*] as well as to the pain of the temporomandibular joint [*Cathomen-Rötheli et al. 1976*] and to denture soreness [*Yemm 1972*]. Myofascial pain is usually a constant dull muscle pain that is typically exacerbated by the use of targeted muscle(s) [*Sarlani et al. 2005/a*]. Major cause of myofascial pain is the overload (spasm and muscle fatigue) of masticatory muscles because of neuromuscular dysfunction (including several forms of bruxism [*Rosetti et al. 2008*]) induced by complex psychogenic processes [*Schwartz 1955, Laskin 1969, Yemm 1972, Cathomen-Rötheli et al. 1976, Lamprecht et al. 1986, Dahlström 1989, Sieber et al. 2003, Sarlani et al. 2005/a*], which may also be elicited under PDI (see also *paragraphs 3.3.3., 3.3.9., 3.3.12.*). Disturbed relationships of the teeth and/or occlusal surfaces [*Lamprecht et al. 1986, Schulte 1988*], altered occlusal guidance [*Okano et al. 2007*] as well as poorly occluding and/or ill fitting dentures [*Sandler et al. 1995, Meehan et al. 1995*] also may trigger neuromuscular malfunctions [*Lamprecht et al. 1986, Schulte 1988, Meehan et al. 1995*]; however such anomalisms are likely not major causative factors of myofascial pain [*Schwartz 1955, Laskin 1969, Winter & Yavelow 1975, Laskin & Block 1986, Auerbach et al. 2001*].

3.2.11. Glossodynia and Oropyrosis (Burning Mouth Sy.)

Burning mouth syndrome (BMS) is a distinct clinical entity characterized by a chief complaint of unremitting oral burning concomitant with no oral mucosal clinically observable lesions [*Trombelli et al. 1994, Grushka & Sessle 1991, Scala et al. 2003*], or other relevant *apparent* organic basis [*van der Bijl 1995, Scala et al. 2003*]. It is characterized by constant, chronic burning pain in clinically normal mucosal sites [*Sarlani et al. 2005/b*]. The anterior third and tip of the tongue are most commonly affected; however, any oral site may be involved, including the alveolar region, the palate, the inner surfaces of the lips, and the buccal mucosa [*Lamey & Lamb 1994, Sarlani et al. 2005/b*]. The burning pain can be unilateral or bilateral or can start on one side and spread to the opposite side. In latter case, pain usually does not respect any recognizable area of innervations [*Sandler et al. 1995*]. It is usually milder upon awakening and progressively increases in the curse of the day [*Sarlani et al. 2005/b*]. Although, insertion of the denture increases the pain intensity in many cases, and burning mouth syndrome can be induced also via PDI related psychogenic pathways; data suggest a complex interaction between several general health factors, psychosocial stressors and denture dysfunction in order to explain burning mouth syndrome in most cases [*Swensson & Kaaber 1995, Aneksuk 1989, Grushka & Sessle 1991*].

Health factors like menopause related hormonal alterations [Aneksuk 1989, Myers & Naylor 1989, Santoro et al. 2005, Nasri et al. 2007], nutritional deficiencies [Aneksuk 1989, Touger-Decker 1998, Scala et al. 2003, Maltsman-Tseikhin et al. 2007], diabetes [Aneksuk 1989, Scala et al. 2003, Maltsman-Tseikhin et al. 2007] and other general conditions like multiple chronic diseases [Swensson & Kaaber 1995, Maltsman-Tseikhin et al. 2007, Nasri et al. 2007], pain symptoms in parts of the body other than the oral cavity [Swensson & Kaaber 1995], psychosocial stress factors [Aneksuk 1989, Swensson & Kaaber 1995, Scala et al. 2003], sleep disturbances [Nasri et al. 2007] as well as local irritative factors of microbial and/or denture origin [Aneksuk 1989, Miyamoto & Ziccardi 1998, Swensson & Kaaber 1995, Scala et al. 2003, Nasri et al. 2007] including especially candidiasis [Taillandier et al. 2000, Satoh 2004] should also be considered carefully. Changes of pain tolerance especially at the tongue tip and also in the lower lip because of certain changes of the peripheral or central sensory functions [Grushka et al. 1987, Gruschka & Sessle 1991, Ito et al. 2002], as well as altered perception (increased sensory and pain thresholds) of nonnociceptive and nociceptive thermal stimuli also likely play a role [Svensson et al. 1993]. Certain salivary factors (including xerostomia) should also be taken into account [Grushka et al. 1987, Aneksuk 1989, Gruschka & Sessle 1991, Niedermeier et al. 2000, Scala et al. 2003, Nasri et al. 2007].

3.2.12. Toot-Located Pain

Although there can be numerous causes of tooth-located pain [*Türp et al. 2009*] (see also in *paragraph 4.4.1.*) the most frequent causes of tooth-located pain are periodontal inflammations as well as caries induced inflammation of the dental pulp (pulpitis) and related periapical inflammatory processes. Although premised inflammations are primarily of somatic origin [*Türp et al. 2009*] (see also in *paragraph 4.4.1.*), psychosocial stress induced alterations of immune/inflammatory processes may also trigger and/or worsen tooth related inflammatory processes and related pain (see *paragraph 3.4.8.*). Tooth-located pain of primarily psychogenic origin called *atypical odontalgia* may also occur [*Ahlberg et al. 2004, Sarlani et al. 2005/b, Dworkin & Sherman 2006, Baad-Hansen 2008*]. The pathomechanism of atypical odontalgia is far not clear yet; however, alteration of catecholamine (epinephrine and norepinephrine) [*Nagy et al. 2000*] and HSP70/HSPA type stress protein [*Fábián et al. 2009/a*] levels in the dental pulp may play an important role. Although there are only few published cases in the literature [*Golan 1997, Fábián 1999, Müller-Fahlbusch 1991, Baad-Hansen 2008*], tooth located pain of psychogenic origin is a rather frequent symptom of PDI patients [*Plainfield 1969, Müller-Fahlbusch 1991, Fábián 1999*]. The pain can be centered on apparently normal teeth, endodontically treated teeth, abutment teeth [*Sarlani et al. 2005/b*] and on dental implants [*Kromminga et al. 1991*]. Extraction site (alveolar bone) of a previously extracted tooth (or removed implant) is also frequently targeted and referred to as *phantom tooth pain* [*Plainfield 1969, Fábián 1999, Sarlani et al. 2005/b*].

The pain of atypical odontalgia (including phantom pain) is typically continuous, dull, aching or burning, and of moderate (but sometimes severe) intensity [*Sarlani et al. 2005/b*]. It can occur in any tooth or teeth group, but most commonly, it involves the maxillary premolar and molar teeth [*Sarlani et al. 2005/b*]. Stress related appearance of pain in relation with *impacted, non-erupted or partially erupted teeth* (most typically wisdom teeth) may also occur. Certain stress conditions (especially with repressed aggression) are likely to enhance eruption tendencies of such teeth, which may lead to local inflammation, tension or pressure of the surrounding bone or neighboring teeth. Although the pathomechanism is not yet clear, stress induced increase of expression [*Blake et al. 1991, Fukodo et al. 1997, Kageyama et al. 2000, Fleshner et al. 2004*] and release [*Fábián et al. 2004, Fleshner et al. 2004*] of HSP70/HSPA type stress proteins and consequent activation of osteoclasts (see *paragraph 3.4.8.*) and bone resorption (a major factor of tooth eruption [*Wise & Lin 1995*]) is rather likely [*Fábián et al. 2009/b*]. (It may also be noted that, aggression related psychological coupling and psychosymbolic function of teeth [*Every 1965, Fábián & Fábián 2000, Fábián et al. 2007/a*] fit perfectly the enhanced eruption tendencies, "resulting" in bigger "teeth-weapons" [*Every 1960, 1965*].)

3.2.13. Temporomandibular Joint Pain

Temporomandibular joint pain may be of psychogenic [Schwartz 1955, Laskin 1969, Hahn 1979, Lamprecht et al. 1986, Schulte 1988, Mairgünther & Dielert 1991, Green & Laskin 2000, Dworkin et al. 1994, Dworkin & Sherman 2006], occlusal [Hahn 1979, Lamprecht et al. 1986, Schulte 1988, Le Bell et al. 2006, Learreta et al. 2007], external traumatic [Schulte 1988] internal degenerative [Mairgünther & Dielert 1991, Zhang et al. 1999, Yamakawa et al. 2002] and tumorous origin. It may also appear as a symptom of a temporomandibular disorder (see also paragraph 3.3.12.), which is currently vied as an interrelated set of clinical conditions presenting with signs and symptoms in masticatory and related muscles of the head and neck, and the soft tissue and bony components of the temporomandibular joint [Dworkin et al. 1994, Sarlani et al. 2005/a, Osterberg & Carlsson 2007]. Disc displacement is not necessarily painful [Sandler et al. 1995, Sarlani et al. 2005/a], although a pain is typically present in the case of acute disc displacement without reduction [Sarlani et al. 2005/a]. Synovitis, capsulitis and osteoarthritis usually present with a constant deep pain, that is exacerbated by mandibular movement as well as with tenderness upon palpation of the joint, crepitus, and restricted mouth opening secondary to pain [Sandler et al. 1995, Sarlani et al. 2005/a] Although the condition of natural dentition or dentures does not necessarily bear on the occurrence of TMD [Graber 1971, Laskin & Block 1986, De Boever & De Boever 1997, Hiltunen et al. 1997, Hagag et al. 2000], PDI cases with significant alteration of the neuromuscular and or immune/inflammatory function can also result in temporomandibular pain (see paragraphs 3.3.12, 3.4.8.).

3.2.14. Neuropathic Pain

Neuropathic mechanisms may also induce severe orofacial pain [*Kromminga et al. 1989, Köling 1998, Pertes 1998, Scardina et al. 2002, Sarlani et al. 2005/a*]. Although neuropathic pain syndromes are rarely related to PDI, in some cases the dental treatment (and/or the inserted denture) may be a cause (i.e. traumatic neuritis) or may trigger (increase the frequency of appearance of) pain attacks [*Tesserioli de Siqueira et al. 2004*]. *Traumatic neuritis* occur following direct neural injury, although occasionally there is a delay of the onset of pain after the injury [*Sandler at el. 1995, Sarlani et al. 2005/a*]. This pain is typically described as constant and burning while superimposed exacerbations may occur [*Sarlani et al. 2005/a*]. Abnormal sensations such as allodynia and hyperalgesia as well as neural sensory or motor deficits often accompany the pain [*Sarlani et al. 2005/a*]. *Trigeminal and glossopharyngeal neuralgia* are relatively rare conditions, which can be characterized by unilateral, episodic, lancinating pain in the distribution of one or more divisions of the trigeminal nerve or the glossopharyngeal nerve [*Kromminga et al. 1989, Pertes 1998, Sarlani et al. 2005/a*]. Trigeminal neuralgia may be accompanied by a contraction of the facial musculature (hence the term tic douloureux) [*Sarlani et al. 2005/a*]. This kind of pain is severe, although usually lasts only for seconds or minutes with asymptomatic periods between the pain attacks. Trigeminal pain may be triggered in trigger zones on the skin (and/or on the oral mucosa [*Tesserioli de Siqueira et al. 2004*]) by nonnoxious stimulation like light touch or vibration [*Sandler et al. 1995, Sarlani et al. 2005/a*], but also by chewing, shaving or exposure to cold wind [*Köling 1998*]. Importantly, trigger zones are not always coinciding with the area of pain [*Sandler et al. 1995, Sarlani et al. 2005/a*]. Glossopharyngeal neuralgia may be triggered by swallowing, chewing, talking, coughing or yawning [*Köling 1998, Sarlani et al. 2005/a*]. *Herpetic and postherpetic neuralgia* appear during or following the outbreak of herpes zoster eruption, and present as continuous severe burning pain with sharp exacerbations [*Sandler et al. 1995, Sarlani et al. 2005/a*]. Tactile allodynia (pain in response to an innocuous stimulus) and hyperalgesia (exaggerated pain in response to a noxious stimulus) are also often present [*Sarlani et al. 2005/a*]. There is also a recurrent form of postherpetic neuralgia with remission phases of months or years. *Eagle's syndrome* (a compression of the glossopharyngeal nerve by an elongated styloid process or ossified stylohyoid ligament) [*Sarlani et al. 2005/a*] usually induce dull and persistent neck and throat pain; however radiation of the pain to the TMJ or the upper limb may also occur. Pain is usually exacerbated by rotation of the head, swallowing, extending the tongue and by palpation of the tonsillar fossa.

3.2.15. Vascular Pain

There is also several pain of vascular origin, which may appear as orofacial pain [*Burton 1969, Köling 1998, Zimmermann 2004, Gratt et al. 2005, Gratt & Anbar 2005, Sarlani et al. 2005/b*]. Although PDI is rarely a reason of vascular pain, however dental treatment (and/or the inserted denture) may provoke vascular pain attack. *Giant cell arteritis* (GCA) is a multifocal granulomatous vasculitis of likely autoimmune origin targeting medium-sized and large cranial arteries especially the extracranial branches of carotid arteries [*Sandler et al. 1995, Sarlani et al. 2005/b*]. The superficial temporal artery is most commonly affected (referred to as *temporal arteritis*), however other arteries including maxillary- and lingual arteries may also be involved [*Sandler et al. 1995, Sarlani et al. 2005/b*]. Depending on the arteries involved, symptoms may include severe throbbing temporal headache which aggravates upon recumbence or palpation (temporal artery), and/or pain of masticatory muscles upon chewing leading to "jaw claudication" (maxillary artery), and/or pain and blanching of the tongue (lingual artery) [*Sandler et al. 1995, Sarlani et al. 2005/b*]. Importantly, *vision loss and cerebrovascular accidents may also occur* as most feared complications of GCA, therefore early diagnosis of this disorder is highly important [*Sandler et al. 1995, Sarlani et al. 2005/b*].

Cluster headache (CH) is characterized by extreme, excruciating and throbbing unilateral pain attack, and by associated autonomic features like conjunctival injection, lacrimation, nasal congestion, rhinorrhoea and sweating of forehead and face [*Köling 1998, Sarlani et al. 2005/b*]. The pain is localized in the orbital, supraorbital (forehead) and temporal region, [*Sarlani et al. 2005/b*] but sometimes also in the jaws or teeth [*Sarlani et al. 2005/b*]. The pain paroxysms last 15 to 180 minutes and occur usually 1 to 2 per day (range: every other day to 8 times daily) [*Sarlani et al. 2005/b*]. Premised paroxysms occur in discrete time periods lasting a few months (cluster period) separated by remission periods lasting months or years [*Sarlani et al. 2005/b*]. *Chronic paroxysmal hemicrania* (CPH) is a rare type of headache that is characterized by daily, multiple, attacks of severe unilateral pain and associated autonomic symptoms including lacrimation, rhinorrhoea, conjunctival injection and nasal congestion [*Sarlani et al. 2005/b*]. Attacks may occur 1 to 40 times per day and last 2 to 120 minutes with a mean of approximately 15 minutes [*Sarlani et al. 2005/b*]. Importantly, CPS shows a very robust response to indomethacine treatment, therefore a drug trial is advocated when the frequency of pain episodes is higher than 4 per day [*Sarlani et al. 2005/b*].

Arterial vasodilatation induced pain may also occur in the orofacial region, because of the consequent stretching of capillaries and small veins following arterial vasodilatation [*Burton 1969, Zimmermann 2004*]. Local increase of nitric oxide (NO) level in the blood may be a cause of such an excessive arterial vasodilatation [*Gratt et al. 2005*]. Importantly, NO may also enhance nociception locally and may contribute to aggravation of pain at the level of central nervous system as a neurotransmitter too [*Gratt & Anbar 2005, Sarlani et al. 2005/b*]. *Arterial vasoconstriction* may also be a reason of vascular pain because of the consequent hypoxia of the supplied area. *Pulpitis of teeth* are also considered as a certain, unique type of vascular pain. In certain cases, *arteriosclerosis* of the carotid arteries [*Kleindienst et al. 1993, Wick et al. 2004*] (likely to be linked also with periodontal disease [*Schett et al. 1997, Wick et al. 2004*]) may be another cause of vascular orofacial pain. Similarly, *embolism* and/or *thrombosis* of carotid arteries (if any) may also lead to orofacial pain of vascular origin.

3.2.16. Other Pain Symptoms

Sensitization induced pain like *nociceptor sensitization* during peripheral inflammation [*Woda & Pionchon 2000*] as well as *central sensitization* (activity dependent neuronal plasticity) maintained by ongoing activity from damaged peripheral tissues, by altered inhibitory control in the brainstem, or by hyper/hypoactivity of descending activator/inhibitory controls [*Woda & Pionchon 2000, 2001*] may also cause orofacial pain [*Woda & Pionchon 2000, 2001*]. *Abnormal sympathetic activity* may also induce pain symptoms also in the orofacial region [*Woda & Pionchon 2000, 2001*]. Role of *female hormones* are also suggested as a cause of pain because of the strong female prevalence of orofacial pain [*Woda & Pionchon 2000, 2001*] and because of the marked prevalence of changes in *estrogen* levels in patients with orofacial idiopathic pain [*Woda & Pionchon 2000, 2001*]. *Paresthesias* and *dysaesthesias* may also appear as pain [*Di Felice et al. 1991, Hampf 1987, Pertes 1998*]. Myositis and myospasm are also possible (although not a common) cause of PDI-related pain. *Myositis* refers to true muscle inflammation that may result from a spreading infection or acute trauma to the muscle tissue [*Sarlani et al. 2005/a*]. This kind of pain is constant and characterized by the presence of the cardinal signs of inflammation such as swelling, erythema, and elevated temperature over the affected muscle [*Sarlani et al. 2005/a*]. *Myospasm* is an acute condition characterized by severe muscle pain, marked limitation of mouth opening and, often, acute malocclusion [*Sarlani et al. 2005/a*]. *Numerous other disorder* including cardiac problems (angina pectoris, myocardial infarction), Paget's disease, migraine, dissection or thrombosis/embolism of extracranial carotid arteries, cerebrovascular processes, cluster headache, multiple sclerosis and seizure disorder can be a cause of orofacial pain as well [*Sandler et al. 1995, Israel & Scrivani 2000, Sarlani et al. 2005/b*]. *Psychogenic origin* of orofacial pain should also be considered certainly [*Sandler et al. 1995, Pertes 1998, Israel & Scrivani 2000, Sarlani et al. 2005/b*].

3.3. NEUROMUSCULAR SYMPTOMS

3.3.1. Specificities of Orofacial Muscles

Masticatory and facial muscles are highly sensitive muscles having a *rather extended representation in the motor cortices* comparing to other muscles [*Sergl 1996*]. Besides motor cortices, other brain centers including limbic system, thalamus, cerebellum, as well as the basal ganglia and brainstem reticular formation are also involved in the neuromuscular regulation of facial and masticatory muscles [*Harris & Griffin 1975*]. In contrast to most other muscles, which are supplied *via* the spinal cord, *motor nervous supplies of masticatory and facial muscles are directly from the brainstem via several cranial nerves*. Brainstem is a structure mediating numerous important psychoemotional processes such as pain, arousal, attention, mood (i.e. depression), anxiety as well as defensive and reproductive behaviors [*Clark et al. 2006*]. Therefore, *brainstem seems to be an ideal structure to regulate muscles having unique functions strongly interrelated with emotions* including speech (chewing muscles, tongue-, lip-, and facial muscles), expressing emotions nonverbally (facial muscles), fighting and aggressiveness (chewing muscle) or sexuality (lips, tongue). Thus, it is no wonder that, facial and masticatory muscles are highly sensitive to psycho-emotional processes [*Heggendorn et al. 1979, Graber 1995, Fuhr & Reiber 1995*], and increase of their tone (muscle tension) occurs rather frequently [*Heggendorn et al. 1979, Graber 1995, Fuhr & Reiber 1995*]. Accordingly, their reaction (increase of tension) to stress is stronger and longer lasting comparing to other muscles of the body [*Heggendorn et al. 1979*].

3.3.2. Motor Nervous Supplies

Motor nervous supplies of the orofacial muscles are conducted by several cranial nerves [*Griffin & Harris 1975, Williams & Warwick 1980*]. *Masticatory muscles* including the masseter, the temporalis, the lateral pterygoid and the medial pterygoid muscles are supplied by the *mandibular nerve* (which is a branch of the *trigeminal nerve*). The anterior belly of digastric muscle, the mylohyoid muscle and the tensor veli palatini muscle are also supplied by the *mandibular nerve* [*Griffin & Harris 1975, Williams & Warwick 1980*]. *Facial muscles* including the epicranial musculature, orbicularis oculi and palpebral musculature, the nasal musculature, the buccolabial musculature, and the platisma are supplied by the *facial nerve*. The posterior belly of digastric muscle and the stylohyoid muscle is also supplied by the *facial nerve* [*Williams & Warwick 1980*]. The geniohyoid muscle is supplied by the *hypoglossal nerve*. Sternocleidomastoid muscle is supplied by the *accessory nerve*. Muscles of the palatine musculature including levator veli palatini, palatoglossus, palatopharingeus muscles and musculus uvulae (but with the exception of tensor veli palatini muscle, see above) are supplied by nerve fibers which leave the brainstem (medulla) in the cranial part of the *accessory nerve*, and which reach the pharyngeal plexus via the *vagus nerve* [*Williams & Warwick 1980*]. Although disturbed regulatory influences of any above nerve may be resulted in oral parafunctions, temporomandibular dysfunction or other neuromuscular manifestation, the malfunction of the trigeminal system may be of particular importance in relation with orofacial symptoms of neuromuscular origin [*Griffin & Harris 1975*].

3.3.3. Motor Units and their Control

The function of masticatory and facial muscles is primarily regulated by the alpha and gamma motoneurons of above listed motor nerves. *Alpha motoneurons* are responsible for the maintenance of muscle tone as well as for the volitional and/or reflex contraction of the muscles [*Graber 1995, Fuhr & Reiber 1995*]. Each of alpha motoneurons usually supplies roughly 15-30 masticatory muscle fibers, forming motor units with a diameter of roughly 5-11 mm [*Graber 1995*]. These can be considered as rather small units comparing to those of bigger muscles containing up to several hundred of muscle fibers [*Silverman 1961*]. (There are roughly 4 motor fibers in motor units of the intrinsic muscles of the eye, which deal with the "finest movements" [*Silverman 1961*]). *Gamma motoneurons* (also referred to as *fusimotor fibers*) are responsible for the "fine tuning" of the muscle spindles which determine the muscle stretch related discharge of afferent fibers leaving the muscle spindles. Since premised afferent fibers bring about monosynaptic facilitation of alpha motoneurons, in this way an alpha-gamma linkage control of muscle tone and muscular contraction develops [*Harris & Griffin 1975*].

Importantly, there is also an *inhibitory control* of muscular contraction due to *Golgi tendon organs*. In this case afferents originating from the Golgi tendon organs bring about synaptic inhibition of the alpha motoneurons via a disynaptic (or may be polysynaptic) nervous path [*Harris & Griffin 1975, Munro 1975/a*]. This reflex provides an important protective function against overtask and/or overload of the muscles. Further, both alpha and gamma motoneurons are also influenced by *afferent sensory fibers*, therefore a wide variety of peripheral stimuli including pain, touch or pressure [*Hunt & Paintal 1958, de Laat et al. 1985, van der Glas et al. 1985, 1988, Munakata & Kasai 1992, Kossioni & Karkazis 1995*] can influence muscle tone and muscle contraction. Premised influence of sensory impulses is responsible also for *pain induced reflex myospasm*, which is a frequent concomitant phenomenon of deep-seated pain symptoms (see also *paragraph 3.2.4.*). Alpha and gamma motoneurons are also influenced by higher brain centers, therefore *psychoemotional and psychosocial stress factors* also significantly influence muscle tone and contraction. Such influences of higher regulatory centers on peripheral motoneurons are responsible for the *stress induced tension of masticatory and facial muscles*, which frequently lead to myofascial pain and parafunction. Similarly, the facial expressions accompanying different moods are the result of such selectively influenced excitation of different muscles or muscle groups too [*Silverman 1961*].

3.3.4. The Rest Position

The *rest position* can be defined as a position, from which all free movements of the jaw start [*Munro 1975/a*]. Although this position seems to be relatively stable in healthy individuals, changes due to age, malocclusion, loss of teeth or wearing dentures may occur. Position of the head as well as inputs from the temporomandibular joints, oral mucosal receptors and psychic centers also mediate rest position [*Kawamura et al. 1958*]. In this position the teeth are not in contact and the interocclusal distance (free way space) averages 1,7 mm clinically [*Garnick & Ramfjord 1962, Munro 1975/a*]. However, under minimum muscle activity (under deep relaxation) the interocclusal distance averages 3,29 mm indicating that, changes of muscle tone and coupled alterations of the neuromuscular regulation significantly influence resting position [*Munro 1975/a*]. Accordingly, psychosocial stress also alter rest position, especially because *stress induced increase of muscle tension is usually higher in elevators comparing to depressors* [*Heggendorn et al. 1979, Graber 1995, Fuhr & Reiber 1995*]. Increased muscular tone of elevators *may lead to the decrease of free way space*; which may trigger parafunction due to the increasing frequency of occurrence of spontaneous contact between antagonist teeth [*Troest 1995*]. *Neuromuscular disregulation* and consequent loss of normal reciprocal actions of the mandibular elevators and depressors [*Kawamura et al. 1957*] may also decrease free way space and trigger parafunction. From this point of view, especially alterations of the jaw closing reflex (jaw jerk) and the inverse stretch reflex as well as their balance may be of particular interest (see below).

3.3.5. The Jaw Closing Reflex

The *jaw closing reflex (jaw jerk)* is a *stretch reflex* of the mandibular elevator muscles acting against gravity and with resulting jaw closure [*Munro 1975/a*]. Because of this reflex, in decerebrate animal the jaws are closed [*Sherrington 1906*], although a free-way space may be present depending on the level of decerebration [*Kawamura et al. 1958*] (indicating the role of brainstem structures in marking out and maintaining rest position). This is a monosynaptic reflex [*Szentágothai 1948*] released by *primary spindle endings* [*Szentágothai*

1948] sensitive to muscle stretch. Coupled facilitation of agonists (other closing muscles) also induced monosynaptically [*Lloyd 1946a,b*], whereas coupled reflex inhibition of antagonists (other opening muscles) require an interneuron [*Eccless 1962*]. Jaw closing reflex can be inhibited by the *inverse stretch reflex* [*Munro 1975/a*]. If the stimulus to the closing muscle nerve is increased in intensity, *Golgi tendon organs* are stimulated, leading to the inhibition of the muscle (and its synergists) and facilitation of antagonists [*Laporte & Lloyd 1952*]. Although the major function of this inhibitory reflex may be the protection against the overload of the muscles (as indicated above), it may also influence muscle tone and muscular contraction as well [*Harris & Griffin 1975, Munro 1975/a*].

3.3.6. The Jaw Opening Reflex

The *jaw opening reflex* operates to protect the masticatory apparatus and to regulate the force and rhythm of chewing [*Sherrington 1917, Hoffmann & Tönnies 1948, Kawamura et al. 1957, Munro 1975/a*]. This is a multisynaptic reflex [*Munro 1975/a*] leading to the inhibition of mandibular elevator muscles (closing muscles) and activation of mandibular depressors (opening muscles) [*Munro 1975/a*]. In decerebrate (and/or narcotized) animal this reflex can be released applying blunt pressure or electric stimulation of teeth, gums and front part of hard palate [*Sherrington 1917*] as well as electric stimulation or pinching of the tongue [*Cardot & Laugier 1922/a,b,c*]. Suddenly appearing foreign bodies between the antagonistic teeth (i.e. a piece of bone during chewing) as well as suddenly appearing nociceptive pain of oral mucosa (i.e. accidental biting on tongue, lip or cheek), also trigger this *protective masticatory muscle reflex* (see also *paragraph 3.2.4.*). Golgi tendon organs, muscle spindle endings and mechanoreceptors of the temporomandibular joint capsule are likely to modulate the reflex and may lead to malfunctions of the reflex in certain cases [*Griffin & Harris 1975*] also in relation with psychosocial stress.

3.3.7. Occlusal Discomfort and Dysesthesia

Occlusal discomfort may be induce by occlusal interferences [*Le Bell et al. 2006, Learreta et al. 2007*] especially in sensitive patients with increased vulnerability [*Le Bell et al. 2006*]. Oral parafunctions and/or increased muscle tension leading to fatigue in masticatory muscles can also result in occlusal discomfort [*Mew 2004, Litter 2005*] because of the failure of proper proprioceptive feedback [*Litter 2005*]. In more severe forms occlusal complaint may appear as an *occlusal dysesthesia* (OD) [*Baba et al. 2005, Clark et al. 2005*], which is a collective noon of several uncomfortable feelings of occlusion despite the *absence* of any observable occlusal anomaly or discrepancy [*Fábián et al. 2005, Baba et al. 2005, Fábián 2007*]. These patients are preoccupied with their dental occlusion, believing that, it is abnormal [*Jagger & Korszun 2004*], therefore occlusal dysesthesia is frequently also referred to as "*phantom bite*" or "*occlusal neurosis*" in the literature. The condition is remarkable for the nature of the involved explanations and interpretations that the patients give and for their persistence in trying to find a "dental" or "occlusal" solution [*Jagger & Korszun 2004*] or a "bite correction" [*Toyofuku & Kikuta 2006*]. However, available evidence suggests that, the symptoms cannot be improved by occlusal treatments; therefore, it is essential to avoid irreversible restorative treatment [*Jagger & Korszun 2004, Toyofuku & Kikuta 2006, Reewes & Merril 2007*].

Although the prognosis for symptom elimination is poor [*Jagger & Korszun 2004*], but need not necessarily be poor for patients' overall functioning and well-being [*Jagger & Korszun 2004, Toyofuku & Kikuta 2006*]. Importantly, sensory perceptive and discriminative abilities of OD patients seems to be different from that of healthy sample, and their occlusal thickness discrimination ability is higher (more sensitive) comparing to that of control [*Baba et al. 2005*]. Accordingly, erroneous integration and consequently increased perception of peripheral signals because of the malfunction of serotonin and norepinephrine systems was hypothesized as a possible pathomechanism behind such symptoms [*Toyofuku & Kikuta 2006*]. Interestingly, majority of patient with occlusal dysesthesia has no history of significant psychiatric illness, and there is an absence of obvious psychosocial problems in many cases [*Toyofuku & Kikuta 2006*]. On the other hand, occlusal dysesthesia may be a symptom of somatoform disorder [*Reeves & Merrill 2007*] or may be of depression [*Toyofuku & Kikuta 2006*]. In certain cases, occlusal dysesthesia may also be a symptom of more severe psychiatric conditions, and may represent a defense against psychiatric decompensation and outbreak of paranoia or other psychotic symptoms [*Marbach 1978*].

3.3.8. Instability of Removable Denture

Stability of dentures is highly important for patient satisfaction with removable dentures; although correlation of patient satisfaction with retention/stability scores assessed by the dentist is much weaker in the case of RPDs [*Wakabayashi et al. 1998*] comparing to full dentures [*Obrez & Grussing 1999*]. Increased vertical dimension and improper determination of the horizontal dimension of occlusion as well as occlusal interferences and unfavorable denture bearing tissues may frequently lead to instability of removable dentures (especially of complete dentures) [*Griffin & Harris 1975, Michman & Anselm 1975, Gonzalez & Desjardins 1983*]. Inadequate border seal [*Kivovics et al. 2007*], overextension or underextension of the denture base as well as the improper relation of teeth to the ridge and inadequate contour of the artificial gingiva may also lead to denture instability [*Gonzalez & Desjardins 1983*]. Use of canine guidance instead of bilateral balanced occlusion may also trigger instability of complete dentures [*Rehmann et al. 2008*]. Certain patients, especially edentulous patients also complain of lack of adequate space of tongue movement and consequent instability of denture [*Griffin & Harris 1975*]. (Interestingly, it appears that, not only decreased space but also facilitation of tongue protrusive muscles and/or inhibition of tongue retrusive muscles caused by occlusal discrepancies may also be responsible for such symptoms; because when the occlusion is corrected, premised tongue space related complaints of patients disappear in certain cases [*Griffin & Harris 1975*]).

Changes of saliva secretion [*Niedermeier & Krämer 1992, Niedermeier et al. 2000, Darwell & Clark 2000, Wolff et al. 2003*] and alterations of neuromuscular function may also be a cause of instability of removable (especially complete) dentures. A significant difference was observed in the flow of minor salivary glands (playing major role in denture base stability [*Niedermeier & Krämer 1992, Niedermeier et al. 2000, Márton et al. 2004*]) among euhydrated, dehydrated and rehydrated subjects [*Niedermeier et al. 2000, Lamey et al. 2007*]; therefore decreased water intake (especially of older patients) should also be considered as a possible cause. Similarly, both saliva secretion [*Zusmann et al. 2007, Fábián et al. 2008/a*] and neuromuscular function [*Michman & Langer 1975*] may be significantly altered with age, or because of systemic diseases or medication, which may also lead to denture instability. Certainly, psychogenic factors including psychosocial stress and other psychoemotional conditions may significantly alter saliva secretion (see *paragraph 3.5.2.*) and neuromuscular function (see *paragraphs 3.3.1., 3.3.3.*) as well, which may lead to an appearance of instability of dentures as a psychogenic symptom of PDI.

3.3.9. Bruxism

Bruxism can be defined as a *nonfunctional contact* of the teeth during *grinding*, *gnashing*, *tapping* or *clenching*. There are at least two EMG patterns responsible for bruxism such as [*Wruble et al. 1989, Glaros 2006*]: (1) high amplitude brief rhythmic EMG bursts that can vary in total duration and are primarily responsible for grinding, gnashing and tapping behavior; (2) arrhythmic, high-amplitude activity typically of short duration, primarily responsible for clenching [*Wruble et al. 1989, Piquero & Sakurai 2000, Glaros 2006*]. Grinding, gnashing and tapping most likely occur at night, whereas clenching may occur during the day and also at night [*Piquero & Sakurai 2000, Glaros 2006*]. Bruxism frequently appears already in the childhood [*Mikami 1977, Ozaki et al. 1990, Glaros 2006*], and family or living environment may influence its incidence [*Mikami 1977, Ozaki et al. 1990*]. Psychosocial factors [*Biondi & Picardi 1993, Kampe et al. 1997*] and psycho-emotional conflicts [*Mikami 1977, Somer 1991, Biondi & Picardi 1993*] may also be responsible for the *rather frequent* appearance of bruxism also in *adults*. Increased level of anxiety and lower level of socialization also increases the incidence of bruxing behavior [*Kampe et al. 1997*]. Recent fMRI study also indicated that, the overall extent of brain motor areas during clenching and grinding task was reduced in subjects with self-reported parafunctional masticatory activity [*Byrd et al. 2009*]. Supplementary motor area data indicated that, motor planning and initiation particularly during the act of clenching are less prominent in individuals with parafunctional behaviors [*Byrd et al. 2009*].

Malocclusions including occlusal early contacts and other occlusal disharmonies [*Glaros 2006*] as well as improper determination of the vertical dimension [*Piquero et al. 1999*] and/or other alterations of the maxillomandibular relationship [*Biondi & Picardi 1993, Le Bell et al. 2006, Learreta et al. 2007*] may also induce bruxism. Ill-fitting removable dentures also frequently induce clenching [*Sandler et al. 1995*]. Malocclusions and denture related discrepancies are likely to trigger *ancient mechanisms* similar to those being responsible for the elimination of impacted occlusal foreign bodies in *animals* (i.e. impacted pieces of bones, or small pebbles) *via* biting on it with strong biting forces (to crush by pressing) and/or *via* intermittent isometric grinding movements (to grind, to „erode" it). It is also likely that there are individual differences in vulnerability to occlusal interferences [*Le Bell et al. 2006*] causing bruxism in a certain proportion (but not in all) of the patients. Accordingly, the minimal detectable thickness of occlusal foreign bodies seems to be decreased in the case of bruxers [*Suganuma et al. 2007*] which refers to increased occlusal sensitivity of bruxism patients. Although masticatory forces appearing under bruxism may overload the teeth and their periodontium, it is likely that, bruxism accounts for a healthy periodontal apparatus when other diseases are not present [*Winter & Yavelow 1975*]. However, tooth wear (attrition) may occur rather frequently [*Glaros 2006*].

3.3.10. Soft Tissue Parafunctions

Inadequacies of dentures including decreased vertical dimension, insufficient horizontal overlap and shaping of teeth, improper position of teeth, and poor location of plane of occlusion may frequently lead to biting of tongue, cheek and lip [*Gonzalez & Desjardins 1983, Piquero et al. 1999*] and mucosa ridging [*Piquero et al. 1999*]. Ill-fitting removable dentures also frequently induce parafunctions, such as tongue thrusting [*Sandler et al. 1995*], and consequent indentation of tongue [*Piquero et al. 1999*]. Storing a thick wedge of tongue in between the teeth with consequent protrusion (or laterotrusion) of the mandible also may occur, especially in patients with occlusal discomfort or dysesthesia [*Mew 2004*]. Similarly, maintenance of an increased lip-seal with increased tension of the orbicularis oris muscle also frequently occur [*Mew 2004*]. Accidental biting on tongue (and other soft tissues) also may occur as soft tissue parafunction of neuromuscular origin (i.e. not necessarily related to the presence or absence of any denture). In such cases malfunction of preventive reflex mechanisms such as the inhibitory influence of jaw muscle proprioceptors on genioglossus activity (which may lead to accidental bite on tongue) [*Sauerland & Mizuno 1970*] as well as a decreased (or absence of) inhibitory effect of the mechanical stimulation of tooth on tongue protrusion [*Schmitt et al 1973*] can be expected as a cause [*Griffin & Harris 1975*]. Similar mechanisms may be responsible for frequent accidental biting on cheek and lip as well. Lack of muscle tone may also lead to biting of soft tissues [*Gonzalez & Desjardins 1983*]. Since soft tissue parafunctions show the highest incidence in the age group of 20 to 29 years [*Piquero et al. 1999*], it is likely that psychosocial stress effects and consequent neuromuscular dysfunction rather than denture mistakes and organic diseases are the major cause of such manifestations.

3.3.11. Overactive Gag Reflex ("Gagging")

The term gagging refers to a defense reflex, which attempts to eject unwanted, irritating, or toxic materials from the upper gastrointestinal tract [*Murphy 1979, Yoshida et al. 2007*]. Although gag reflex is a normal defense function of human, overactive gag reflex ("gagging") may be rather disadvantageous for denture wearers, especially for those wearing removable dentures [*Murphy 1979, Barsby 1994, 1997, Gáspár et al. 2002*]. Gagging may also lead to failure to tolerate making impression and/or other routine dental procedures [*Murphy 1979, Yoshida et al. 2007*]. In certain cases gagging may also be triggered by feel, touch, taste, smell, sight or thought of certain nondental factors [*Murphy 1979*] like appearance of a hair, a piece of eggshell, a piece of bone (etc.) in the mouth as well as by the smell of certain biological products and the sight of other people gagging or the sight of blood (etc.) [*Murphy 1979*]. There can be numerous mechanisms behind gagging including several gastrointestinal and central nervous defense pathways [*Friedman & Isselbacher 1991*]; but denture related gagging are primarily induced by either several (basically classic [*Hilgard & Marquis 1940*] and operant [*Skinner 1938*]) conditioning processes, or several neurotic psychological pathways [*Savage & McGregor 1970, Newton 1984, Gáspár et al. 2002*]. Conditioning processes are typical of gagging caused by learned avoidance reactions originating from former aversive encounters with dental treatment [*Eli & Kleinhauz 1997*]; whereas neurotic psychological pathways are typical of gagging caused by deep-seated defense mechanisms, which serve as inadequate solutions to several psychodynamic conflicts [*Eli & Kleinhauz 1997, Gáspár et al. 2002*].

3.3.12. Temporomandibular Joint Symptoms

Temporomandibular disorder (TMD) is currently viewed as an interrelated set of clinical conditions presenting with signs and symptoms in masticatory and related muscles of the head and neck, and the soft tissue and bony components of the temporomandibular joint (TMJ) [*Dworkin et al. 1994, Sarlani et al. 2005/a, Osterberg & Carlsson 2007*]. Symptoms of TMD can be various. *Disc displacement with reduction* is characterized by improvement of the position of the displaced disc during opening. An opening joint clicking occurs as the condyle positions itself under the posterior band of the disc; whereas closing joint clicking can be heard as the condyle slips off the disc. Pain may or may not be present [*Sandler et al. 1995, Sarlani et al. 2005/a*], and patient may complain of episodic and momentary catching of the jaw movement during opening [*Sarlani et al. 2005/a*]. *Disc displacement without reduction* refers to an altered disc-condyle relation that is not improved during mouth opening. There is frequently a sudden onset, the displaced disc blocks the condylar movement, resulting in limited (25-30 mm) mouth opening with deflection to the affected site and restricted lateral excursion to the contralateral side [*Sarlani et al. 2005/a*]. Pain is typically present in the acute condition, while chronic dislocation may be nonpainful, and there is a gradual increase in the mandibular range of motion. *Synovitis and capsulitis* of TMJ are characterized by constant deep pain in the TMJ, tenderness to palpation and restricted mouth opening secondary to pain [*Sarlani et al. 2005/a*]. Acute malocclusion of the posterior teeth may also occur [*Sarlani et al. 2005/a*]. *Osteoarthritis* of TMJ is characterized by deterioration of the articular surfaces, and consequent pain that is exacerbated by mandibular movement as well as by tenderness upon palpation, crepitus, and limited range of mandibular movement [*Sarlani et al. 2005/a*].

Epidemiologic and clinical studies of TMD confirm its status as a chronic pain problem [*Dworkin et al. 1994, Molin 1999, Dworkin & Sherman 2006*]. Studies also confirm that, the condition of natural dentition or dentures does not necessarily bear on the occurrence of TMD [*Schwartz 1955, Laskin 1969, Graber 1971, de Laat et al. 1986, Witter et al. 1994, De Boever & De Boever 1997, Hiltunen et al. 1997, Hagag et al. 2000, Green & Laskin 2000, Auerbach et al. 2001*]. However, in *certain* cases malocclusion may contribute to the appearance of the disorder [*Hahn 1979, Lamprecht et al. 1986, Schulte 1988, Zhang et al. 1999, Gleissner et al. 2003, Oizumi 2008*]. Loss of posterior occlusal support (shortened dental arches) [*Costen 1934, Hahn 1979, Sandler et al. 1995, Ciancaglini et al. 1999, Oizumi 2008*], deep overbite [*Costen 1934, Hahn 1979*], occlusal/cuspal interferences [*Hahn 1979, Sandler et al. 1995, Hagag et al. 2000, Le Bell et al. 2006, Learreta et al. 2007*], defects in anterior guidance [*Hagag et al. 2000, Oizumi 2008*] or alterations of the maxillomandibular relationship [*Biondi & Picardi 1993, Hagag et al. 2000, Oizumi 2008*] *may* induce TMD related problems in *certain* cases.

Importantly, *open-close-clench cycle* coupled EMG pattern of TMD related muscle dysfunction patients shows certain alterations such as: (1) increased duration of muscle contraction before initial tooth contact [*Munro 1975/b*]; (2) increased activity of temporalis and masseter muscles in the opening phase [*Munro 1975/b*]; (3) absence or incompleteness of the inhibitory response following initial tooth contact [*Munro 1975/b*]; (4) absence of the correlations of the phases of the cycle [*Griffin et al. 1975*]. Further, an abnormally lengthened inhibitory response ("silent period") of TMD patients was also found under *chin tapping* experiments [*Bessette et al. 1971, Dahlström 1989*]. Following making and insertion of dentures significant improvement may occur including recovery of inhibitory response and recovery of correlations of the phases of *open-close-clench cycle* [*Griffin et al. 1975*]. However a worsening of the increased activity of the mandibular elevator (jaw closing) muscles during mouth opening [*Tsuru & Kawamura 1962*] and a worsening of the increased duration of muscle contraction before initial tooth contact [*Griffin et al. 1975*] may also occur following insertion of dentures, which may predispose to PDI related TMJ problems. Thus, TMD related symptoms may also induced by dentures without any significant occlusal or other inadequacies in the case of PDI patients. In such cases neuromuscular dysfunction caused by psychosocial or psychoemotional stress factors rather than dental status or malocclusion are the major cause of denture related TMJ symptoms [*Schwartz 1955, Laskin 1969, Graber 1971, Hahn 1979, Biondi & Picardi 1993, Dworkin et al. 1994, Molin 1999, Green & Laskin 2000, Auerbach et al. 2001, Ahlberg et al. 2004, Osterberg & Carlsson 2007*]. Stress induced *pro*inflammatory changes of immune/inflammatory processes may also predispose to the appearance of TMJ symptoms also in PDI cases (see *paragraph 3.4.8.*).

3.4. IMMUNE- AND INFLAMMATORY REACTIONS

3.4.1. Central Nervous Control of Immunity

Highest central components, which significantly influence immunity, are located in *higher cortical-, limbic-* and *neurosensory systems* receiving and integrating a great diversity of signals arising from inside and outside the body [*Chrousos 1998, Ligier & Sternberg 2000*]. Influence of personality, cognitions and certain psychoemotional states on immune responses also occur due to this structures. The *lateralized cortical control of immunity*, resulting in the upregulation during left hemispheric and downregulation during right hemispheric activity are likely to occur also due to certain cortical areas [*Gruzelier et al.*

1998, Clow et al. 2003]. Other highly important central components influencing immune response significantly are located in the *hypothalamus*. Especially important are the parvonuclear neurons of *paraventricular nuclei* (PVN), which release corticotrophin-releasing hormone (CRH) leading to the production of adrenocorticotrop hormone (ACTH) in the *anterior pituitary gland* and consequent release of glucocorticoids in the *adrenal cortex* (referred to as *hypothalamic-pituitary adrenocortical axis*, HPA axis) [*Chrousos 1998, Ligier & Sternberg 2000, Krahwinkel et al. 2004*]. Another key elements are located in the *brain stem*, including the *locus ceruleus* and other mostly noradrenergic cell groups of the pons and medulla as well as the *paragigantocellular* and *parabrachial nuclei* of the medulla [*Chrousos 1998, Ligier & Sternberg 2000*], which elements influence the immune reactions primarily due to the activation of the *sympathetic nervous system*. (Besides HPA axis, this latter system of sympathetic autonomic response is also under the control of hypothalamus certainly [*Weinberg 1977*].)

3.4.2. Hormonal and Autonomic Control of Immunity

As indicated above, the most important effector arms of the central nervous regulation of immunity are the hypothalamic-pituitary adrenocortical axis (HPA axis) and the efferent sympathetic-adrenomedullary system [*Cannon 1939, Selye 1955, Weinberg 1977, Breivik et al. 1996, Chrousos 1998*]. *Activation of the HPA axis* has profound effects on the immune- and inflammatory response, because glucocorticoids (i.e. *cortisol, corticosterone*) alter leukocyte trafficking and function, decrease production of pro-inflammatory cytokines and several other mediators of inflammation, as well as inhibit the latter's' effect on numerous target tissues [*Breivik et al. 1996, Chrousos 1998, Szabó 1998, Ligier & Sternberg 2000*]. Glucocorticoids also suppress the expression of inducible nitric oxide synthase (iNOS) that producing nitric oxide (NO) [*Szabó 1998*], which is a free radical with various controlling functions in most tissues [*McCann 2000*] and a common inflammatory mediator during various forms of inflammation including inflammatory response to bacterial lipopolysaccharide (LPS) [*Szabó 1998, McCann 2000, Fábián et al. 2009/b*]. Glucocorticoids also appear to cause a shift from a Th1-type CD4$^+$cell response (favoring cellular over humoral immune response) to a Th2-type CD4$^+$cell response, favoring humoral over cellular immune response [*Chrousos 1998, Ligier & Sternberg 2000*].

The *sympathetic nervous system* modulates the immune- and inflammatory response *via* regional innervations of immune organs, including bone marrow, spleen, thymus, lymph nodes, Peyer's patches, tonsils, adenoid and appendix [*Breivik et al. 1996, Chrousos 1998, Ligier & Sternberg 2000*]. The sympathetic nervous system also reaches all sites of inflammation via the postganglionic sympathetic neurons; therefore, function of immune cells and immune accessory cells containing receptors for neurotransmitters or neuropeptides secreted by postganglionic sympathetic neurons can also be regulated locally due sympathetic activation [*Chrousos 1998, Ligier & Sternberg 2000*]. The sympathetic nervous system also reaches the salivary glands and likely influence the level of salivary immunoglobulin A (sIgA) [*Gruzelier et al. 1998*]. The sympathetic *activation of adrenal medulla* leads to the release of catecholemines (i.e. epinephrine, norepinephrine and dopamine) into the blood, from which release of norepinephrine seems to be of particular *immunological* importance (notwithstanding that epinephrine is considered as the "main hormone" of adrenal medulla [*Goldstein   2000*]). *Norepinephrine* exerts similar (but systemic) effects like neurotransmitters of the postganglionic sympathetic neurons (i.e. primarily norepinephrine [*Goldstein 2000*]). Further, increase of norepinephrine in the blood seems to be responsible for the release of immune activator/modulator chaperokines (*HSP70/HSPA type stress proteins*) into the blood [*Fleshner et al. 2004, Johnson & Fleshner 2006*] and likely into the saliva [*Fábián et al. 2003, 2004, 2009/a*] (see also *paragraph 3.4.7.*).

3.4.3. Executive Elements of the Immune System

The immune system consists of immune organs, immune cells, cytokines [*Dhabhar 2000/b, Ligier & Sternberg 2000*] and defense molecules of the innate immunity [*Fábián et al. 2008/a*]. *Immune organs* include bone marrow, thymus, spleen, lymph nodes and other specialized tissues such as small intestinal Peyer's patches, tonsils, adenoid and appendix [*Dhabhar 2000/b, Ligier & Sternberg 2000*] *Bone marrow* and *thymus* are primarily responsible for production and maturation of immune cells [*Ligier & Sternberg 2000*]. Most important immunological function of *spleen* is to serve as a "meeting place" for immune cells and target antigens present in the *blood*; consequently, spleen is an organ of *general* immune defense. Most important immunological function of *lymph nodes, Peyer's patches, tonsils, adenoid* and *appendix* is to serve as "meting place" of immune cells and target antigens present in the *lymphatic fluid* [*Ligier & Sternberg 2000*]; therefore, these organs are responsible rather for a *local* than a general screening function.

Immune cells include T and B lymphocytes, plasmacells, natural killer (NK) lymphocytes, monocytes/macrophages, dendritic cells (DC), neutrophile granulocytes, eosinophile granulocytes, basophile granulocytes, and mast cells [*Dhabhar 2000/b, Ligier & Sternberg 2000*]. *T cells* are primarily responsible for the governing of immune reactions (CD4$^+$ T-helper cells) as well as for direct killing of MHC-signal bearing infected cells (CD8$^+$ T-killer cells). Some T cells are also responsible for immune memory (CD45RO$^+$ memory T-cells) [*Dhabhar 2000/b, Ligier & Sternberg 2000*]. *B cells* are primarily responsible for antibody production due to differentiation into antibody producing *plasmacells*. B cells are also responsible for immune memory (memory B cells) [*Ligier & Sternberg 2000*]. *Natural killer (NK) cells* are responsible for direct killing of those infected or tumoric cells which *do not* bear MHC signals [*Fábián et al. 2009/a,b*]. *Monocytes* and *macrophages* are phagocytes and antigen presenting cells (APCs) of the blood and other tissues respectively [*Ligier & Sternberg 2000, Fábián et al. 2009/a*]. *Dendritic cells* are antigen presenting cells of the lymphoid organs but may also be present in other tissues (i.e. especially in the oral mucosa) [*Ito et al. 1998, Cutler & Jotwani 2006, Fábián et al. 2007/b, 2009/a*]. *Neutrophile granulocytes* are primarily responsible for the phagocytosis and elimination of microbes and cellular debris in the blood. They also produce significant amount of cytokines [*Ligier & Sternberg 2000*]. *Eosinophile granulocytes* produce high amount of several immune inflammatory mediators and are responsible for the elimination of parasitic infections. *Basophile granulocytes* produce high amount of immune inflammatory signal molecules including histamine, and are involved in several allergic and irritative reactions. *Mast cells* are rather similar to basophile granulocytes and are involved primarily in several allergic and irritative reactions triggered by the degranulation of these cells [*Ligier & Sternberg 2000*].

Cytokines are molecules primarily used for communication of several immune cells with each other. Further, cytokines can cross the blood-brain barrier at leaky points and *via* specific active transport [*Ligier & Sternberg 2000*]; therefore, another important function of cytokines is to *influence central nervous functions* including stress response [*Ligier & Sternberg 2000, Amar 2006*] as well as other psychoemotional functions [*Amar 2006*]. There are several subtypes of cytokines like several *interleukins* (IL), *interferons, growth factors, tumor necrosis factors* (TNF), and several *other molecules* like *chaperokines* [*Ligier & Sternberg 2000, Fábián 2009/a*]. Cytokines may be either *proinflammatory* or *regulatory*. Those cytokines, which exert chemotactive properties, are also referred to as *chemokines*. *Chaperokines* are unique molecules, which are able to function as both cytokine and molecular chaperone [*Asea 2005, Fábián 2009/a*].

Defense molecules of the innate immunity include the complement system and several other nonspecific defense molecules [*Dalmadi & Fábián 2004, Fábián et al. 2008/a,d*]. The *complement system* primarily responsible for the lysis of bacteria (or any other nonviral microbes) as well as virus infected cells due to lysis of the microbial (cellular) membrane. There are also several other *nonspecific defense molecules* such as *cystatines, calprotectine, lactoferrine, lysozyme, defensins, mucins, peroxidases* (etc.) which may either destroy microbes or at least inhibit their growth or colonization due to various pathways [*Dalmadi & Fábián 2004, Fábián et al. 2008/a,d*]. Antibody-catalyzed ozone formation is another important defense pathway of innate immunity, which also leads to efficient killing of bacteria (and other microbes) [*Nathan 2002, Wentworth Jr. et al. 2002*].

3.4.4. Major Pathways of Immune Response

There are two major facets of immune response including innate immunity and acquired immunity [*Dhabhar 2000/b, Ligier & Sternberg 2000*]. *Innate immune response* (also referred to as "*nonspecific*", "*native*" or "*natural*" immunity) is carried out primarily by monocytes/macrophages, neutrophile granulocytes, NK cells, as well as the complement system and several nonspecific defense molecules (see above). It is regulated primarily by macrophage-derived cytokines [*Dhabhar 2000/b*]. This response represents a "first-line defense" against pathogens [*Ligier & Sternberg 2000*], however it does not discriminate against antigens, and it is not enhanced by repeated exposure to a certain antigen [*Dhabhar 2000/b*]. *Acquired immune response* (also referred to as "adaptive" or "specific" immunity) is carried out primarily by T and B cells (including plasmacells, see above) and is regulated primarily by lymphocyte derived cytokines [*Dhabhar 2000/b*]. However, the antigen presenting function of monocytes/macrophages as well as dendritic cells is also highly important [*Ligier & Sternberg 2000*]. Primary effector arms of acquired immune response are either the T-killer (CD8$^+$) cells (*cell mediated response* of acquired immunity) or the plasmacells and their major products the antibodies (*humoral response* of acquired immunity). The acquired immune response is directed against specific antigens and is often enhanced following repeated exposure to antigen [*Dhabhar 2000/b*]. Although reactions of immune response can be classified into premised major categories; it is highly important to note that, *immune response is a mixture of innate and acquired immunity in most cases* [*Dhabhar 2000/b*].

3.4.5. Acute Stress Related Changes of Immunity

Despite of the general assumption that stress suppresses immune function; *acute* stress (lasting for a period of a *few minutes* to a *few hours* [*Dhabhar 2000/b*]) is likely to induce *an adaptive redistribution* rather than a general suppression and/or destruction of immune system in short run [*Dhabhar et al. 1995, Gruzelier et al. 1998, Dhabhar 2000/a,b*]. Acute stress induced sympathetic activation leads to an increase of salivary immunoglobulin A (sIgA) [*Gruzelier et al. 1998*] that is interestingly influenced by a *lateralized* cortical control [*Gruzelier et al. 1998, Clow et al 2003*]. Acute stress induced increase of blood glucocorticoids is known to alter *leukocyte trafficking* [*Chrousos 1998, Ligier & Sternberg 2000*] that is a regular circulating patrol of immune cells between immune and nonimmune organs. Alteration of trafficking is likely to be mediated by glucocorticoid-induced changes in either the expression or the affinity of adhesion molecules on the surface of leukocytes and/or endothelial cells [*Dhabhar 2000/a*]. *Acute* stress induced alteration of trafficking results in *prompt* and *selective retention* of several leukocytes in *certain* organs [*Fauci & Dale 1974, Fauci 1975*] such as the skin, gastrointestinal mucosa (including oral mucosa), urogenital epithelia, air way (lung) epithelia, liver, lymph nodes and bone marrow [*Fauci et al. 1974, 1975, Dhabhar et al. 1996, Dhabhar 2000/a,b*]; however there is a consequent *decrease* of *total leukocyte number* in the *blood* and also in the spleen [*Dhabhar et al. 1995, Dhabhar 2000/a*]. The decrease of number of T cells, B cells, NK cells, and monocytes in the blood can be rather drastic (40-70% lower than baseline) [*Dhabhar et al. 1995, Dhabhar 2000/a*]; whereas the number of neutrophile PMN cells usually do not change (moreover even may increases) [*Dhabhar 2000/a*].

Importantly, the leukocyte redistribution is likely to *enhance the immune activity of those organs in which the leukocytes are accumulated* [*Dhabhar et al. 1996, Dhabhar 2000/a,b*], whereas immune function of the *blood* and *spleen is likely to be suppressed*. Furthermore, the cumulation of leukocytes is *selective* resulting in *specific selection patterns* of leukocytes in several tissues. Therefore not only *quantitative*, but also *qualitative* and *tissue specific changes* of immune reactivity (including *upregulation* as well as *downregulation* of *certain* immune functions in *certain* tissues) also may occur [*Fleshner et al. 1992, Dhabhar 2000/a,b*]. For example, stress related increase of blood glucocorticoid level induce a *general shift* from a Th1-type response to a Th2-type response (see above) [*Chrousos 1998, Ligier & Sternberg 2000*]; nevertheless, because of a *specific selection pattern* there is an *increased predisposition* to Th1 mediated delayed-type hypersensitivity (DTH) response in the *skin* [*Dhabhar 2000/a*]. (Please note that: similar mechanisms may be responsible for stress induced increase of oral mucosal DTH as well.) Please also consider that, a general shift from a Th1-type CD4$^+$cell response to a Th2-type CD4$^+$cell response can be adaptive for short run against external (extracellular) infectious agents but causes vulnerability to certain infectious agents (and also tumors) *already existing* in the body [*Chrousos 1998*]. Please consider that, in latter case, the infecting agents exist intracellular; thus, efficient cellular immune responses would be needed for their proper elimination. Therefore it is highly important fact that, acute stress induced redistribution of leukocytes is *reversed promptly* upon the cessation of acute stress [*Dhabhar et al. 1995, Dhabhar 2000/a*].

3.4.6. Chronic Stress Related Changes of Immunity

In contrast to acute stress, longer run *chronic* stress (that persist *at least* for several hours per day for *at least* several days [*Dhabhar 2000/b*]) clearly leads to a *maladaptive decrease of immune-inflammatory defense* [*Dhabar McEwen 1997; Dhabhar 2000/b, Chiapelli & Hodgson 2000*]. In contrast to *acute* stress which may induce either an *increase* or a *decrease* of certain immune functions (see above); there is a *general suppression* of various immune parameters under *chronic* stress. There is a significant decrease of lymphocyte response to mitogen stimulation, a decrease of total number of cytotoxic T cells as well as a decreased activity of NK cells and other cellular immune responses [*Chiapelli & Hodgson 2000*] and cytokine production [*Dhabhar 2000/b*].

A redistribution of the immune system also occur in the case of chronic stress, however it is likely to be different from that of acute stress [*Dhabhar 2000/a*]. (For example, the spleen is likely to be relatively enriched in leukocytes, which is not the case under acute stress [*Dhabhar 2000/a*].) There is also an increased susceptibility to microbial infection and tumor growth under chronic stress [*Chiapelli & Hodgson 2000*]. Importantly, there is a more or less *continuous* and *long run* enhance of both *sympathetic activity* and exposure to *glucocorticoid hormones* overall in the body; with a consequent disruption of the circadian autonomic and corticosterone rhythms. Therefore, the *chronic stress response may persist long after the primary (triggering) stress factor has subsided* [*Dhabhar 2000/b*]. (Simply to say: fixation of a "pathological balance" occurs, which „the body gets used with".).

3.4.7. Role of HSP70/HSPA Type Stress Proteins

Although, there is a significant amount of data related to major pathways of stress induced immune- and inflammatory changes (outlined above), much less is known about the concrete pathways leading to orofacial symptoms. There is likely to be a key role of the *HSP70/HSPA type stress proteins* (being immune activator/modulator chaperokines [*Asea 2005*]) in this relation; because these molecules are present in any orofacial cells and psychosocial stress induces their intracellular expression [*Blake et al. 1991, Fukodo et al. 1997, Kageyama et al. 2000, Fleshner et al. 2004*] as well as extracellular release [*Fábián et al. 2004, Fleshner et al. 2004*] due to glucocorticoid and/or epinephrine and/or norepinephrine hormones [*Fleshner et al. 2004*]. Further, their level also increases in the blood [*Fleshner et al. 2004*] and the saliva [*Fábián et al. 2004*] under psychosocial stress; very likely because of the increased blood level of norepinephrine *via* an alpha1-adrenerg-receptor pathway [*Fleshner et al. 2004, Johnson & Fleshner 2006*]. Moreover, HSP70/HSPA type stress proteins play important role in the stress adaptation of dental pulp, periodontal tissues, bone and oral mucosa [*Fábián et al. 2007/b, 2008/b,c, 2009/a,b*]. They are likely to play a role also in the disadvantageous amplification of several immune/inflammatory reactions of the oral (orofacial) tissues [*Fábián et al. 2007/b, 2008/b,c, 2009/a,b*], as well as in the mucosal allergic and autoimmune reactions [*Fábián et al. 2007/b, 2008/b,c, 2009/a,b*] (see also *paragraph 3.4.8.*).

3.4.8. Chronic Inflammations

There is a high number of several inflammatory processes, which may occur in the orofacial region. Many of them is of particular diagnostic interest (see *paragraphs 3.2.14, 3.2.15, 3.2.16, 4.4.1, 4.4.2, 4.4.4.*), whereas some of them frequently appear also as a *major symptom* of PDI patients. *Psychosocial stress induced* chronic inflammations of the oral mucosa, temporomandibular joint, dental pulp, periapical tissues and periodontal tissues belong to this group primarily. *Stress induced activation of HSP70/HSPA type stress proteins* (see *paragraph 3.4.7.*) *are likely to play pivotal role* in premised stress induced oral inflammatory processes [*Fábián et al. 2007/b, 2008,b,c, 2009/a,b*]; notwithstanding that *HSP70/HSPA proteins* also play a highly important role in the maintenance of orofacial tissues' health [*Fábián et al., 2007/b, 2008,b,c, 2009/a,b*].

Oral mucosal inflammation may occur because of cross reactivity of specific antibodies against *microbial* HSP70 type stress proteins with *human* HSP70/HSPA proteins and/or because of autoantibodies against HSP70/HSPA proteins. Despite the expected role of HSP70/HSPA in the oral tolerance (see *paragraph 3.4.9.*) data in the literature suggest that overexpression of HSP70/HSPA may also play a role in the appearance of *mucosal allergic reactions*, because HSP70/HSPA proteins are likely to play a role in haptenation and consequent sensitization [*Fábián et al. 2009/a*]. Highly frequent occurrence of premised autoantibodies against HSP70/HSPA type proteins was also reported in the serum of metal-allergic patients [*Jin et al. 2003*]. *Inflammation of TMJ* (see also *paragraph 3.2.13, 3.3.12*) may also worsen on the basis of stress induced alteration of inflammatory processes [*Fábián et al. 2009/a,b*]. Although HSP70/HSPA proteins may control spondyloarthropathic disease progression via inhibition of HLA-B27 protein accumulation and alteration of endoplasmic reticulum (ER) stress signaling [*Fábián et al. 2009/b*]; on the other hand, uncomplexed extracellular HSP70/HSPA molecules induces the secretion of proinflammatory cytokines playing mayor role in the progression of inflammatory bone loss [*Fábián et al. 2009/b*]. Because of this "Janus-faced" character of HSP70/HSPA proteins in this respect, they may play a role in both improvement and worsening of the disease, depending on the properties of a given concrete case [*Fábián et al. 2009/a,b*].

Inflammatory processes of the dental pulp can also be triggered or worsened due to the overexpression of HSP70/HSPA proteins under stress. Disadvantageous *amplification of inflammatory response* to bacteria (i.e. carious dentine) and/or to several dental materials as well as to tooth preparation due to the immune enhancing effect of HSP70/HSPA proteins could be expected as a possible pathway [*Fábián et al. 2009/a*]. *Flare up or formation of periapical lesions* may also be triggered and or worsened due to stress induced overexpression of HSP70/HSPA molecules [*Fábián et al. 2009/a*]. The expression of

HSP70/HSPA proteins was increased in lymphocytes and endothelial cells of inflammatory granulation tissues, as well as in lining epithelium of radicular and residual cysts [*Suzuki et al. 2002*]. HSP70/HSPA proteins also induce bone resorption [*Nair et al. 1999*], due to proinflammatory cytokines, which are known activators of osteoclasts [*Fábián et al. 2009/b*]. All these findings are strong indications of an important role of HSP70/HSPA proteins in the flare up and/or progression of periapical inflammatory processes [*Fábián et al. 2009/a*]. *Exacerbations of periodontal inflammations* are also likely to occur due to premised bone resorptive effects [*Fábián et al. 2009/a,b*]; after the turning of gingivitis into a more severe inflammation (i.e. periodontitis) with pocket formation and irreversible destruction of the periodontal bone. Similarly, stress induced overexpression of HSP70/HSPA molecules is likely to play a role in the accelerated loss of periodontal bone of patients with spondyloarthropathies [*Fábián et al. 2009/a,b*].

3.4.9. Mucosal Allergy and Irritation

Allergic and/or irritative reactions of the oral mucosa primarily occur due to wearing fixed- and/or removable dentures prepared from *dental cast alloys* [*Borelli et al. 1988, Garhammer et al. 2001, Schmalz & Garhammer 2002*] and/or *acrylate* resins [*Nealey & del Rio 1969, Borelli et al. 1988, Wöstmann 1996*]. Other dental materials like amalgam (see also *paragraph 3.5.9.*) and rarely composites may also induce such reactions. The most frequent *objective intraoral symptoms* of such reactions are gingival redness, more severe gingivitis (erythema and swelling), tongue anomalies (lingua geographica, redness of tongue), redness of palate, more severe inflammation of palate (erythema and swelling), gingival and/or other mucosal ulceration, and lichenoid lesions [*Bánóczy et al. 1979, Borelli et al. 1988, Garhammer et al. 2001, Schmalz and Garhammer 2002, Vamnes et al. 2004, Garau et al. 2005, Namikoshi 2006*]. The most frequent *subjective intraoral complaints* include glossodynia, burning mouth, "electrical" sensation, saliva related complaints (see *paragraph 3.5.2.*), metal taste and/or other alteration of taste sensation (see *paragraph 3.5.4.*), mucosal itching, paresthesias and other pseudoneurological symptoms (see also *paragraph 3.5.7.*) [*Borelli et al. 1988, Garhammer et al. 2001, Vamnes et al. 2004*]. The most frequent general complaints (see also *paragraph 3.5.8. 3.5.9.*) include headache, weakness, paresthesia, joint pain, fatigue, appearance of blisters and intestinal problems [*Garhammer et al. 2001, Vamnes et al. 2004*], however a history and/or coexistence of local or general eczema, allergic dermatitis, rhinitis, urticaria, allergic type asthma bronchiale, angiooedema, lip swelling and facial swelling may also appear [*Borelli et al. 1988, Gawkrodger 2005*].

There are four major subtypes of *allergic reactions* based on the traditional classification of *Coombs and Gell*, from which especially immediate IgE mediated (type I) and delayed type (type IV) reactions are of particular interest for dentists [*Borelli et al. 1988*]. However, it should be also emphasized that, most allergic manifestations are a certain "mixture" of several reactions traditionally classified as distinct subtypes [*Borelli et al. 1988, Martin 2004, Usmani & Wilkinson 2007, Vojdani et al. 2008*]. *Immediate, IgE mediated (type I) reactions* primarily occur due to cell surface binded IgE antibodies inducing degranulation of basophile granulocytes and mast cells and consequent release of histamine and several other bioactive substances [*Borelli et al. 1988, Mallo-Pérez & Díaz-Donado 2003, Vojdani et al. 2008*]. Such reactions are responsible for numerous severe or even life dangerous allergic reactions such as *allergic type asthma bronchiale, angiooedema, food hypersensitivity reaction* and *anaphylactic shock* [*Borelli et al. 1988, Mallo-Pérez & Díaz-Donado 2003, Vojdani et al. 2008*].

The *delayed type (type IV) allergic reactions* develop in three major phases as follows: (1) metal ions or other small molecule allergens (referred to as *haptens*) bind to proteins and hapten-protein-complexes develop [*De Rossi & Greenberg 1998, Büdinger & Hertl 2000, Martin 2004*]; (2) hapten-protein-complexes are presented by antigen presenting cells inducing T-lymphocyte activation and consequent proliferation/accumulation of a specific T-lymphocyte population in lymph nodes [*De Rossi & Greenberg 1998, Büdinger & Hertl 2000, Martin 2004*] (see also *paragraph 3.4.3.*). Premised T-lymphocyte population is specifically *sensitized* and possess *hapten-protein-complex*-specific antigenreceptors on their surfaces [*De Rossi & Greenberg 1998, Büdinger & Hertl 2000, Martin 2004*]; therefore, this phase is referred to as *sensitization phase*; (3) if hapten-protein-complexes at issue appear again, trafficking (recirculating) sensitized T-lymphocytes become reactivated and start to release proinflammatory cytokines and chemokines (see also *paragraph 3.4.3.*) which lead to cellular immune-inflammatory reactions in the tissue [*De Rossi & Greenberg 1998, Büdinger & Hertl 2000, Martin 2004*]. Accordingly, this phase is referred to as *effector phase* [*Borelli et al. 1988*]. The occurrence of premised effector phase is the primary cause of most denture related mucosal allergic reactions, as well as for various allergic reactions including contact eczemas, allergic dermatitis and certain granulomatous reactions [*De Rossi & Greenberg 1998, Büdinger & Hertl 2000, Borelli et al. 1988, Martin 2004*].

Mucosal irritation can be divided into several subgroups including mechanical, microbial, chemical and electrical. *Mechanical irritations* may be caused by several parafunctions (see *paragraphs 3.3.9., 3.3.10.*) and due to instability of dentures (see *paragraph 3.3.8.*). *Microbial irritations* are caused by the fermentation products and/or toxins of various microbes accumulated on the surfaces of teeth and/or dental restorations (i.e. bacterial biofilm, plaque) [*Schmalz & Garhammer 2002, Chen & Zirwas 2007*] as well as in the periodontal pocket. *Chemical irritations* may occur because of the release of several acrylic monomers [*Geurtsen 2000, Lassila & Vallittu 2001*] from acrylic resins of removable dentures [*Borelli et al. 1988, Wöstmann 1996*] and resin-based filling materials [*Geurtsen 2000*] as well as because of the degradation or erosion of several acrylic resins leading to the appearance of several unbound resin components [*Geurtsen 2000, Ortengren 2000*]. Similarly, chemical irritation may also occur because of corrosion of dental alloys [*Wirz et al. 1987, Schmalz et al. 1998, Garhammer et al. 2001, Schmalz & Garhammer 2002*]. (*Corrosion* is a release of metallic derivatives as a result of several chemical (or electrochemical) reactions of alloys being in touch with saliva, gingival crevicular fluid, immune cells and oral microbes [*Wirz et al. 1987, Schmalz et al. 1998, Pfeiffer & Schwickerath 1991, Garhammer et al. 2001, Geurtsen 2002, House et al. 2008*].) Although release of acrylic monomers and corrosion of metals are primarily responsible for irritation, they may also increase the *risk* of allergic reactions, because significant amount of acrylic or metallic derivatives can be released from the intraorally placed resins and/or alloys (which may lead to allergic reactions).

Electric irritation may occur because of *potential differences* between several alloys placed into the mouth (saliva), which may lead to the appearance of an electric potential of mV order of magnitude resulting in *galvanic electric current*. Although in some cases the galvanic electric current may rise even up to roughly 100 μA [*Sutow et al 2004*], it is generally below 15 μA [*Sutow et al 2004*]. Notwithstanding that, this value is rather low, galvanic currents may exert significant biological effects on the oral mucosa resulting in gingival swelling, erythema, mucosal pain and lichenoid reactions [*Bánóczy et al. 1979, Schmalz and Garhammer 2002*]. Although galvanic current induced symptoms should be clearly distinguished from chemical irritative and allergic reactions, increased galvanic currents may indicate higher *risk* of chemical irritative and/or allergic reactions in sensitive patients, because of the significant amount of ions released from dental alloy surfaces.

Importantly, oral mucosa is less sensitive to allergens [*Borelli et al. 1988, Holmstrup 1992, De Rossi & Greenberg 1998, Spiechowicz et al. 1999*] but more sensitive to toxic or irritative agents [*Borelli et al. 1988, Huang et al. 2001*] comparing to skin in most cases. Therefore the incidence of irritative reactions is comparatively high, whereas "real" allergic reactions rarely occur [*Borelli et al. 1988, Wöstmann 1996, Spiechowicz et al. 1999, Garhammer et al. 2001*]. The proportion of verified allergic reactions is not more than 10% [*Garhammer et al. 2001*] in a selected group of patients with oral mucosal symptoms of *either* irritative *or* allergic origin [*Garhammer et al. 2001*]. There are several reasons behind the *relative resistance of the oral mucosa against allergens*. First of all, oral mucosa exerts several specific immunological properties [*Novak et al. 2008*], which are likely to be responsible for the *"oral tolerance"* phenomenon. Further, decreased ceratinization of the oral mucosa makes haptenization (binding of haptens) due to keratin-derived proteins less likely comparing to skin [*De Rossi & Greenberg 1998*]. Moreover, *saliva* is likely to *dilute and/or entrap haptens* appearing in the mouth [*De Rossi & Greenberg 1998, Fábián et al. 2007/b, 2008/a,b, 2009/a*] *leading to their elimination* and consequent prevention of delayed type (type IV) allergic reactions.

There are also *immune regulatory proteins* present in the saliva such as HSP70/HSPA type salivary molecular chaperones (see *paragraphs 3.4.7., 3.4.8.*). These proteins were expected to function as *"natural occurring vectors" for physiological desensitization processes* [*Fábián et al. 2009/a*] similarly as described in relation with "oral-tolerance"-based *sublingual immunotherapeutic approaches* [*Novak et al. 2008*]. (However their role may be "Janus faced" under certain conditions, because HSP70/HSPA proteins may also play a role in haptenation induced sensitization [*Fábián et al. 2009/a*]; and autoantibodies against HSP70/HSPA type proteins also frequently appear in the serum of certain metal-allergic patients [*Jin et al. 2003*].).

Although denture related allergic reactions are fortunately rare and primarily belong to the delayed type (type IV) reactions [*Garhammer et al. 2001*], occasionally rather severe and dangerous denture-related allergic reactions may also occur [*Hansen & West 1997*]. Therefore, great care should be taken about patients with *severe local reactions* as well as with a history of *urticaria, allergic type asthma bronchiale, angiooedema, anaphylactic shock or any other IgE mediated (type I) reactions*. Patients with premised pathologies are of *higher risk* of the appearance of *life dangerous* IgE mediated (type I) *allergic reaction*. Importantly, dangerous allergic reactions may appear either immediately (in few minutes) or in a few hours after the treatment (i.e. after the insertion of a new denture [*Hansen & West 1997*]). Therefore, patients should be informed about possible delayed complications; and continuous observation of risk patients for at least 4 to 6 hours (occasionally up to three days in a hospital) following hazardous dental treatments (i.e. local anesthesia, insertion of new denture etc.) may also be needed.

Dentists should also be prepared for first aid interventions against severe anaphylactic reactions especially if dealing with such patients. Please note that: mild symptoms such as pruritus or urticaria can be controlled by administration of 0.2 to 0.5 mL of 1:1000 epinephrine subcutaneously, with repeated doses as required at 3-min intervals for a severe reactions. An intravenous infusion should be initiated to provide a route for administration of epinephrine, (diluted 1:50.000) and volume expanders if intractable hypotension occurs [*Austen 1991*]. Laryngotomy may also be needed if laryngeal angiooedema appear.

3.5. OTHER SYMPTOMS

3.5.1. Cognitive-Behavioral Symptoms

Besides various cognitive-behavioral symptoms caused by any psychiatric conditions of PDI patients, the most important behavioral symptom of PDI patient is *overcriticism*. It frequently appears as *esthetical* complaints of *overcritical patients* [*Ma et al. 2008*]. Overcritical patients usually demands extraordinary efforts (and/or previous guarantees of treatment outcome) at no additional cost [*Ma et al. 2008*], and expect treatment goals, which are very difficult or impossible to achieve [*Ma et al. 2008*]. Although appearance of esthetic complaints may be the most frequent, *overcriticism* may also occur in relation with any other aspect of denture and dental treatment certainly. Importantly, failure to recognize psychogenic factors in such cases, together with prolonged unsuccessful somatic/operative dental therapy may induce profound behavioral changes, and incite certain patients to seek relief through litigation [*Harris et al. 1993*].

3.5.2. Salivation Problems

Saliva is a major determinant of the oral environment and oral comfort [*Dalmadi & Fábián 2004*]. Salivary components can originate from several sources including the major and minor salivary glands, the blood, the oral mucosal cells and the oral microbes, which leads to a rather complex collection of molecules [*Fábián et al. 2008/a,d*]. Saliva constituents play major role in several oral processes, including formation of acquired pellicle on tooth surfaces, bacterial adhesion and biofilm (plaque) formation, crystal growth homeostasis of teeth, mucosal surface protection, hard tissue surface protection and antimicrobial defense [*Guggenheimer & Moore 2003, Fábián et al. 2008/a,d*]. Saliva also play important role in the oral wound healing, dental caries formation, calculus formation and gingival inflammation [*Fábián et al. 2008/a,d*]. Quantitative and/or qualitative changes of saliva are also major cause of both subjective dry mouth sensation (xerostomia) and ptyallorhea (ptyalismus)

[*Fábián et al. 2008/a,d*]. Salivary changes may also lead to halithosis (see *paragraph 3.5.3.*) alteration of taste perception (see *paragraph 3.5.4.*) and alteration of phonation (see *paragraph 3.5.5.*).

Based on above data it is obvious that, salivary changes are major determinant of the oral milieu; and qualitative or quantitative alterations of saliva secretion may lead to general oral discomfort as well as specific oral symptoms. There can be many causes behind alterations of salivary secretion including several *systemic diseases* and/or their *medication* [*Locker 1993, Friedlander et al. 2002, Fábián et al. 2008/a,d*]. Insertion of new dentures (especially but not exclusively removable dentures) also frequently leads to significant changes of salivary secretion [*Gonzalez & Desjardins 1983, Niedermeier et al. 2000, Wolff et al. 2004, Nikolopoulou & Tzortzopoulou 2007*], even if such changes do not necessarily occur in all cases [*Márton et al. 2004*]. Improper (deep) bite registration can lead to "*pseudo*ptyalismus", because of a consequent occurrence of ptyallorhea in the angle of mouth.

Importantly, occurrence of psychosocial and/or psychoemotional stress also strongly influence salivary secretion [*Locker 1993*], and therefore may lead to the appearance of several saliva related manifestations including saliva related symptoms of PDI. *Anxiety* [*Somer et al. 1993*] and *depression* [*Bushfield et al. 1961, Gottlieb et al. 1961*] may lead to rather significant decrease of salivary flow rate. *Acute stress conditions* induce significant elevation of salivary amylase [*Fábián et al. 2004, Nater et al. 2005*] and salivary molecular chaperone HSP70/HSPA level [*Fábián et al. 2004*] as well as prompt changes of bacterial adherence to salivary mucins [*Bosch et al. 2000*]. Acute stress conditions usually increase the level of salivary sIgA [*Stone et al. 1994, Zeier et al. 1996, Gruzelier et al. 1998*], however acute stress effects coupled with *negative emotions* may also decrease it [*Stone et al. 1994, Zeier et al. 1996, Deinzer & Schuller 1998*]. Importantly, there is also a *lateralized cortical control* of salivary sIgA [*Gruzelier et al. 1998, Clow et al. 2003*], resulting in the upregulation during left hemispheric and downregulation during right hemispheric psychological activity [*Gruzelier et al. 1998, Clow et al. 2003*]. *Severe psychiatric disorders* as well as neurological conditions appearing with sensory hallucinations or paranoid events may also lead to rather "strange" saliva related complaints of patients.

3.5.3. Halithosis (Oral Malodor, Foetor Ex Ore)

The most plausible causes of oral malodor (halitosis) are insufficient oral hygiene, periodontal disease, carious lesions [*Yaegaki & Coil 1999/a,b, 200/b, Lang & Filippi 2004, Nalcaci & Baran 2008*] or non-oral causes like nose-throat disorders, several medical conditions, several drugs, or nutritional habits [*Yaegaki & Coil 2000/a,b, Lang & Filippi 2004, van der Broek et al. 2007*]. However, in some cases there are several *psychological* or *psychopathological* causes behind the appearance of oral malodor [*Yaegaki & Coil 1999/a,b Lang & Filippi 2004*]. Wearing of removable dentures may also induce self reported halithosis [*van der Broek et al. 2007, Nalcaci & Baran 2008*] *either* because of a bacterial biofilm accumulation on dentures [*van der Broek et al. 2007, Nalcaci & Baran 2008*] *or* may be because of an interference of removable dentures with retronasal smell recognition (see *paragraph 3.5.4.*). Since the bacterial decomposition processes and resulted volatile sulfur compounds are decisively responsible for the appearance of malodor in most cases [*Rosenberg et al. 1995, Sanz et al. 2001, Lang & Filippi 2004*], *stress induced deterioration of salivary defense functions* (and consequent changes of oral microbiota) may also lead to oral malodor [*Fábián et al. 2008/a,d*]. It may also occur that, patients expect but do *not* exhibit own oral malodor (also referred to as "*pseudohalitosis*" or "*halitofobia*") [*Rosenberg et al. 1995, Yaegaki & Coil 1999/b, 2000/a,b, Giddon & Anderson 2006*], which may also appear as a symptom of PDI. Although elimination of gingival bleeding, periodontal pockets or carious lesions, and also professional dental hygiene and proper individual dental hygiene including tongue brushing are crucial to control oral malodor (halitosis) [*Sanz et al. 2001*], in cases of psychogenic origin psychosomatic therapy of patients is also needed [*Yaegaki & Coil 1999/a, 2000, Lang & Filippi 2004*].

3.5.4. Alteration of Taste Sensation

Denture induced oral inflammations, bacterial biofilm accumulation because of wearing dentures [*Nalcaci & Baran 2008*] or release of chemical components from dentures (i.e. acrylate monomer [*Har-zion et al. 2004*], nickel [*Pfeiffer & Schwickerath 1991*]) may appear as *real taste stimuli*. However, dentures may induce a "real" *alteration of taste sensation* as well. Such denture induced alterations of taste sensation may occur primarily due to six major pathways as follows: (1) prevention of contact between receptor sites and food [*Laney & Gibilisco 1983, Har-zion et al. 2004, Nalcaci & Baran 2008*]; (2) prevention of contact of the tongue with the palatal rugae, which is considered as highly important for dispersing the food and bringing it into more intimate contact with the taste buds [*Steas 1997, Har-zion et al. 2004*]; (3) entrapment of a part of the food between the mucosa and the baseplate [*Har-zion et al. 2004*]; (4) interference with chewing and usual mobility of the tongue and cheeks and consequently decreased release of taste and smell flavor stimuli [*Har-zion et al. 2004*]; (5) interference with the free movement of humid and warm air in the oral and nasal cavities and consequent affection of retronasal olfaction; (6) appearance of pain and pressure or alteration of mucosal touch experience, which also may lead to taste alterations [*Har-zion et al. 2004*].

Alteration of taste sensation is more frequently a complaint of removable denture wearers [*Taylor & Doku 1963, Henkin & Christiansen 1967/a, Bates & Murphy 1968, Yoshinaka et al. 2007, Nalcaci & Baran 2008*]. The most frequent form of taste alteration is coupled with the elevation of taste threshold for *bitter* and especially *sour* in complete denture wearers [*Henkin & Christiansen 1967/a, Yoshinaka et al. 2007*]. However, the role of prostheses as a major initiating factor of such alteration of taste sensation not entirely substantiated yet [*Laney & Gibilisco 1983, Har-Zion et al. 2004, Hedge & Dwivedi 2007*]. Upper removable dentures may prevent regular contact between the *palatal receptor sites* and the taste stimuli (i.e. food) [*Har-zion et al. 2004, Yoshinaka et al. 2007 Nalcaci & Baran 2008*]. Further, upper removable dentures might affect the natural air flow (evoked during mastication) between the oral and nasal cavities being essential for the identification of *retronasal flavor* (*smell*) stimuli [*Har-zion et al. 2004*]. Lower removable denture may interfere with the function of *taste receptors of the tongue and the pharynx* [*Har-zion et al. 2004*] (located near to the root of the tongue [*Henkin & Christiansen 1967/b*]).

Psychological stress factors may also lead to the alteration of taste sensation. There can be numerous central nervous mechanisms considered behind psychological alteration of taste sensation including conditioned learning processes [*Chang & Scott 1984*] and modulation of glutamate-, GABA- or substance-P related orosensory (taste related) synaptic transmission of the rostral nucleus of the solitary tract (rNST) in brainstem [*Smith et al. 1998, Grabauskas & Bradley 1998*]. (Latter may occur via local changes in brainstem, or via descending regulatory cortical connections of rNST from the insula [*Shipley 1982, Smith et al. 1998*] and the amygdala [*Halsell 1998*].) Since taste and olfaction (especially *retronasal* stimuli) are complex sensory functions being in strong interrelationship with each other [*Rolls & Baylis 1994, Rolls et al. 1997, Rolls et al. 1998*]; taste alteration may also occur because of the alteration of olfactory function [*Rolls et al. 1998*].

Recent data indicated alteration of evoked olfactory cortex activity via modulation of glutamatergic synaptic transmission induced by increased extracellular HSP70/HSPA stress protein level in the brain [*Mokrushin & Pavlinova 2008*]. This latter finding indicate that, stress induced release of HSP70/HSPA proteins (see also *paragraph 3.4.7.*) into the extracellular space in the brain [*Guzhova et al. 2001, Lancaster et al. 2004, Mokrushin & Pavlinova 2008*] likely alter central nervous mechanisms of flavor discrimination. Since glutamatergic synaptic transmission is also strongly involved in taste pathways [*Bradley & Grabauskas 1998, Smeraski et al. 1998, Smith et al. 1998*]; premised stress induced release of HSP70/HSPA in the brain is likely to modulate taste sensation also by direct means (i.e. not only via alteration of olfaction). Although influence of HSP70/HSPA proteins on glutamatergic receptors was studied in relation with central nervous synaptic transmission only [*Mokrushin & Pavlinova 2008*], similar influence of *salivary* HSP70/HSPA on receptor binding of major umami taste inducer glutamate to expected umami taste receptors in the mouth may also be possible. Please consider that, premised expected intraoral receptors of glutamate [*Yamaguchi & Kimizuka 1979*] may be similar in this respect to those of the central nervous system.

Although all above findings clearly indicate a possible significant influence of dentures and psychosocial stress effects on taste and alterations of taste, there are certain severe diseases, which may also induce alteration of taste sensation. Nasal and sinus diseases [*Bromley 2000*], sensory neuropathy [*Scardina et al. 2002*] and/or several neurological processes of the brain [*Bromley 2000*] as well as medication [*Bromley 2000, Friedlander et al. 2002*] and psychiatric problems should also be considered when taste related complaints appear. Low concentration of gustin (the major zinc-containing salivary protein) in the saliva [*Law et al. 1987*] as well as zinc deficiency [*Law et al. 1987, Pfeiffer & Schwickerath 1991*] may also lead to the appearance of metallic taste [*Pfeiffer & Schwickerath 1991*] or other taste disturbances. There are also age-related changes of taste recognition [*Winkler et al. 1999*], however they are much less dramatic than commonly occurs with other senses such as sight and hearing [*Easterby-Smith et al. 1994*].

3.5.5. Alteration of Speech

Speech may be altered in some patients after insertion of a new prosthesis, especially (but not exclusively) in the case of complete denture patients [*Darley 1983, Gonzalez &*

Desjardins 1983, Mazurat & Mazurat 2003]. Obviously, it is more difficult to adapt pronunciation of consonants to a new oral situation than vocals; because of the crucial impact of morphology and position of lips, teeth, palatal gingiva, palate and tongue during pronunciation of consonants [*Molly et al. 2008*]. Artificial teeth (of any dentures) *primarily* disturb the production of plosives and fricatives [*Molly et al. 2008*], whereas removable dentures (including RPDs and especially full dentures) frequently make the pronunciation of labio-dental and apico-alveolar consonants difficult [*Lundqvist 1993, Jacobs et al. 2001, Manders et al. 2003, Molly et al. 2008*]. However *any other consonants* [*Kaán et al. 1993*] (i.e. bilabial-, palatal- velar- and glottal- consonants [*Molly et al. 2008*]) or *vocals* [*Seifert et al. 1999/a,b*] may also be distorted following insertion of a new denture. Moreover the voice itself, and the range of the voice may also be changed because of insertion of new dentures [*Seifert et al. 1999/a,b*].

Improper placement of teeth in the vertical, horizontal, and frontal planes usually contributes to speech changes to which the patient cannot accommodate [*Darley 1983, Gonzalez & Desjardins 1983*]. Improper determination of vertical and/or horizontal dimension(s) may also lead to significant alteration of speech [*Seifert et al. 1999/a,b, Rodrigues-Garcia et al. 2003*]. Palatopharingeal overextension of removable dentures may also be a cause of speech related problems [*Darley 1983*]. Decrease of the adequate space (to allow of tongue movements) provided within the dental arch [*Gonzalez & Desjardins 1983*], and the palatal thickness [*Gonzalez & Desjardins 1983, Seifert et al. 1999/a,b*] as well as the design, contour, and thickness of connector elements of RPDs [*Hörschgen et al. 2004*] may also induce speech alterations. Shaping of oral surfaces of dentures (i.e. smooth versus meshy) may also have some significance [*Kivovics et al. 1990*]. It should be also considered that, tongue play a major role in stabilizing lower complete dentures, and this "new" (not natural) function of tongue may interfere with (and disturb) its phonetic function [*Bohnenkamp & Garcia 2007*]. Disregulations of saliva secretion [*Gonzalez & Desjardins 1983, Guggenheimer & Moore 2003, Wolff et al. 2003*] and psychomotor function [*Gonzalez & Desjardins 1983*] may also induce significant alterations of speech. Importantly, stress and other psychoemotional factors also strongly influence both saliva secretion (see *paragraph 3.5.2.*) and psychomotor function (see *paragraphs 3.3.1., 3.3.3.*); therefore, alteration of speech may also appear as a primarily psychogenic symptom of PDI.

3.5.6. Tinnitus

Tinnitus is an auditory phantom phenomenon characterized by the sensation of sounds without objectively identifiable sound sources [*Kahlbrock & Weisz 2008*]. The underlying physiological mechanisms are still unknown. Although a hearing damage frequently implied, it is also likely that, tinnitus is not solely produced in the periphery of the auditory system [*Baguley et al. 2002, Weisz et al. 2006, Kahlbrock & Weisz 2008*]. Altered, abnormal oscillatory patterns of spontaneous brain activity are also likely to play a role in the appearance of tinnitus [*Weisz et al. 2005, Kahlbrock & Weisz 2008*]. Tinnitus may also appear due to TMJ disorder [*Chole & Parker 1992, Henderson et al. 1992, Kempf et al. 1993, Peroz 2003*]. Possible role of a compression of the Eustachian tube due to dorsocranial displacement of the mandible [*Goodfriend 1936, Shapiro & Truex 1943, Peroz 2003*] as well as alteration of pressure in the middle ear *via* tagging of the "tiny ligament" (ligamentum discomalleolare [*Pinto 1962*]) due to disc displacement [*Chole & Parker 1992, Henderson et al. 1992, Peroz 2003*] may be expected in such cases. Tinnitus may also appear as an additional symptom of neuromuscular dysfunctions of orofacial muscles [*Myrhaug 1969, Kempf et al. 1993, Peroz 2003*], especially as the *stapedius muscle* is supplied by the facial nerve, and the *tensor tympani* and *tensor veli palatini muscles* are supplied by the trigeminal nerve [*Peroz 2003*]. Occasionally trigger points of the masseter and medial pterygoid muscles may also induce ear symptoms including tinnitus (see *paragraph 4.2.4.*). Psychosocial stress factors (including PDI) may also play significant role in the appearance of certain tinnitus symptoms [*Peroz 2003, Tönnies 2006*].

3.5.7. Pseudoneurological Symptoms

Pseudoneurological symptoms are symptoms appearing as if they would be caused by any neurological disorder; however without any detectable somatic/neurological background. Several sensory disturbances such as hypoaesthesia, hyperaesthesia, anaesthesia, paresthesia and dysaesthesia as well as facial palsy are the most important such symptoms in the orofacial region. Certain pain symptoms (see *paragraphs 3.2.9., 3.2.11, 3.2.12.*), taste related phenomena (see *paragraph 3.5.4.*) and tinnitus (see *paragraph 3.5.6.*) as well as certain autonomic (i.e. salivation problems, see *paragraph 3.5.2.*) and motor symptoms (i.e. facial tic, oral parafunctions see *paragraphs 3.3.9, 3.3.10.*) may also be classified as a member of this group. Although pseudoneurological symptoms are of psychogenic origin and may be a psychogenic symptom of PDI patients [*Di Felice et al. 1991, Hampf 1987*]; any possible somatic causes including both local (peripheral) and central nervous causes should also be considered and ruled out very carefully.

Edentulous patients may experience sensory disturbances (especially paresthesia or dysaesthesia) of the mental nerve (lower lip), caused by pressure of an ill-fitting lower denture on the mental foramen, and/or on the alveolar nerve itself (especially in the case of severe bone loss of the alveolar ridge) [*Rashid & Yusuf 1997, Wismeijer et al. 1997*]. Decreased flow rate of salivary glands (especially decreased palatal secretion) may also induce oral dysaesthesias [*Niedermeier et al. 2000*]. Strongly compromised failing teeth [*Dale & Amonett 1983*] and periapical infections [*Elliston & Hoen 1996, Di Lenarda et al. 2000*] may also cause such symptoms especially in the mandible. Sensory disturbances may also appear because of endodontic treatment of mandibular teeth [*Morse 1997, Knowles et al. 2003, Vasilakis & Vasilakis 2004*] and surgical interventions [*Wismeijer et al. 1997, Goodacre et al. 2003*] in the mandible. Denture induced irritative reactions may also coupled with paresthesia, mucosal itching or other pseudoneurological symptoms [*Garhammer et al. 2001*]. Oral motor symptoms of somatic origin may appear as a focal manifestation of general dyskinesias or because of medications [*Clark 2006, Lobbezoo & Naeije 2007, Balasubramaniam & Ram 2008*]. Similarly, specific orofacial movement disorders such as orofacial dyskinesia [*Lobbezzo & Naeije 2007, Balasubramaniam & Ram 2008*] and oromandibular dystonia [*Lobbezzo & Naeije 2007, Balasubramaniam & Ram 2008*] may also appear. There are also various severe disorders including cerebrovascular processes, neurodegenerative disorders, multiple sclerosis [*Scardina et al. 2002*], neuropathies [*Scardina et al. 2002*], various somatic pain manifestations (see *paragraphs 3.2.14., 3.2.15., 3.2.16.*), seizure disorder, insufficient local blood circulation (etc.) all of which may also be responsible for the appearance of such symptoms.

3.5.8. General Health Symptoms

Some general symptoms including *fatigue, weakness, headache, dizziness, nausea, emotional tension* and *irritability* may occur rather frequently in relation with denture intolerance. Although premised symptoms are primarily caused by the psychoemotional condition (including psychiatric disorders) of denture intolerance patients; such symptoms may be triggered by local disturbing factors too [*Eidelman 1979, 1982, Amar 2006*]. Perturbations in the communication of immune system towards the brain due to several inflammatory mediators and cytokines (see *paragraph 3.4.3.*) could theoretically also lead to affective manifestations such as *depressive symptoms* [*Amar 2006*]. Denture induced nocturnal bruxism may be coupled with *sleep disturbances* and with consequent psycho-vegetative and psycho-emotional symptoms [*Ieremia et al. 1989*]. *Psychogenic fever* a common psychosomatic disease with acute or persistent body temperature above normal range under psychosocial stress may also appear as a symptom of orofacial psychosomatic manifestations [*Oka & Oka 2007*] including also PDI. *Aerophagia* (chronic air swallowing) may also be associated with frequent saliva swallowing [*Ogami et al. 2005*] caused by PDI induced ptyalismus. Complaints by patients who attribute their symptoms to *dental alloys* or *other dental materials* (see also *paragraphs 3.4.9. and 3.5.9.*) are also often general in nature [*Garhammer et al. 2001*]; and may include various symptoms like headache, weakness, paresthesia as well as appearance of *blisters* and *intestinal problems* [*Garhammer et al. 2001*]. In certain cases *headache* (occasionally mimicking migraine type headache) may also appear in relation with denture wearing [*Melis & Secci 2006*].

3.5.9. "Amalgam Illness"

Possible adverse health effects due to mercury released by amalgam fillings have been discussed in several studies of patients who attribute various symptoms to the effects of amalgam fillings [*Lindberg et al. 1994, Malt et al. 1997, Bailer 2001, Vamnes et al. 2004*]. Although the frequency of occurrence of amalgam related symptoms is rather frequent [*Lygre et al. 2003, Scott et al. 2004*], in general, no systematic relation of specific symptoms to increased mercury levels could be established in such cases [*Herrström & Högstedt 1993, Lindberg et al. 1994, Malt et al. 1997, Melchart et al. 1998, Osborne & Albino 1999, Bailer 2001*]. Although in *certain* cases the toxic/irritative effects may not be excluded [*Melchart et al. 1998, Strömberg et al. 1999, Issa et al. 2004, Scott et al. 2004, McCullough & Tyas 2008*], there are primarily psychological and/or pathopsychological causes behind the "amalgam illness" [*Herrström & Högstedt 1993, Lindberg et al. 1994, Malt et al. 1997, Osborne &*

Albino 1999, Bailer 2001]. In the absence of any clear toxicological and/or allergological evidence (see also *paragraph 3.4.9.*), "amalgam illness" may be seen as a label for a general tendency toward somatization [*Lindberg et al. 1994, Malt et al. 1997, Bailer 2001*]. There is a strict similarity with the *idiopathic environmental intolerance* (formerly: "*multiple chemical sensitivity*") [*Malt et al. 1997*], but in this case the multiple somatic and/or mental symptoms are attributed specifically to amalgam fillings [*Schuurs et al. 2000, Garhammer et al. 2001*]. (The *idiopathic environmental intolerance* is a disorder likely to be of primarily psychogenic origin [*Bornschein et al. 2001, 2002, Bailer et al. 2005, 2008, Hausteiner et al. 2007*] characterized by various somatic symptoms which cannot be explained organically, but are attributed to the influences of potentially toxic environmental chemicals in low, usually harmless doses [*Bornschein et al. 2001, 2002, Bailer et al. 2005, 2008, Hausteiner et al. 2007*].)

3.6. CONCLUSION

There are various symptoms which may occur in relation with psychogenic denture intolerance [*Fábián & Fábián 2000, Fábián et al. 2006, 2007/a*]. Their pathomechanisms may include both somatic and psychogenic mechanisms. PDI related symptoms are usually multifactorial (multicausal) [*Fábián & Fábián 2000, Fábián et al. 2006, 2007/a*], therefore both somatic and psychogenic pathways of pathomechanism should be considered carefully for both diagnosis and treatment. It is also highly important to recognize the "point of attack" at which psychogenic pathways join major somatic pathways of pathomechanisms. Especially, because somatic type treatment modalities (i.e. physiotherapy, medication therapy, diet- or medicinal herb therapy etc.) may be introduced most efficiently at that particular point of pathomechanism (and along) within the frame of multimodal therapies [*Fábián et al. 2007/a*] utilizing both somatic type and psychological approaches.

REFERENCES

[1]   Ahlberg, J; Nikkilä, H; Könönen, M; Partinen, M; Lindholm, H; Sarna, S; Savolainen, A. Associations of perceived pain and painless TMD-related symptoms with alexithymia and depressive mood in media personnel with or without irregular shift work. *Acta Odontol Scand*, 2004 62, 119-123.

[2]   Amar, S. Stress and inflammation: A bidirectional relationship. In: Mostofsky DI, Forgione AG, Giddon, DB. *Behavioral dentistry*. Ames (Iowa): Blackwell Munksgaard; 2006; 29-36.

[3]   Aneksuk, V. Burning mouth syndrome. *J Dent Assoc Thai*, 1989 39, 251-258.

[4]   Asea, A. Stress proteins and initiation of immune response: Chaperokine activity of Hsp70. *Exerc Immunol Rev*, 2005 11, 34-35.

[5]   Auerbach, SM; Laskin, DM; Frantsve, LME; Orr, T. Depression, pain, exposure to stressful life events, and long-term outcomes in temporomandibular disorder patients. *J Oral Maxillofac Surg*, 2001 59, 628-633.

[6]   Austen, KF. Diseases of immediate type hypersensitivity. In: Wilson JD, Braunwald E, Isselbacher KJ, Petersdorf RG, Martin JB, Fauci AS, Root RK (eds.) *Harrison's Principles of Internal Medicine Vol. 2. (Twelfth Edition)*. New York: McGraw-Hill; 1991; 1422-1428.

[7]   Baad-Hansen, L. Atypical odontalgia - pathophysiology and clinical management. *J Oral Rehabil*, 2008 35, 1-11.

[8]   Baba, K; Aridome, K; Haketa, T; Kino, K; Ohyama, T. Sensory perceptive and discriminative abilities of patients with occlusal dysesthesia. *Nihon Hoteshu Shika Gakki Zasshi*, 2005 49, 599-607.

[9]   Baguley, DM; Axon, P; Winter, IM; Moffat, DA. The effect of vestibular nerve section upon tinnitus. *Clin Otolaringol Allied Sci*, 2002 27, 219-226.

[10]   Bailer, J; Rist, F; Rudolf, A; Staehle, HJ; Eickholz, P; Triebig, G; Bader, M; Pfeifer, U. Adverse health effects related to mercury exposure from dental amalgam fillings: toxicological or psychological causes? *Psychol Med*, 2001 31, 255-263.

[11]   Bailer, J; Witthöft, M; Paul, C; Bayerl, C; Rist, F. Evidence for overlap between idiopathic environmental intolerance and somatoform disorders. *Psychosom Med*, 2005 67, 921-929.

[12]   Bailer, J; Witthöft, M; Rist, F. Psychological predictors of short- and medium term outcome in individuals with idiopathic environmental intolerance (IEI) and individuals with somatoform disorders. *J Toxicol Environ Health A*, 2008 71, 766-775.

[13]   Balasubramaniam, R. & Ram, S. Orofacial movement disorders. *Oral Maxillofac Surg Clin North Am*, 2008 20, 273-285.

[14]   Baldry, PE. *Acupuncture, trigger points and musculoskeletal pain. (Third edition)*. Edinburgh - London - New York - Philadelphia - San Francisco - Toronto: Elsevier; 2005; 45-72.

[15]   Bánóczy, J; Roed-Petersen, B; Pindborg, JJ; Inovay, J. Clinical and hystologic studies on electrogalvanically induced oral white lesions. *Oral Surg Oral Med Oral Pathol*, 1979 48, 319-323.

[16]   Barsby, MJ. The use of hypnosis in the management of "gagging" and intolerance to dentures. *Brit Dent J*, 1994 176, 97-102.

[17]   Barsby, MJ. Hypnosis in the management of denture intolerance. *Hypn Int Monographs*, 1997 3, 71-78.

[18]   Bates, JF. & Murphy, WM. A survey of an edentulous population. *Brit Dent J*, 1968 124, 116-121.

[19]   Bessette, R; Bishop, B; Mohl, N. Duration of masseteric silent period in patients with TMJ syndrome. *J Appl Physiol*, 1971 30, 864-869.

[20]   Besson, JM. The neurobiology of pain. *Lancet*, 1999 353, 1610-1615.

[21]   Biondi, M. & Picardi, A. Temporomandibular joint pain-dysfunction syndrome and bruxism: etiopathogenesis and treatment from a psychosomatic integrative viewpoint. *Psychother Psychosom*, 1993 59, 84-98.

[22]   Blake, MJ; Udelsman, R; Feulner, GJ; Norton, DD; Holbrook, NJ. Stress-induced heat shock protein 70 expression in adrenal cortex: an adrenocorticotropic hormone-sensitive, age-dependent response. *Proc Natl Acad Sci USA*, 1991 88, 9873-9877.

[23]   Bohnenkamp, DM. & Garcia, LT. Phonetics and tongue position to improve mandibular denture retention: A clinical report. *J Prosthet Dent*, 2007 98, 344-347.

[24] Borelli, S; Seifert, HU; Seifert, B. Sensibilisierung und allergische Reaktionen. In: hupfauf L (ed.) *Teilprothesen.* München: Urban & Schwarzenberg; 1988; 247-263.

[25] Bornschein, S; Förstl, H; Zilker, T. Idiopathic environmental intolerances (formerly multiple chemical sensitivity) psychiatric perspectives. *J Intern Med,* 2001 250, 309-321.

[26] Bornschein, S; Hausteiner, C; Zilker, T; Förstl, H. Psychiatric and somatic disorders and multiple chemical sensitivity (MCS) in 264 "environmental patients". *Psychol Med,* 2002 32, 1387-1394.

[27] Bosch, JA; De-Geuss, EJC; Ligtenberg, TMJ; Nazmi, K; Veerman, ECI; Hoogstraten, J; Amerogen, AVN. Salivary MUC5B-mediated adherence (ex vivo) of Helicobacter Pilory during acute stress. *Psychosom Med,* 2000 62, 40-49.

[28] Bradley, RM. & Grabauskas, G. Neural circuits for taste. Excitation, inhibition, and synaptic plasticity in the rostral gustatory zone of the nucleus of the solitary tract. *Ann NY Acad Sci,* 1998 855, 467-474.

[29] Breivik, T; Thrane, PS; Murison, R; Gjermo, P. Emotional stress effects on immunity, gingivitis and periodontitis. *Eur J Oral Sci,* 1996 104, 327-334.

[30] Bromley, SM. Smell and taste disorders: a primary care approach. *Am Fam Physician,* 2000 61, 427-438.

[31] Burton, RC. The problem of facial pain. *JADA,* 1969 79, 93-101.

[32] Bushfield, BL; Wechsler, H; Barnum, WJ. Studies of salivation in depression. *Arch Gen Psych,* 1961 5, 472-477.

[33] Büdinger, L. & Hertl, M. Immunologic mechanisms in hypersensitivity reactions to metal ions: an overview. *Allergy,* 2000 55, 108-115.

[34] Byrd, KE; Romito, LM; Dzemidzic, M; Wong, D; Talavage, TM. fMRI study of brain activity elicited by oral parafunctional movements. *J Oral Rehabil,* 2009 36, 346-361.

[35] Cannon, WB. *The wisdom of the body.* New York: Norton; 1939.

[36] Cardot, H. & Laugier, H. Le réflexe linguo-maxillare. *C R Soc Biol,* 1922/a 86, 529-530.

[37] Cardot, H. & Laugier, H. Anesthésie et réflexe linguomaxillare. *C R Soc Biol,* 1922/b 87, 215-219.

[38] Cardot, H. & Laugier, H. Le réflexe linguomaxillare (ultime réflexe) *C R Acad Sci D,* 1922/c 174, 1368-1369.

[39] Carli, G. An update on pain physiology: the relevance of Craig's and Jäning's hypotheses for hypnotic analgesia. *Contemp Hypnosis,* 2009 26, 4-14.

[40] Cathomen-Rötheli, M; Hobi, V; Graber, G. Studies on the personality structure of patients with myoartropathy. *SSO Schweiz Monatsschr Zahnheilkd,* 1976 86, 29-40.

[41] Chang, FCT. & Scott, TR. Conditioned taste aversions modify neuronal responses to gustatory stimuli. *J Neurosci,* 1984 4, 1850-1862.

[42] Chen, AY. & Zirwas, MJ. Denture stomatitis. *Skinmed,* 2007 6, 92-94.

[43] Chiapelli, F. & Hodgson, D. Immune suppression. In: Fink G, editor in chief. *Encyclopedia of stress. (vol. 2.).* San Diego: Academic Press; 2000; 531-536.

[44] Chole, RA. & Parker, WS. Tinnitus and vertigo in patients with temporomandibular disorders. *Arch Otolaryngol Head Neck Surg,* 1992 118, 817-821.

[45] Chrousos, GP. Stressors, stress, and neuroendocrine integration of the adaptive response. The 1997 Hans Selye memorial lecture. *Ann NY Acad Sci,* 1998 851, 311-335.

[46] Ciancaglini, R; Gherlone, EF; Radaelli, G. Association between loss of occlusal support and symptoms of functional disturbances of the masticatory system. *J Oral Rehabil*, 1999 26, 248-253.

[47] Clark, GT. Medical management of oral motor disorders: dystonia, dyskinesia, and drug-induced dystonic extrapiramidal reactions. *J Calif Dent Assoc*, 2006 34, 657-667.

[48] Clark, GT; Minakuchi, H; Lotaif, AC. Orofacial pain and sensory disorders in the elderly. *Dent Clin North Am*, 2005 49, 343-362.

[49] Clark, DL; Boutros, NN; Mendez, MF. *The brain and behavior. An introduction to behavioral neuroanatomy*. Cambridge: Cambridge University Press; 2006; 165-177.

[50] Clow, A., Lambert, S; Evans, P; Hucklebridge, F; Higuchi, K. An investigation into asymmetrical cortical regulation of salivary sIgA in conscious man using transcranial magnetic stimulation. *Int J Psychophysiol*, 2003 47, 57-64.

[51] Costen, JB. A syndrome of ear and sinus symptoms dependent upon disturbed function of the temporomandibular joint. *Annals Otol Rhinol Laringol*, 1934 43, 1-15.

[52] Cutler, CW. & Jotwani, R. Dendritic cells at the oral mucosal interface. *J Dent Res*, 2006 85, 678-689.

[53] Dahlsröm, L. Electromyographic studies of craniomandibular disorders: a review of the literature. *J Oral Rehabil*, 1989 16, 1-20.

[54] Dale, RA. & Amonett, R. Paresthesia from an overdenture abutment: report of a case. *JADA*, 1983 107, 943-944.

[55] Dalmadi, L. & Fábián, TK. The role of saliva in the oral defence mechanisms. *Fogorv Szle*, 2004 97, 199-203.

[56] Darley, FL. Speech pathology. In: Laney WR, Gibilisco JA (eds.) *Diagnosis and treatment in prosthodontics*. Philadelphia: Lea & Febiger; 1983; 346-376.

[57] Darvell, BW. & Clark, RK. The physical mechanisms of complete denture retention. *Brit Dent J*, 2000 189, 248-252.

[58] De Boever, JA. & De Boever, AM. Dental aspects of the treatment of temporomandibular joint disorders. *Rev Belge Med Dent*, 1997 52, 258-273.

[59] Deinzer, R. & Schuller , N. Dynamics of stress-related decrease of salivary immunoglobulin A (sIgA): Relationship to symptoms of the common cold and studying behavior. *Behav Med*, 1998 23, 161-169.

[60] de Laat, A; van der Glas, HW; Weytjens, JLF; van Steenberghe, D. The masseteric post-stimulus electromyographic-complex in people with dysfunction of the mandibular joint. *Arch Oral Biol*, 1985 30, 177-180.

[61] de Laat, A; van Steenberghe, D; Lesaffre, E. Occlusal relationships and temporomandibular joint dysfunction. Part II: Correlations between occlusal and articular parameters and symptoms of TMJ dysfunction by means of stepwise logistic regression. *J Prosthet Dent*, 1986 55, 116-121.

[62] De Rossi, SS. & Greenberg, MS. Intraoral contact allergy: A literature review and case reports. *JADA*, 1998 129, 1435-1441.

[63] Dhabhar, FS. Effects of stress on immune cell distribution. In: Fink G, editor in chief. *Encyclopedia of stress. (vol. 2.)*. San Diego: Academic Press; 2000/a; 507-514.

[64] Dhabhar, FS. Stress-induced enhancement of immune function. In: Fink G, editor in chief. *Encyclopedia of stress. (vol. 2.)*. San Diego: Academic Press; 2000/b; 515-523.

[65] Dhabhar, FS. & McEwen, BS. Acute stress enhances while chronic stress suppresses immune function in vivo: A potential role for leukocyte trafficking. *Brain Behav Immunol*, 1997 11, 286-306.

[66] Dhabhar, FS; Miller, AH; McEwen, BS; Spencer, RL. Effects of stress on immune cell distribution - dynamics and hormonal mechanisms. *J Immunol*, 1995 154, 5511-5527.

[67] Di Felice, R; Samson, J; Carlino, P; Giuliani, M; Fiore-Donno, G. Psychogenic oral paresthesia. *Rev Odontostomatol (Paris)*, 1991 20, 189-194.

[68] Di Lenarda, R; Cadenaro, M; Stacchi, C; Paresthesia of the mental nerve induced by periapical infection. *Oral Surg Oral Med Oral Pathol Oral Radiol Endod*, 2000 90, 746-749.

[69] Dworkin, SF. & Sherman J. Chronic orofacial pain: biobehavioral perspectives. In: Mostofsky DI, Forgione AG, Giddon DB editors. *Behavioral dentistry*. Ames (Iowa): Blackwell Munksgaard; 2006; 99-113.

[70] Dworkin, SF; Turner, JA; Wilson, L; Massoth, D; Whitney, C Huggins, Burgess, J; Sommers, E; Truelove, E. Brief group cognitive-behavioral intervention for temporomandibular disorders. *Pain*, 1994 59, 175-187.

[71] Easterby-Smith, V; Besford, J; Heath, R. The effect of age on the recognition thresholds of three sweeteners: sucrose, saccharin and aspartame. *Gerodontology*, 1994 11, 39-45.

[72] Eccles, JC; Central connections of muscle afferent fibers. In: Baker H, editor. *Symposion of Muscle Receptors*. Hong Kong: Hong Kong University Press; 1962; 81-101.

[73] Eidelman, D. "Fatigue or rest" and associated symptoms (headache, vertigo, blurred vision, nausea, tension and irritability) due to locally asymptomatic, unerupted, impacted teeth. *Med Hypothesis*, 1979 5, 339-346.

[74] Eidelman, D. Pathology in the lower half of the functional face - its significance in clinical medicine. *Med Hypothesis*, 1982 8, 149-154.

[75] Eli, I. & Kleinhauz, M. Hypnosis and dentistry. *Hypn Int Monographs*, 1997 3, 59-69.

[76] Elliston, NK. & Hoen, MM. Infectious transient dental-related paresthesia. *Gen Dent*, 1996 44, 66-69.

[77] Every, RG. The significance of extreme mandibular movements. Lancet, 1960 2, 37-39.

[78] Every, RG. The teeth as weapons. their influence on behaviour. Lancet, 1965 27, 685-688.

[79] Fábián G. Psychosomatic aspects of orthodontics. [Az orthodontia pszichoszomatikus vonatkozásai]. In: Fábián TK, Vértes G editors. *Psychosomatic dentistry [Fogorvosi pszichoszomatika]*. Budapest: Medicina; 2007; 137-146.

[80] Fábián, G; Bálint, M; Fábián, TK. Psychology and psychosomatics of the orthodontic treatment. *Fogorv Szle*, 2005 98, 113-119.

[81] Fábián, TK. Treatment possibilities of denture intolerance. Use of photo-acoustic stimulation and hypnotherapy in a difficult clinical case. [Adalékok a protézis intolerancia gyógyításához. Fény-hang kezeléssel kombinált hipnoterápia alkalmazásának szokatlan módja egy eset kapcsán.] *Hipno Info*, 1999 38, 81-88.

[82] Fábián, TK. & Fábián, G. Dental stress. In: Fink G, editor in chef. *Encyclopedia of Stress. Vol. 1.* San Diego: Academic Press; 2000; 657-659.

[83] Fábián, TK; Gáspár, J; Fejérdy, L; Kaán, B; Bálint, M; Csermely, P; Fejérdy, P. Hsp70 is present in human saliva. *Med Sci Monitor*, 2003 9, BR62-65.

[84] Fábián, TK; Tóth, Zs; Fejérdy, L; Kaán, B; Csermely, P; Fejérdy, P. Photo-acoustic stimulation increases the amount of 70 kDa heat shock protein (Hsp70) in human whole saliva. A pilot study. *Int J Psychophysiol*, 2004 52, 211-216.

[85] Fábián, TK; Mierzwińska-Nastalska, E; Fejérdy P. Photo-acoustic stimulation. A suitable method in the treatment of psychogenic denture intolerance. *Protet Stomatol*, 2006 56, 335-340.

[86] Fábián, TK; Fábián, G; Fejérdy, P. Dental Stress. In: Fink G editor in chef. *Encyclopedia of Stress. 2-nd enlarged edition, Vol. 1.* Oxford: Academic Press; 2007/a; 733-736.

[87] Fábián, TK; Fejérdy, P; Nguyen, MT; Sőti, Cs; Csermely, P. Potential immunological functions of salivary Hsp70 in mucosal and periodontal defense mechanisms. *Arch Immunol Ther Exp*, 2007/b 55, 91-98.

[88] Fábián, TK; Fejérdy, P; Csermely, P. Chemical biology of saliva in health and disease. In: Begley T, editor in chief. Wiley encyclopedia of chemical biology. Hoboken: John Wiley & sons; 2008/a. DOI: 10.1002/9780470048672.wecb643

[89] Fábián, TK; Sőti, Cs; Nguyen, MT; Csermely, P; Fejérdy, P. Expected functions of salivary HSP70 in the oral cavity. (Review article). In: Morell E, Vincent C editors. *Heat shock proteins: New research.* Hauppauge: Nova Science Publishers; 2008/b; 321-340.

[90] Fábián, TK; Sőti, Cs; Nguyen, MT; Csermely, P; Fejérdy, P. Expected functions of salivary HSP70 in the oral cavity. *Int J Med Biol Frontier*, 2008/c; 289-308.

[91] Fábián, TK; Fejérdy, P; Csermely, P. Salivary genomics, transcriptomics and proteomics: The emerging concept of the oral ecosystem and their use in the early diagnosis of cancer and other diseases. *Current Genomics*, 2008/d 9, 11-21.

[92] Fábián, TK; Gótai, L; Beck, A; Fábián, G; Fejérdy, P. The role of molecular chaperones (HSPAs/HSP70s) in oral health and oral inflammatory diseases: A review. *Eur J Inflammation*, 2009/a 7, 53-61.

[93] Fábián, TK; Csermely, P; Fábián, G; Fejérdy, P. Spondyloarthropathies and bone resorption: A possible role of heat shock protein (Hsp70). (Review). *Acta Physiol Hungarica*, 2009/b 96, 149-155.

[94] Fauci, AS. Mechanisms of corticosteroid action on lymphocyte subpopulations. I. Redistribution of circulating T and B lymphocytes to the bone marrow. *Immunology*, 1975 28, 669-680.

[95] Fauci, AS. & Dale, DC. The effect of in vivo hydrocortisone on subpopulations of human lymphocytes. *J Clin Invest*, 1974 53, 240-246.

[96] Fields, HL. *Pain.* New York: McGraw - Hill; 1987; 216.

[97] Fields, HL. & Basbaum, AI. Central nervous system mechanisms of pain modulation. In: Wall PD, Melzack R editors. *Textbook of pain. (Third edition).* Edinburgh: Churchill Livingstone; 1994; 243-257.

[98] Fleshner, M; Watkins, LR; Lockwood, LL; Laudeslager, ML; Maier, SF. Specific changes in lymphocyte subpopulations: a potential mechanism for stress-induced immunomodulation. *J Neuroimmunol*, 1992 41, 131-142.

[99] Fleshner, M; Campisi, J; Amiri, L; Diamond, DM. Cat exposure induces both intra- and extracellular Hsp72: the role of adrenal hormones. *Psychoneuroendocrinology*, 2004 29, 1142-1152.

[100] Friedlander, AH; Friedlander, IK; Marder, SR. Bipolar I disorder. Psychopathology, medical management and dental implications. *JADA*, 2002 133, 1209-1217.

[101] Friedman, LS. & Isselbacher, KJ. Anorexia, nausea, vomiting and indigestion. In: Wilson JD, Braunwald E, Isselbacher KJ, Petersdorf RG, Martin JB, Fauci AS, Root RK editors. *Harrison's principles of internal medicine.* (International edition). New York: McGraw-Hill; 1991; 251-253.

[102] Fuhr, K. & Reiber, T. Klinische Funktionsdiagnostik. In: Koeck B, editor. *Funktionsstörungen des Kauorgans.* München - Wien - Baltimore: Urban & Schwarzenberg; 1995; 75-78.

[103] Fukodo, S; Abe, K; Hongo, M; Utsumi, A; Itoyama, Y. Brain-gut induction of heat shock protein (HSP) 70 mRNA by psychophysiological stress in rats. *Brain Res*, 1997 16, 146-148.

[104] Ganong, WF. *Review of medical physiology. (Hungarian edition).* Budapest: Medicina; 1990; 140-148.

[105] Garau, V; Masala, MG; Cortis, MC; Pittau, R. Contact stomatitis due to palladium in dental alloys: A clinical report. *J Prosthet Dent*, 2005 93, 318-320.

[106] Garhammer, P; Schmalz, G; Hiller, KA; Reitinger, T; Stolz, W. Patients with local adverse effects from dental alloys: frequency, complaints, symptoms, allergy. *Clin Oral Invest*, 2001 5, 240-249.

[107] Garnick, J. & Ramfjord, SP. Rest position. An electromyographic and clinical investigation *J Prosthet Dent*, 1962 12, 895-911.

[108] Gáspár, J; Fejérdy, L; Fábián, TK. The psychical aspects of overactive gag reflex (gagging): a case report. *Fogorv Szle*, 2002 95, 199-203.

[109] Gawkrodger, DJ. Investigation of reactions to dental materials. *Brit J Dermatol*, 2005 153, 479-485.

[110] Gebhardt, GF; Sandkühler, J; Thalhammer, JG; Zimmermann, M. Inhibition of spinal cord of nociceptive information by electrical stimulation and morphine microinjection at identical sites in midbrain of the cat. *J Neurophysiol*, 1984 51, 75-89.

[111] Gerbershagen, HU. *Die schwierige Schmerzpatient in der Zahnmedizin.* Stuttgart: Thieme; 1995; 2-15, 27, 39, 116-117.

[112] Geurtsen, W. Biocompatibility of resin-modified filling materials. *Crit Rev Oral Biol Med*, 2000 11, 333-355.

[113] Geurtsen, W. Biocompatibility of dental casting alloys. *Crit Rev Oral biol Med*, 2002 13, 71-84.

[114] Giddon, DB. & Anderson, NK. The oral and craniofacial area and interpersonal attraction. In: Mostofsky DI, Forgione AG, Giddon DB editors. *Behavioral dentistry.* Ames (Iowa): Blackwell Munksgaard; 2006; 3-17.

[115] Gill, HI. Muscle spindles in the lateral pterygoid muscle. *J Dent Res*, 1969 48, 1084.

[116] Glaros, AG. Bruxism. In: Mostofsky DI, Forgione AG, Giddon DB editors. *Behavioral dentistry.* Ames (Iowa): Blackwell Munksgaard; 2006; 127-137.

[117] Gleissner, C; Kaesser, U; Dehne, F; Bolten, WW; Willershausen, B. Temporomandibular joint function in patients with longstanding rheumatoid arthritis - I. Role of periodontal status and prosthetic care - a clinical study. *Eur J Med Res*, 2003 27, 98-108.

[118] Golan, HP. The use of hypnosis in the treatment of psychogenic oral pain. *Am J Clin Hypn*, 1997 40, 89-96.

[119] Goldstein, DS. Sympathetic Nervous System. In: Fink G, editor in chef. *Encyclopedia of Stress. Vol. 1.* San Diego: Academic Press; 2000; 558-565.

[120] Gonzalez, JB. & Desjardins, RP. Management of patients with new prostheses. In: Laney WR, Gibilisco JA editors. *Diagnosis and treatment in prosthodontics.* Philadelphia: Lea & Febiger; 1983; 506-535.

[121] Goodacre, CJ; Bernal, G; Rungcharassaeng, K; Kan, YKK. Clinical complications with implant and implant prostheses. *J Prosthet Dent*, 2003 90, 121-132.

[122] Goodfriend, DJ. Symptomatology and treatment of abnormalities of the mandibular articulation. *Dent Cosmos*, 1936 78, 844-852, 947-960.

[123] Gottlieb, G; Paulson, G; Raleigh, NC. Salivation in depressed patients. *Arch Gen Psych*, 1961 5, 468-471.

[124] Grabauskas, G. & Bradley, R. Ionic mechanisms of GABA$_A$ biphasic synaptic potentials in gustatory nucleus of the solitary tract. *Ann NY Acad Sci*, 1998 855, 486-487.

[125] Graber, G. Neurologische und psychosomatische Aspekte der Myoarthropathien des Kauorgans. *Zahnärztl Welt Rundschau*, 1971 21, 997-1000.

[126] Graber, G. Der Einfluss von Psyche und Stress bei dysfunktionsbedingten Erkrankungen des stomatognathen Systems. In: Koeck B, editor. *Funktionsstörungen des Kauorgans.* München - Wien - Baltimore: Urban & Schwarzenberg; 1995; 50-69.

[127] Gratt, BM. & Anbar, M. A pilot study of nitric oxide blood levels in patients with chronic orofacial pain. *Oral Surg Oral Med Oral Pathol Oral Radiol Endod*, 2005 100, 441-448.

[128] Green, CS. & Laskin, DM. Temporomandibular disorders: Moving from a dentally based to a medically based model. *J Dent Res*, 2000 79, 1736-1739.

[129] Griffin, CJ. & Harris, R. The regulatory influences of the trigeminal system. In: Griffin CJ, Harris R editors. *The temporomandibular joint syndrome. The masticatory apparatus of man in normal and abnormal function.* (Monographs in oral science, Vol. 4.) Basel - München - Paris - London - New York - Sydney: Karger; 1975; 65-86.

[130] Griffin, CJ, Watson, JE; Marshall, WG: Electromyographic analysis of the effects of treatment in patients with the temporomandibular joint syndrome. In: Griffin CJ, Harris R editors. *The temporomandibular joint syndrome. The masticatory apparatus of man in normal and abnormal function.* (Monographs in oral science, Vol. 4.) Basel - München - Paris - London - New York - Sydney: Karger; 1975; 188-200.

[131] Grushka, M; Sessle, BJ; Howley, TP. Psychophysical assessment of tactile, pain and thermal sensory functions in burning mouth syndrome. *Pain*, 1987 28, 169-184.

[132] Grushka, M. & Sessle, BJ. Burning mouth syndrome. *Dent Clin North Am*, 1991 35, 171-184.

[133] Gruzelier, J; Clow, A; Evans, P; Lazar, I; Walker, L. Mind-body influences on immunity: Lateralized control, stress, individual difference predictors and prophylaxis. *Ann NY Acad Sci*, 1998 851, 487-494.

[134] Guggenheimer, J. & Moore, PA. Xerostomia. Etiology, recognition and treatment. *JADA*, 2003 134, 61-69.

[135] Guzhova, I; Kislyakova, K; Moskaliova, O; Fridlanskaya, I; Tytell, M; Cheetham, M; Margulis, B. In vitro studies show that HSP70 can be released by glia and that exogenous HSP70 can enhance neuronal stress tolerance. *Brain Res*, 2001 914, N1, 66-73.

[136] Hahn, W. Results of a clinicopsychological study of diseases of the temporomandibular joint. *Int Dent J*, 1979 29, 260-268.

[137] Hagag, G; Yoshida, K; Miura, H. Occlusion, prosthodontic treatment, and temporomandibular disorders: a review. *J Med Dent Sci*, 2000 47, 61-66.

[138] Halsell, CB. Differential distribution of amygdaloid input across rostral solitary nucleus subdivisions in rat. *Ann NY Acad Sci*, 1998 855, 482-485.

[139] Hansen, K. & Schliack, H. *Segmentale Innervation*. Stuttgart: Thieme, 1962.

[140] Hansen, PA. & West, LA. Allergic reaction following insertion of a Pd-Cu-Au fixed partial denture: a clinical report. *J Prosthodont*, 1997 6, 144-148.

[141] Hampf, G. Dilemma in treatment of patients suffering from orofacial dysaesthesia. *Int J Oral Maxillofac Surg*, 1987 16, 397-401.

[142] Harris, M; Feinmann, C; Wise, M; Treasure, F. Temporomandibular joint and orofacial pain: clinical and medicolegal management problems. *Brit Dent J*, 1993 174, 129-136.

[143] Harris, R. & Griffin, CJ. Neuromuscular mechanisms and the masticatory apparatus. In: Griffin CJ, Harris R editors. *The temporomandibular joint syndrome. The masticatory apparatus of man in normal and abnormal function.* (Monographs in oral science, Vol. 4.) Basel - München - Paris - London - New York - Sydney: Karger; 1975; 45-64.

[144] Har-Zion, G; Brin, I; Steiner, J. Psychophysiological testing of taste and flavour reactivity in young patients undergoing treatment with removable orthodontic appliances. *Eur J Orthodontics*, 2004 26, 73-78.

[145] Hausteiner, C; Bornschein S; Zilker, T; Henningsen, P; Förstl, H. Dysfunctional cognitions in idiopathic environmental intolerances (IEI) - An integrative psychiatric perspective. *Toxicology Letters*, 2007 171, 1-9.

[146] Hedge, AM. & Dwivedi, S. Effect of removable orthodontic appliance on taste and flavor perception - a clinical study. *J Clin Pediatr Dent*, 2007 32, 79-82.

[147] Heggendorn, H; Voght, HP; Graber, G. Experimentelle Untersuchungen über die orale Hyperaktivität bei psychischer belastung, im besonderen bei Aggression. *Schweiz Mschr Zahnheilk*, 1979 89, 1148-1161.

[148] Henderson, DH; Cooper, JCJ; Bryan, GW; Van Sickels, JE. Otologic complaints in temporomandibular joint syndrome. *Arch Otolaryngol Head Neck Surg*, 1992 118, 1208-1213.

[149] Henkin, RI. & Christiansen, RL. Taste thresholds in patients with dentures. *JADA*, 1967/a 75, 118-120.

[150] Henkin, RI. & Christiansen, RL. Taste localization on the tongue, palate, and pharinx of normal man. *J Appl Physiol*, 1967/b 22, 316-320.

[151] Herrström, P. & Högstedt, B. Clinical study of oral galvanism: no evidence of toxic mercury exposure but anxiety disorder is an important background factor. *Scand J Dent Res*, 1993 1011, 232-237.

[152] Hilgard, ER. & Marquis, DM. *Conditioning and learning.* New York: Appleton-Century-Crofts; 1940.

[153] Hiltunen, K; Vehkalahti, M; Ainamo, A. Occlusal imbalance and temporomandibular disorders in the elderly. *Acta Odontol Scand*, 1997 55, 137-141.

[154] Hoffmann, P. & Tönnies, JF. Nachweis des völlig konstanten Vorkommens des Zungen-Kieferreflexes beim Menschen. *Pflugers Arch ges Physiol*, 1948 250, 103-108.

[155] Holmstrup, P Oral mucosa and skin reactions related to amalgam. *Adv Dent Res*, 1992 6, 120-124.

[156] House, K; Sernetz, F; Dymock, D; Sandy, JR; Ireland, AJ. Corrosion of orthodontic appliances - should we care? *Am J Orthod Dentofacial Orthop*, 2008 133, 584-592.

[157] Hörschgen, J; Wisser, W; Berger, R; Lotzmann, U. Der Einfluss der grossen Verbinder von Zahnärztlichen Teilprothesen auf die Lautbildung. *Folia Phoniatr Logop*, 2004 56, 114-156.

[158] Huang, FM; Tai, KW; Hu, CC; Chang, YC. Cytotoxic effects of denture base materials on a permanent human oral epithelial cell line and on primary human oral fibroblasts in vitro. *Int J Prosthodont*, 2001 14, 439-443.

[159] Hunt, CC. & Paintal, AS. Spinal reflex regulation of fusimotor neurones. *J Physiol Lond*, 1958 143, 195-212.

[160] Hunt, SP; Pini, A; Evan, G. Induction of c-fos-like proteins in spinal cord neurons following sensory stimulation. *Nature*, 1987 328, 632-634.

[161] Ieremia, L; Popoviciu, L; Balas, M; Dodu, S Gábor, D. Nocturnal bruxism. Contributions to the detection and assessment of involvement in the craniomandibular pain dysfunction syndrome. *Rev Med Interna Neurol Psihiatr Neurochir Dermatovenerol Neurol Psihiatr Neurochir*, 1989 34, 307-316.

[162] Israel, HA. & Scrivani, SJ. The interdisciplinary approach to oral, facial and head pain. *JADA*, 2000 131, 919-926.

[163] Issa, Y; Brunton, PA; Glenny, AM; Duxbury, AJ. Healing of oral lichenoid lesions after replacing amalgam restorations: A systematic review. *Oral Surg Oral Med Oral Pathol Oral Radiol Endod*, 2004 98, 553-565.

[164] Ito, H; Takekoshi, T; Miyauchi, M; Ogawa, I; Takata, T; Nikai, H; Takemoto, K. Three-dimensional appearance of Langerhans cells in human gingival epithelium as revealed by confocal laser scanning microscopy. *Arch Oral Biol*, 1998 43, 741-744.

[165] Ito, M; Kurita, K; Ito, T; Arao, M. Pain threshold and pain recovery after experimental stimulation in patients with burning mouth syndrome. *Psychiatr Clin Neurosci*, 2002 56, 161-168.

[166] Jacobs, R; Manders, E; Van Looy, C; Lembrechts, D; Naert, I; van Steenberghe, D. Evaluation of speech in patients rehabilitated with various oral implant-supported prostheses. *Clin Oral Implant Res*, 2001 12, 167-173.

[167] Jagger, RG; Korszun, A. Phantom bite revised. *Br Dent J*, 2004 197, 241-243.

[168] Jin, GB; Nakayama, H; Shmyhlo, M; Inoue, S; Kondo, M; Ikezawa, Z; Ouchi, Y; Cyong, JC; High positive frequency of antibodies to methallothionein and heat shock protein 70 in sera of patients with metal allergy. *Clin Exp Immunol*, 2003 131, 275-279.

[169] Johnson, JD. & Fleshner, M. Releasing signals, secretory pathways, and immune function of endogenous extracellular heat shock protein 72. *J Leukoc Biol*, 2006 79, 425-434.

[170] Kaán, M; Bolla, K; Keszler, B. Speech characteristics of persons wearing full upper and lower prostheses. *Fogorv Szle*, 1993 86, 45-53.

[171] Kalbrock, N; Weisz, N. Transient reduction of tinnitus intensity is marked by concomitant reductions of delta band power. *BMC Biology*, 2008 6, 4.

[172] Kampe, T; Edman, G; Bader, G; Tagdae, T; Karlsson, S. Personality traits in a group of subjects with long-standing bruxing behaviour. *J Oral Rehabil*, 1997 24, 588-593.

[173] Kageyama, H; Suzuki, E; Kashiva, T; Kanazawa, M; Osaka, T; Kimura, S; Namba, Y; Inoue, S. Sucrose-diet feeding induces gene expression of heat shock protein in rat brain under stress. *Biochem Biophy Res Commun*, 2000 274, 355-358.

[174] Kawamura, Y; Kishi, K; Nobuhara, M; Fujimoto, J. Studies on masticatory function. I. An electromyographic analysis of the chewing pattern of the normal occlusion and malocclusion. *Med J Osaka Univ*, 1957 8, 229-239.

[175] Kawamura, Y; Funakoshi, M; Tsukamoto, S. Brain-stem representation of jaw muscle activites of the dog. *Jap J Physiol*, 1958 8, 292-304.

[176] Kempf, HG; Roller, R; Mühlbrandt, L. Correlation between inner ear disorders and temporomandibular joint diseases. *HNO*, 1993 41, 7-10.

[177] Kivovics, P; Sajgó, P; Herendi, G; Hermann, P. Evaluation of comfort, sound formation and food relations of the oral surface of mould cast metal plates, based on patient questionnaires. *Fogorv Szle*, 1990 83, 371-373.

[178] Kivovics, P; Jáhn, M; Borbély, J; Márton, K. Frequency and location of traumatic ulcerations following placement of complete dentures. *Int J Prosthodont*, 2007 20, 397-401.

[179] Kleindienst, R; Xu, Q; Willeit, J; Waldenberger, FR; Weimann, S; Wick, G. Immunology of atherosclerosis. Demonstration of heat shock protein 60 expression and T lymphocytes bearing alpha/beta or gamma/delta receptor in human atherosclerotic lesions. *Am J Pathol*, 1993 142, 1927-1937.

[180] Knowles, KI; Jergenson, MA; Howard, JH. Paresthesia associated with endodontic treatment of mandibular premolars. *J Endod*, 2003 29, 768-770.

[181] Kossioni AE. & Karzakis, HC. Variation in the masseteric silent period in older dentate humans and in denture wearers. *Arch Oral Biol*, 1995 40, 1143-1150.

[182] Köling, A. Neurologist, otolaryngologist...? Which specialist should treat facial pain? *Lakartidningen*, 1998 95, 2320-2325.

[183] Krahwinkel, T; Nastali, S; Azrak, B; Willershausen, B. The effect of examination stress conditions on the cortisol content of saliva - a study of students from clinical semesters. *Eur J Med Res*, 2004 28, 256-260.

[184] Kromminga, R; Müller-Fahlbusch, H; Habel, G. Interdisciplinary investigations on the critcism of the therm "anesthesia dolorosa". *Dtsch Zahnärztl Z*, 1989 44, 960-961.

[185] Kromminga, R; Habel, G; Müller-Fahlbusch, H. Failure of dental implants following psychosomatic disturbances in the stomatognathic system - a clinical-catamnestic study. *Dtsch Stomatol*, 1991 41, 233-236.

[186] Lamey, PJ. & Lamb, AB. Lip component of burning out syndrome. *Oral Surg Oral Med Oral Pathol*, 1994 78, 590-593.

[187] Lamey, PJ; Biagioni, PA; AlHashimi, I. The feasibility of using infrared thermography to evaluate minor salivary gland function in euhydrated, dehydrated and rehydrated subjects. *J Oral Pathol Med*, 2007 36, 127-131.

[188] Lamprecht, F; Demmel, HJ; Riehl, A. Psychosomatic findings in orofacial pain dysfunction syndrome. *Z Psychosom Med Psychoanal*, 1986 32, 382-393.

[189] Lancaster, GI; Moller, K; Nielsen, B; Secher, NH; Febbraio, MA; Nybo, L. Exercise induces the release of heat shock protein 72 from the human brain *in vivo*. *Cell Stress Chaperones*, 2004 9, 276-280.

[190] Laney, WR. & Gibilisco, JA. History, laboratory data and physical examination. In: Laney WR, Gibilisco JA editors. *Diagnosis and treatment in prosthodontics*. Philadelphia: Lea & Febiger; 1983; 26-72.

[191] Lang, B; Filippi, A. Halitosis -- Part 1: epidemiology and pathogenesis. *Schweiz Monatsschr Zahnmed*, 2004 114, 1037-1050.

[192] Laporte, Y. & Lloyd, DPC. Nature and significance of the reflex connections established by large afferent fibers of muscular origin. *Amer J Physiol*, 1952 169, 609-621.

[193] Laskin, DM. Etiology of the pain-dysfunction syndrome. *JADA*, 1969 79, 147-153.

[194] Laskin, DM. & Block, S. Diagnosis and treatment of myofacial pain-dysfunction (MPD) syndrome. *J Prosthet Dent*, 1986 56, 75-84.

[195] Lassila, LV. & Vallittu, PK. Denture base polymer Alldent Sinomer: mechanical properties, water sorption and release of residual compounds. *J Oral Rehabil*, 2001 28, 607-613.

[196] Law, JS; Nelson, N; Watanabe, K; Henkin, RI. Human salivary gustin is a potent activator of calmodulin-dependent brain phosphodiesterase. *Proc Natl Acad Sci USA*, 1987 84, 1674-1678.

[197] Learreta, JA; Beas J; Bono, AE; Durst A. Muscular activity disorders in relation to intentional occlusal interferences. *Cranio*, 2007 25, 193-199.

[198] Le Bell, Y; Niemi, PM; Jämsä, T; Kylmälä M; Alanen, P. Subjective reactions to intervention with artificial interferences in subjects with and without a history of temporomandibular disorders. *Acta Odontol Scand*, 2006 64, 59-63.

[199] Ligier, S. & Stenberg, EM. Immune response. In: Fink G, editor in chief. *Encyclopedia of stress. (vol. 2.).* San Diego: Academic Press; 2000; 523-530.

[200] Lindberg, NE; Lindberg, E; Larsson, G. Psychologic factors in the etiology of amalgam illness. *Acta Odontol Scand*, 1994 52, 219-228.

[201] Litter, B. Phantom bite revisited. *Brit Dent J*, 2005 198, 149.

[202] Lloyd DPC. Facilitation and inhibition of spinal motoneurons. *J Neurophysiol*, 1946/a 9, 421-438.

[203] Lloyd, DPC. Integrative pattern of excitation and inhibition in two-neuron reflex arcs. *J Neurophysiol*, 1946/b 9, 439-444.

[204] Lobbezoo, F. & Naeije, M. Dental implications of some common movement disorders: A concise review. *Arch Oral Biol*, 2007 52, 395-398.

[205] Locker, D. Subjective reports of oral dryness in an older adult population. *Community Dent Oral Epidemiol*, 1993 21, 165-168.

[206] Lundqvist, S. *Speech and other oral functions. Clinical and experimental studies with special reference to maxillary rehabilitation on osseointegrated implants. (Ph.D. thesis).* Göteborg, 1993.

[207] Lygre, GB; Gjerdet, NR; Grønningsæter, AG; Björkman, L. Reporting on adverse reactions to dental materials - intraoral observations at a clinical follow-up. *Community Dent Oral Epidemiol*, 2003 31, 200-206.

[208] Ma, H; Sun, HQ, Ji, P. How to deal with esthetically overcritical patients who need complete dentures: A case report. *J Contemp Dent Pract*, 2008 9, 22-27.

[209] Mairgünther, R. & Dielert, E. Temporomandibular joint examination under general anesthesia - a case report. *Dtsch Stomatol*, 1991 41, 393-395.

[210] Malasubramaniam, R. & Ram, S. Orofacial movement disorders. *Oral Maxillofac Surg Clin North Am*, 2008 20, 273-285.

[211] Mallo-Pérez, L. & Díaz-Donado, C. Intraoral contact allergy to materials used in dental practice. A critical review. *Med Oral*, 2003 8, 334-347.

[212] Malt, UF; Nerdrum, P; Oppedal, B; Gundersen, R; Holte, M; Löne, J. Physical and mental problems attributed to dental amalgam fillings: A descriptive study of 99 self-referred patients compared with 272 controls. *Psychosom Med*, 1997 59, 32-41.

[213] Maltsman-Tseikin, A; Moricca, P. Niv, D. Burning mouth syndrome: will better understanding yield better management? *Pain Pract*, 2007 7, 151-162.

[214] Manders, E; Jacobs, R; Nackaerts, O; Van Looy, C; Lembrechts, D. The influence of oral implant-supported prostheses on articulation and myofunction. *Acta Otorhinolaryngologica Belgica*, 2003 57, 73-77.

[215] Marbach, JJ. Phantom bite syndrome. *Am J Psychiatry*, 1978 135, 476-479.

[216] Martin, SF. T lymphocyte-mediated immune responses to chemical haptens and metal ions: Implications for allergic and autoimmune disease. *Int Arch Allergy Immunol*, 2004 134, 186-198.

[217] Márton, K; Boros, I; Fejérdy, P; Madléna, M. Evaluation of unstimulated flow rates of whole and palatal saliva in healthy patients wearing complete dentures and in patients with Sjögren's syndrome. *J Prosthet Dent*, 2004 91, 577-581.

[218] Mazurat, NM. & Mazurat, RD. Discuss before fabricating: Communicating the realities of partial denture therapy. Part II: Clinical outcomes. *J Can Dent Assoc*, 2003 69, 96-100.

[219] McCann, SM. Nitric oxide. In: Fink G, editor in chief. *Encyclopedia of stress. (vol. 3.).* San Diego: Academic Press; 2000; 53-61.

[220] McCullough, MJ. & Tyas, MJ. Local adverse effects of amalgam restorations. *Int Dent J*, 2008 58, 3-9.

[221] Meehan, S; DeNucci, DJ; Guckes, AD. Orofacial pain resulting from ill-fitting dentures. *Mil Med*, 1995 160, 366-367.

[222] Melchart, D; Wühr, E; Weidenhammer, W; Kremers, L. A multicenter survey of amalgam fillings and subjective complaints in non-selected patients in the dental practice. *Eur J Oral Sci*, 1998 106, 770-777.

[223] Melic, M. & Secci, S. Migraine with aura and dental occlusion: a case report. *J Mass Dent Soc*, 2006 54, 28-30.

[224] Melzack, R. & Wall, PD. *The challenge of pain. (Second edition).* Harmondsworth, Middlessex: Penguin; 1988; 118.

[225] Merskey, H. Pain terms: a list with definitions and notes on usage. Recommended by the IASP sub-committee on taxonomy. *Pain*, 1979 6, 249-252.

[226] Mew, J. Phantom bite. *Brit Dent J*, 2004 197, 660.

[227] Michman, J. & Langer, A. Postinsertion changes in complete dentures. *J Prosthet Dent*, 1975 34, 125-134.

[228] Mikami, DB. A review of psychogenic aspects and treatment of bruxism. *J Prosthet Dent*, 1977 37, 411-419.

[229] Miyamoto, SA. & Ziccardi, VB. Burning mouth syndrome. *Mt Sinai J Med*, 1998 65, 343-347.

[230] Mokrushin, A. & Pavlinova, L. Heat shock protein (Hsp70) modifies evoked activity of olfactory cortex cells in vitro and protects them from acute anoxia, from glutamate excitotoxicity and epilepsy. Morel E, Vinvent C editors. *Heat Shock Proteins: New research.* New York: Nova Sci Publisher; 2008; 275-297.

[231] Molin, C. From bite to mind: TMD -- a personal and literature review. *Int J Prosthodont*, 1999 12, 279-288.

[232] Molly, L; Nackaerts, O; Vandewiele, K; Manders, E; van Steenberghe, D; Jacobs, R. Speech adaptation after treatment of full edentulism through immediate loaded implant protocols. *Clin Oral Implant Res*, 2008 19, 86-90.

[233] Morse, DR. Infection-related mental and inferior alveolar nerve paresthesia: literature review and presentation of two cases. *J Endod*, 1997 23, 457-460.

[234] Munakata, Y. & Kasai, S. Contribution of the mucosal tactile information to the mandibular position sense in patients wearing dentures. *J Oral Rehabil*, 1992 19, 649-654.

[235] Munro, RR. Electromyography of the muscles of mastication. In: Griffin CJ, Harris R editors. *The temporomandibular joint syndrome. The masticatory apparatus of man in normal and abnormal function.* (Monographs in oral science, Vol. 4.) Basel - München - Paris - London - New York - Sydney: Karger; 1975/a; 87-116.

[236] Munro, RR. Electromyography of the masseter and anterior temporalis muscles in the open-close-clench cycle in temporomandibular joint dysfunction. In: Griffin CJ, Harris R editors. *The temporomandibular joint syndrome. The masticatory apparatus of man in normal and abnormal function.* (Monographs in oral science, Vol. 4.) Basel - München - Paris - London - New York - Sydney: Karger; 1975/b; 117-125.

[237] Murphy, WM. A clinical survey of gagging patients. *J Prosthet Dent*, 1979 42, 145-148.

[238] Müller-Fahlbusch, H. Psychogenic pain sensation in teeth, mouth and jaws. *Dtsch Zahnärztl Z*, 1991 46, 109-111.

[239] Myers, A. & Naylor, GD. Glossodynia as an oral manifestation of sex hormone alterations. *Ear Nose Throat J*, 1989 68, 786, 789-790.

[240] Myrhaugh, H. Parafunktionen im Kauapparat als Ursache eines otodentalen Syndroms (I). *Quintessenz*, 1969 20, 89-94, 117-121.

[241] Nagy, G; Bartha, Y; Keresztes, T; Olveti, E; Madléna, M. Quantitaive analyis of cathecolamines in human dental pulp. *J Endod*, 2000 26, 596-598.

[242] Nair, SP; Meghji, S; Reddi, K; Poole, S; Miller, AD; Henderson, B. Molecular chaperones stimulate bone resorption. *Calcif Tissue Int*, 1999 64, 214-218.

[243] Namikoshi, T. Case of oral lichen planus due to dental metal allergy. *Nihon Hotetsu Shika Gakkai Zasshi*, 2006 50, 461-463.

[244] Nalcaci, R. & Baran, I. Factors associated with self-reported halithosis (SRH) and perceived taste disturbance (PTD) in elderly. *Arch Gerontol Geriatr*, 2008 46, 307-316.

[245] Nasri, C; Teixeira, MJ; Okada, M; Formigoni, G, Heir, G; de Siqueira, JTT. Burning mouth complaints: clinical characteristics of a Brazilian sample. *Clinics*, 2007 62, 561-566.

[246] Nater, UM; Rohlender, N; Gaab, J; Berger, S; Jud, A; Kirschbaum, C; Ehlert, U. Human salivary alpha amylase reactivity in a psychosocial stress paradigm. *Int J Psychophysiol.* 2005 55, 333-342.

[247] Nathan, C. Catalytic antibody bridges innate and adaptive immunity. *Science*, 2002 298, 2143-2144.

[248] Nealey, ET. & del Rio, CE. Stomatitis Venenata: Reaction of a patient to acrylic resin. *J Prosthet Dent*, 1969 21, 480-484.

[249] Newton, AV. The psychosomatic component in prosthodontics. *J Prosthet Dent*, 1984 52, 871-874.

[250] Niedermeier, WH. & Krämer, R. Salivary secretion and denture retention. *J Prosthet Dent*, 1992 67, 211-216.

[251] Niedermeier, W; Huber, M; Fischer, D; Beier, K; Müller, N; Schuler, R; Brinninger, A; Fartasch, M; Diepgen, T; Matthaeus, C; Meyer, C; Hector, MP. Significance of saliva for the denture-wearing population. *Gerodontology*, 2000 17, 104-118.

[252] Nikolopoulou, F. & Tzortzopoulou E. Salivary pH in edentulous patients before and after wearing conventional dentures and implant overdentures: a clinical study. *Implant Dent*, 2007 16, 397-403.

[253] Novak, N; Haberstok, J; Bieber, T; Allam, JP. The immune privilege of the oral mucosa. *Trends Mol Med*, 2008 14, 191-198.

[254] Obrez, A. & Grussing, PG. Opinions and feelings on eating with complete dentures: a qualitative inquiry. *Spec Care Dentist*, 1999 19, 225-229.

[255] Ogami, J; Ono, S; Naka, N; Watanuki, K; Ishida, S. X-ray examination of the stomac bubble after frequent experimental swallowing of saliva: the mechanism of aerophagia. *J Med Dent Sci*, 2005 52, 171-175.

[256] Ogawa, T; Tanaka, M; Ogimoto, T; Okushi, N; Koyano, K; Takeuchi, K. Mapping, profiling and clustering of pressure pain threshold (PPT) in edentulous oral mucosa. *J Dentistry*, 2004 32, 219-228.

[257] Oizumi, M. Case report of occlusal treatment with full mouth reconstruction. *Nihon Hotetsu Shika Gakkai Zasshi*. 2008 52, 396-399.

[258] Oka, T. & Oka, K. Age and gender differences of psychogenic fever: a review of the Japanese literature. *BMC BioPsychoSocial Med*, 2007 1, 11.

[259] Okano, N; Baba, K; Igarashi, Y. Influence of altered occlusal guidance on masticatory muscle activity during clenching. *J Oral Rehabil*, 2007 34, 679-684.

[260] Ortengren, U. On composite resin materials. Degradation, erosion and possible adverse effects in dentists. *Swed Dent J Suppl*, 2000 141, 1-61.

[261] Osborne, JW. & Albino, JE. Psychological and medical effects of mercury intake from dental amalgam. A status report for the American Journal of Dentistry. *Am J Dent*, 1999 12, 151-156.

[262] Osterberg, T. & Carlsson, GE. Relationship between symptoms of temporomandibular disorders and dental status, general health and psychosomatic factors in two cohorts of 70-year-old subjects. *Gerodontology*, 2007 24, 129-135.

[263] Ozaki, M; Ishii, K; Ozaky, Y; Hayashida, H; Motokawa, W. Psychosomatic study on the relation between oral habits and personality characteristics of the children in a mountain village. *Shoni Shikagaku Zassi*, 1990 28, 699-709.

[264] Pertes, RA. Differential diagnosis of orofacial pain. *Mt Sinai J Med*, 1998 65, 348-354.

[265] Peroz, I. Funktionsstörungen des Kauorgans bei Tinnituspatienten im Vergleich zu einer Kontrollgruppe. *HNO*, 2003 51, 544-549.

[266] Peyron, R; Laurent, B; Garcia-Larrea, L. Functional imaging of brain responses to pain. A review and meta-analysis. *Neurophysiol Clin*, 2000 30, 63-88.

[267] Pfeiffer, P. & Schwickerath, H. Nickel solubility and metallic taste. *ZWR*, 1991 100, 762-770.

[268] Pinto, OF. A new structure related to the temporomandibular joint and middle ear. *J Prosthet Dent*, 1962 12, 95-103.

[269] Piquero, K. & Sakurai, K. A clinical diagnosis of diurnal (non-sleep) bruxism in denture wearers. *J Oral Rehabil*, 2000 27, 473-482.

[270] Plainfield, S. Communication distortion. The language of patients and practitioners of dentistry. *J Prosthet Dent*, 1969 22, 11-19.

[271] Piquero, K; Ando, T; Sakurai, K. Buccal mucosa ridging and tongue indentation: incidence and associated factors. *Bull Tokyo Dent Coll*, 1999 40, 71-78.

[272] Rashid, N. & Yusuf, H. Intermittent mental paresthesia in an edentulous mandible. *Br Dent J*, 1997 182, 189-190.

[273] Reeves 2nd, JL. & Merrill, RL. Diagnostic and treatment challenges in occlusal dysesthesia. *J Calif Dent Assoc*, 2007 35, 198-207.

[274] Rehmann, P; Balkenhol, M; Ferger, P; Wöstmann, B. Influence of the occlusal concept of complete dentures on patient satisfaction in the initial phase after fitting: bilateral balanced occlusion vs. canine guidance. *Int J Prosthodont*, 2008 21, 60-61.

[275] Rodrigues Garcia, RC Oliveira, VM; Del Bel Cury, AA. Effect of new dentures on interocclusal distance during speech. *Int J Prosthodont*, 2003 16, 533-537.

[276] Rolls, ET. & Baylis, LL. Gustatory, olfactory and visual convergence within the primate orbitofrontal cortex. *J Neurosci*, 1994 14, 5437-5452.

[277] Rolls, ET; Francis, S; Bowtell, R; Browning, D; Clare, S; Smith, E; McGlone, F. Taste and olfactory activation of the orbitofrontal cortex. *Neuroimage*, 1997 5, S199.

[278] Rolls, ET; Critchley, HD; Browning, A; Hernadi, I. The neurophysiology of taste and olfaction in primates, and umami flavor. *Ann NY Acad Sci*, 1998 855, 426-437.

[279] Rosenberg, M; Kozlovsky, A; Gelernter, I; Cherniak, O; Gabbay, J; Bath, R; Eli, I. Self-estimation of oral malodor. *J Dent Res*, 1995 74, 1577-1582.

[280] Rosetti, LM; Pereira de Araujo Cdos, R; Rosetti, PH; Conti, PC. Association between rhythmic masticatory muscle activity during sleep and masticatory myofascial pain: a polysomnographic study. *J Orofac Pain*, 2008 22, 190-200.

[281] Sandler, NA; Ziccardi, V; Ochs, M. Differential diagnosis of jaw pain in the elderly. *JADA*, 1995 126, 1263-1272.

[282] Santoro, V; Caputo, G; Peluso, F. Clinical and therapeutic experience in twenty eight patients with burning mouth syndrome. *Minerva Stomatol*, 2005 54, 489-496.

[283] Sanz, M; Roldán, S; Herrera, D. Fundamentals of breath malodor. *J Contemp Dent Pract*, 2001 2, 1-17.

[284] Sarlani, E; Balciunas, BA; Grace, EG. Orofacial pain - Part I. Assessment and management of musculoskeletal and neuropathic causes. *AACN Clin Issues*, 2005/a 16, 333-346.

[285] Sarlani, E; Balciunas, BA; Grace, EG. Orofacial pain - Part II. Assessment and management of vascular, neurovascular, idiopathic, secondary, and psychogenic causes. *AACN Clin Issues*, 2005/b 16, 347-358.

[286] Satoh, T. Clinical and fundamental investigations on recurrent glossodynia. *Nippon Ishinkin Gakkai Zasshi*, 2004 45, 233-237.

[287] Sauerland, EK. & Mizuno, N. A protective mechanism for the tongue. Suppression of the genioglossal activity induced by stimulation of trigeminal proprioceptive afferents. *Experientia*, 1970 26, 1226-1227.

[288] Savage, RD. & MacGregor, AR. Behavior therapy in prosthodontics. *J Prosthet Dent*, 1970 34, 126-132.

[289] Scala, A; Checchi, L; Montevecchi, M; Marini, I; Giamberardino, MA. Update on burning mouth syndrome: overview and patient management. *Crit Rev Oral Biol Med*, 2003 14, 275-291.

[290] Scardina, GA; Mazzulo, M; Messina, P. Early diagnosis of progressive systemic sclerosis: the role of orofacial phenomena. *Minerva Stomatol*, 2002 51, 311-317.

[291] Schett, G; Metzler, B; Kleindienst, R; Moschen, I; Hattmannsdorfer, R; Wolf, H; Ottenhoff, T; Xu, Q; Wick, G. Salivary anti-hsp65 antibodies as a diagnostic marker for gingivitis and a possible link to atherosclerosis. *Int Arch Allergy Immunol*, 1997 114, 246-250.

[292] Schmalz, G. & Garhammer, P. Biological interactions of dental cast alloys with oral tissues. *Dental Materials*, 2002 18, 396-406.

[293] Schmalz, G; Langer, H; Schweikl, H. Cytotoxicity of dental alloy extracts and corresponding metal salt solution. *J Dent Res*, 1998 77, 1772-1778.

[294] Schmitt, A; Yu, SKJ; Sessle, BJ. Excitatory and inhibitory influences from laryngeal and orofacial areas on tongue position in the cat. *Arch Oral Biol*, 1973 18, 1121-1130.

[295] Schulte, W. Conservative treatment of occlusal dysfunction. *Int Dent J*, 1988 38, 28-39.

[296] Schuurs, AHB; Exterkate, RAM; Ten, CJ. Biological mercury measurements before and after administration of a chelator (DMPS) and subjective symptoms allegedly due to amalgam. *Eur J Oral Sci*, 2000 108, 511-522.

[297] Schwartz, LL. Pain associated with the temporomandibular joint. *JADA*, 1955 51, 394-397.

[298] Scott, A; Egner, W; Gawkrodger, DJ; Hatton, PV; Sherriff, M; van Noort, R; Yeoman, C; Grummit, J. The national survey of adverse reactions to dental materials in the UK: a preliminary study by the UK Adverse Reactions Reporting Project. *Brit Dent J*, 2004 196, 471-477

[299] Seifert, E; Runte, C; Selders, D; Lamprecht-Dinnesen, A; Bollmann, F. Der Einfluss der Zahnprothese auf die Stimme. *HNO*, 1999/a 47, 485-489.

[300] Seifert, E; Runte, C; Riebandt, M; Lamprecht-Dinnesen, A; Bollmann, F. Can dental prostheses influence vocal parameters? *J Prosthet Dent*, 1999/b 81, 579-585.

[301] Selye, H. Stress and disease. *Science*, 1955 122, 625-631.

[302] Sergl, HG. Der Erlebnisraum Mund. In: Sergl HG, editor. *Psychologie ung Psychosomatik in der Zahnheilkunde.* München - Wien - Baltimore: Urban & Schwarzenberg; 1996; 3-9.

[303] Shapiro, HH. & Truex, RC. The temporomandibular joint and the auditory function. *JADA*, 1943 30, 1147-1168.

[304] Sherrington, CS. *The integrative action of the nervous system.* New Haven: Yale University Press; 1906.

[305] Sherrington, CS. Reflexes elicitable in the cat from pinna, vibrissae and jaws. *J Physiol Lond*, 1917 51, 404-431.

[306] Shipley, MT. Insular cortex projections to the nucleus of the solitary tract and brainstem visceromotor nuclei in the mouse. *Brain Res Bull*, 1982 8, 139-148.

[307] Sieber, M; Grubenmann, E; Ruggia, GM; Palla, S. Relation between stress and symptoms of craniomandibular disorders in adolescents. *Schweiz Monatsschr Zahnmed*, 2003 113, 648-654.

[308] Silverman, SI. *Oral physiology.* St Louis: Mosby; 1961; 134, 146.

[309] Skinner, BF. *The behavior of organism.* New York: Appleton-Cntury-Crofts; 1938.

[310] Smeraski, CA; Dunwiddie, TV; Diao, L; Finger, TE. Excitatory amino acid neurotransmission in the primary gustatory nucleus of the goldfish *Carassius Auratus*. *Ann NY Acad Sci*, 1998 855, 442-449.

[311] Smith, DV; Li, CS; Davis, BJ. Excitatory and inhibitory modulation of taste responses in the hamster brainstem. *Ann NY Acad Sci*, 1998 855, 450-456.

[312] Somer, E. Hypnotherapy in the treatment of the chronic nocturnal use of a dental splint prescribed for bruxism. *Int J Clin Exp Hypn*, 1991 39, 145-154.

[313] Somer, E; Ben-Aryeh, H; Laufert, D. Salivary composition, gender, and psychosocial stress. *Int J Psychosom*, 1993 40, 17-21.

[314] Spiechowicz, E; Glantz, PO; Axell, T; Grochowski, P. A long-term follow-up of allergy to nickel among fixed prostheses wearers. *Eur J Prosthodont Restor Dent*, 1999 7, 41-44.

[315] Stone, AA; Neale, JM; Cox, DS; Napoli, A; Valdimarsdottir, H; Kennedy-Moore, E. Daily events are associated with a secretory immune response to an original antigen in men. *Health Psyhol*, 1994 13, 440-446.

[316] Strasbaugh, HJ; Levine, JD. Pain. In: Fink G, editor in chief. *Encyclopedia of stress (Vol. 3)*. San Diego: Academic Press; 2000; 115-118.

[317] Strömberg, R; Langworth, S; Söderman, E. Mercury inductions in persons with subjective symptoms alleged to dental amalgam fillings. *Eur J Oral Sci*, 1999 107, 208-214.

[318] Suganuma, T; Ono, Y; Shinya, A; Furuya, R. The effect of bruxism on periodontal sensation in the molar region: A pilot study. *J Prosthet Dent*, 2007 98, 30-35.

[319] Sutow, EJ; Maillet, WA; Taylor, JC; Hall, GC. In vivo galvanic currents of intermittently contacting dental amalgam and other metallic restorations. *Dent Mater*, 2004 20, 823-831.

[320] Suzuki, T; Kumamoto, H; Ooya, K; Motegi, K. Expression of inducible nitric oxide synthase and heat shock proteins in periapical inflammatory lesions. *J Oral Pathol Med*, 2002 31, 488-493.

[321] Svensson, P; Bjerring, P; Arendt-Nielsen, L; Kaaber, S. Sensory and pain thresholds to orofacial argon laser stimulation in patients with chronic burning mouth syndrome. *Clin J Pain*, 1993 9, 207-215.

[322] Svensson, P. & Kaaber, S. General health factors and denture function in patients with burning mouth syndrome and matched control subjects. *J Oral Rehabil*, 1995 22, 887-895.

[323] Szentágothai, J. Anatomical considerations of mono-synaptic reflex arcs. *J Neurophysiol*, 1948 11, 445-454.

[324] Szabó Cs. Regulation of the expression of the inducible isoform of nitric oxide synthase by glucocorticoids. *Ann NY Acad Sci*, 1998 851, 336-341

[325] Taillandier, J; Esnault, Y; Alemanni, M. A comparison of fluconazole oral suspension and amphotericin B oral suspension in older patients with oropharyngeal candidosis. Multicentre Study Group. *Age Aging*, 2000 29, 117-123.

[326] Taylor, RG; Doku, CH. Dental survey of healthy old persons. *JADA*, 1963 67, 62-70.

[327] Tesserioli de Siqueira, SRD; Nóbrega, JCM; Valle, LBS; Teixeira, MJ; Tesserioli de Siqueira, JT. Idiopathic trigeminal neuralgia: Clinical aspects and dental procedures. *Oral Surg Oral Med Oral Pathol Oral Radiol Endod*, 2004 98, 311-315.

[328] Touger-Decker, R. Oral manifestations of nutrient deficiencies. *Mt Sinai J Med*, 1998 65, 355-361.

[329] Toyofuku, A. & Kikuta, T. Treatment of phantom bite syndrome with milnacipran - a case series. *Neuropsych Dis Treatment*, 2006 2, 387-390.

[330] Tönnies, S. Entspannung für Tinnitusbetroffene durch Photostimulation. *HNO*, 2006 54, 481-486.

[331] Treede, RD. & Magerl, W. Zentrale nozizeptive Neurone und Bahnen. In: Egle UT, Hoffmann SO, Lehmann KA, Nix WA editors. *Handbuch Chronischer Schmerz. Grundlagen, Pathogenese, Klinik und Therapie aus bio-psychosozialer Sicht.* Stuttgart: Schattauer; 2003; 34-44.

[332] Troest, T. Form und Funktion im stomatognathen System. In: Koeck B, editor. *Funktionsstörungen des Kauorgans.* München - Wien - Baltimore: Urban & Schwarenberg; 1995; 11-26.

[333] Trombelli, L; Zangari, F; Calura, G. The burning mouth syndrome. A clinical study. *Minerva Stomatol*, 1994 43, 49-55.

[334] Tsuru, H. & Kawamura, Y. Cuspal inclination and denture function. *J Osaka Univ Dent School*, 1962 2, 89-104.

[335] Türp, JC; Hugger, A; Löst, C; Nilges, P; Schindler, HJ; Staehle, HJ. Vorschlag einer Klassifikation der Odontalgien. *Schmerz*, 2009 23, 448-460.

[336] Usmani, N. & Wilkinson, SM. Allergic skin disease: investigation of both immediate- and delayed-type hypersensitivity is essential. *Clin Exp Allergy*, 2007 37, 1541-1546.

[337] Vamnes, JS; Lygre, GB; Grönningsæter, AG, Gjerdet, NR. Four years of clinical experience with an adverse reaction unit for dental biomaterials. *Community Dent Oral Epidemiol*, 2004 32, 150-157.

[338] van der Bijl, P. Psychogenic pain in dentistry. *Compendium*, 1995 16, 46, 48, 50-54.

[339] van der Broek, AMWT; Feenstra, L; de Baat, C. A review of the current literature on etiology and measurement methods of halithosis. *J Dentistry*, 2007 35, 627-635.

[340] van der Glas, HW; de Laat, A; van Steenberghe, D. Oral pressure mediate a series of inhibitory and excitatory periods in the masseteric poststimulus EMG complex following tapping of a tooth in man. *Brain Res*, 1985 337, 117-125.

[341] van der Glas, HW; de Laat, A; Carels, C; van Steenberghe, D. Interactive periodontal and acoustic influences on the masseteric post-stimulus electromyographic complex in man. *Brain Res*, 1988 444, 284-294.

[342] Vanhaudenhuyse, A; Boly, M; Laureys, S; Faymonville, ME. Neurophysiological correlates of hypnotic analgesia. *Contemp Hypnosis*, 2009 26, 15-23.

[343] Vasilakis, GJ. & Vasilakis, CM. Mandibular endodontic-related paresthesia. *Gen Dent*, 2004 52, 334-338.

[344] Vojdani, A; O'Bryan, T; Kellermann, GH. The immunology of immediate and delayed hypersensitivity reaction to gluten. *Eur J Inflammation*, 2008 6, 1-10.

[345] Wakabayashi, N; Yatabe, M; Ai, M; Sato, M; Nakamura, K. The influence of some demographic and clinical variables on psychosomatic traits of patients requesting replacement removable partial dentures. *J Oral Rehabil*, 1998 25, 507-512.

[346] Weinberg, LA. An evaluation of stress in temporomandibular joint dysfunction-pain syndrome. *J Prosthet Dent*, 1977 38, 192-207.

[347] Weisz, N; Moratti, S; Meinzer, M; Dohrmann, K; Elbert, T. Tinnitus perception and distress is related to abnormal spontaneous brain activity as measured by magnetoencephalography. *PLoS Medicine*, 2005 2, e153, 546-553.

[348] Weisz, N; Hartmann, T; Dohrmann, K; Schlee, W; Norena, A. High-frequency tinnitus without hearing loss does not mean absence of deafferentation. *Hear Res*, 2006 222, 108-114.

[349] Wentworth Jr., P; McDunn, JE; Wentworth, AD; Takeuchi, C; Nieva, J; Jones, T; Bautista, C; Ruedi, JM; Gutierrez, A; Janda, KD; Babior, BM; Eschenmoser, A; Lerner, RA. Evidence for antibody-catalyzed ozone formation in bacterial killing and inflammation. *Science*, 2002 298, 2195-2199.

[350] Wick, G; Knoflach, M; Xu, Q. Autoimmune and inflammatory mechanisms in atherosclerosis. *Annu Rev Immunol*, 2004 22, 361-403.

[351] Williams, PL. & Warwick, R. editors. *Gray's anatomy. (36th edition).* Edinburgh - London - Melburne - New York: Churchill and Livingstone; 1980. 529-540, 1271-1272.

[352] Winkler, S; Garg, AK; Mekayarajjananonth, T; Bakaeen, LG; Khan, E. Depressed taste and smell in geriatric patients. *JADA*, 1999 130, 1759-1765.

[353] Winter, AA. & Yavelow, I. Oral considerations of the myofascial pain dysfunction syndrome. *Oral Surg Oral Med Oral Pathol*, 1975 40, 720-727.

[354] Wirz, J; Jäger, K; Schmidli, F. Klinische Korrosion. *Schweiz Monatschr Zahnmed*, 1987 97, 1151-1156.

[355] Wise, GE. & Lin, F. The molecular biology of initiation of tooth eruption. *J Dent Res*, 1995 74, 303-306.

[356] Wismejer, D; van Waas, MA; Vermeeren, JI; Kalk, W. Patients' perception of sensory disturbances of the mental nerve before and after implant surgery: a prospective study of 110 patients. *Br J Oral Maxillofac Surg*, 1997 35, 254-259.

[357] Witter, DJ; De Haan, AF; Käyser, AF; Van Rossum, GM. A 6-year follow up study of oral function in shortened dental arches. Part II: Craniomandibular dysfunction and oral comfort. *J Oral Rehabil*, 1994 21, 353-366.

[358] Woda, A. & Pionchon, P. A unified concept of idiopathic orofacial pain: pathophysiologic features. *J Orofac Pain*, 2000 14, 196-212.

[359] Woda, A. & Pionchon, P. Orofacial idiopathic pain: clinical signs, causes and mechanisms. *Rev Neurol Paris*, 2001 157, 265-283.

[360] Wolff, A; Gadre, A; Begleiter, A; Moskona, D; Cardash, H. Correlation between patient satisfaction with complete dentures and denture quality, oral condition, and flow rate of submandibular/sublingual salivary glands. *Int J Prosthodont*, 2003 16, 45-48.

[361] Wolff, A; Ofer, S; Raviv, M; Helft, M; Cardash, HS. The flow rate of whole and submandibular/sublingual gland saliva in patients receiving replacement complete dentures. *J Oral Rehabil*, 2004 31, 340-343.

[362] Woolf, CJ. Evidence of central components of post-injury pain. *Nature*, 1983 306, 686-688.

[363] Wöstmann, B. Psychogene Zahnersatzunverträglichkeit. In: Sergl HG, editor. *Psychologie und Psychosomatik in der Zahnheilkunde.* München - Wien - Baltimore: Urban & Schwarzenberg; 1996; 187-213.

[364] Wruble, MK; Lumley, MA; McGlynn, FD. Sleep related bruxism and sleep variables: a critical review. *J Craniomandibular Dis*, 1989 3, 152-158.

[365] Yaegaki, K. & Coil, JM. Clinical application of a questionnaire for diagnosis and treatment of halithosis. *Quintessence Int*, 1999/a 30, 302-306.

[366] Yaegaki, K. & Coil, JM. Clinical dilemmas posed by patients with psychosomatic halithosis. *Quintessence Int*, 1999/b 30, 328-333.

[367] Yaegaki, K. & Coil, JM. Genuine halithosis, pseudo-halithosis, and halithophobia: classification, diagnosis, and treatment. *Compend Contin Educ Dent*, 2000/a 21, 880-886, 888-889, 890.

[368] Yaegaki, K. & Coil, JM. Examination, classification, and treatment of halithosis; Clinical perspectives. *J Can Dent Assoc*, 2000/b 66, 257-261.

[369] Yamaguchi, S. & Kimizuka, A. Psychometric studies on the taste of monosodium glutamate. In: Filer LJ, Garattini S, Kare MR, Reynolds AR, Wurtman RJ editors. *Glutamic acid: Advances in biochemistry and physiology*. New York: Raven Press; 1979; 35-54.

[370] Yamakawa, M; Ansai, T; Kasai, S; Ohmaru, T; Takeuchi, H; Kawaguchi, T; Takehara, T. Dentition status and temporomandibular joint disorders in patients with rheumatoid arthritis. *Cranio*, 2002 20, 165-171.

[371] Yemm, R. Stress-induced muscle activity: A possible etiologic factor in denture soreness. *J Prosthet Dent*, 1972 28, 133-140.

[372] Yoshida, H; Ayuse, T; Ishizaka, S; Ishitobi, S; Nogami, T; Oi, K. Management of exaggerated gag reflex using intravenous sedation in prosthodontic treatment. *Tohuku J Exp Med*, 2007 212, 373-378.

[373] Yoshinaka, M; Yoshinaka, MF; Ikebe, K; Shimanuki, Y; Nokubi, T. Factors associated with taste dissatisfaction in the elderly. *J Oral Rehabil*, 2007 34, 497-502.

[374] Zeier, H; Brauchli, P; Joller-Jemelka, HI. Effects of work demands on immunoglobulin A and cortisol in air traffic controllers. *Biol Psychol*, 1996 42, 413-423.

[375] Zhang, ZK; Ma, XC; Gao, S; Gu, ZY; Fu, KY. Studies on contributing factors in temporomandibular disorders. *Chin J Dent Res*, 1999 2, 7-20.

[376] Zimmermann, M. Physiologie von Nozizeption und Schmerz. In: Basler HD, Franz C, Kröner-Hervig B, Rehfisch HP editors. *Psychologische Schmerztherapie*. Berlin: Springer; 2004; 17-58.

[377] Zusmann, E; Yarin, AL; Nagler, RM. Age- and flow-dependency of salivary viscoelasticity. *J Dent Res*, 2007 86, 281-285.

Chapter 4

DIAGNOSIS AND DIFFERENTIAL DIAGNOSIS

ABSTRACT

One of the most important goals of the diagnosis of psychogenic denture intolerance (PDI) is the early recognition of the disorder and the avoidance of further useless invasive dental treatment, especially because aggravation or spread of symptoms following invasive dental interventions is not uncommon. Early diagnosis (or assumption) of PDI is also crucial for the prevention of symptom chronification which frequently render pain and other symptoms intractable. The most important diagnostic tool for such purposes is collecting detailed patient's history and careful evaluation of *all* relevant *psychosocial*, *medical* and *dental* anamnestic data including their understanding in a context of a *biopsychosocial model* of orofacial disorders. Careful clinical examination of the oral and orofacial region and general health status as well as X-ray, MRI and other specific examinations are also cornerstones of a proper diagnostic process certainly. Referral to other professionals may also be needed, and especially recommended in the case of pain and other (pseudo)neurological symptoms. Since psychogenic symptoms may mimic a great variety of somatic symptoms, a clear-cut diagnosis and proper differential diagnosis of PDI could be rather difficult. Therefore, it should be emphasized that, *the diagnosis of PDI is a presumptive one in many cases*. The diagnosis may change later in the course of the disease as the clinical findings change and/or stabilize, therefore continuous monitoring and evaluation of the patient over time is essential. A detailed differential diagnosis considering possible disorders of the teeth, and/or oral- and maxillofacial tissues should also be carried out, and *any other possible somatic causes behind the symptoms should also be excluded*. Fundamentals of the complex diagnostic process and the use of several diagnostic tools will be introduced in this chapter.

4.1. INTRODUCTION

Early diagnosis (or assumption) of PDI is crucial for the prevention of symptom chronification which frequently render pain and other symptoms intractable. The avoidance of further useless dental treatment is also highly important, because aggravation or spread of symptoms following invasive dental interventions frequently occurs. The most important diagnostic tool for early recognition of the disorder is collecting detailed patient's history [*Ross et al. 1953, Barsby 1994, Pertes 1998*]. A careful evaluation of *all* relevant *psychosocial, medical* and *dental* anamnestic data including their understanding in a context of a *biopsychosocial model* of orofacial disorders is also crucial [*Engel 1977, Freeman 1999, Bensing 2000, Green & Laskin 2000, Derra 2002, Dworkin & Sherman 2006*]. Careful clinical examination of the oral and orofacial region and general health status as well as X-ray, MRI and other specific examinations are also cornerstones of a proper diagnostic process. Referral to other professionals may also be needed, and especially recommended in the case of (pseudo)neurological symptoms and pain.

4.2. DIAGNOSTIC TOOLS

4.2.1. Patient's History (Anamnesis)

As previously mentioned, one of the most important (if not the most important) diagnostic tool for making diagnosis of PDI is collecting detailed patient's history [*Ross et al. 1953, Barsby 1994, Pertes 1998*] including a careful evaluation of *all* relevant *psychosocial, medical* and *dental* anamnestic data [*Ross et al. 1953, Pertes 1998, Dworkin & Sherman 2006*]. History taking is an art in the subtle direction of conversation with the patient. As the interview develops and the data accumulate, insight into the patient's problems becomes more apparent to the dentist, further enabling him to direct the interview along the most useful lines [*Laney & Gibilisco 1983*]. History-taking is a process usually extending over a number of patient's visit to reach adequate amount of data related to the *dental-, medical-,* and *psychosocial* life events [*Fábián & Fábián 2000, Fábián et al. 2007/b*]. Correlation may exist between the degree of satisfaction with dentures and the patient's ability to adjust to general health problems [*Emerson & Giddon 1955, Tickle et al. 1997*] and/or psychosocial problems. Therefore, interrelations between psychosocial- medical- and dental history should be evaluated carefully [*Ross et al. 1953, Dworkin & Sherman 2006*], and the data should be understand in a context of a *biopsychosocial model* of disorders [*Engel 1977, Freeman 1999, Bensing 2000, Green & Laskin 2000, Derra 2002, Dworkin & Sherman 2006*].

History of symptoms that are inconsistent with physical findings and history of a *precipitating life event* after which the symptom began [*Müller-Fahlbusch & Sone 1982, Bálint et al. 2003, Brodine & Hartshorn 2004, Dworkin & Sherman 2006*] are hallmarks of PDI cases [*Müller-Fahlbusch & Sone 1982, Brodine & Hartshorn 2004, Fábián et al. 2004/b*]. Moreover, as a result of apparent shortcomings in primary care and preliminary diagnostics, many PDI patients typically look back on long and complicated case histories with numerous negative examinations and futile attempts at somatic therapies and/or somatic interventions [*Marxkors & Müller-Fahlbusch 1981, Kreyer 2000, Dworkin & Sherman 2006*]. Increased number of dental clinics and hospitals visited by the patient in the previous time also refers to an increased risk of PDI [*Miyachi et al. 2007*]. History of any dental or facial trauma may also be a sign of increased risk of appearance of psychogenic orofacial symptoms [*Lesse, 1956, Müller-Fahlbusch & Sone 1982, Macfarlane et al. 2003, Brodine & Hartshorn 2004*]. Similarly, head and neck traumas especially survived head and/or neck cancer [*Duke et al. 2005*] as well as whiplash trauma [*Salé & Isberg 2007*] may also increase the risk of such manifestations significantly. History of symptom substitutions (turning of a symptom into an other one) also frequently appear in the history of PDI patients; however the role of possible environmental or other psychosocial changes should also be considered carefully before assuming an underlying pathopsychological background [*Gale & Carlsson 1976*].

4.2.2. Evaluation of Medical and Psychosocial Status

Besides orofacial status (including intraoral and dental status, see below), there are two other major facets of patients' status namely the medical- and the psychosocial status. *Medical status* may strongly influence both diagnostic and treatment procedures as well as the prognosis of PDI. Importantly, there is a strong association between *self-reported* general health status and the *subjectively* evaluated oral health status [*Emerson & Giddon 1955, Tickle et al. 1997*] indicating that, lower level of *self reported* general health may predispose to oral discomfort and consequent oral psychosomatic manifestations [*Emerson & Giddon 1955, Tickle et al. 1997*]. *Depression, anxiety disorder, somatization* and other *psychiatric disorders* as well as any other diseases leading to significant suffering and/or limitations of psychosocial functioning may lead to significant treatment difficulties and poor prognosis [*Dworkin & Sherman 2006*].

Psychosocial status also strongly influences both treatment possibilities and the prognosis of the offered treatment. Psychosocial conditions may trigger the appearance and/or may lead to the fixation of orofacial psychosomatic problems [*Ross et al. 1953, Nakaminami et al. 1989, Dworkin & Sherman 2006*]. Fixation of a *sick role* of the patients may also be rooted in several psychosocial causes [*Dworkin & Sherman 2006*]. Accordingly, both treatment possibilities and their prognosis are more guarded when self reported activity limitations are high. The prognosis is especially poor, if the medical and/or dental symptoms interferes appreciable with ability to discharge responsibilities (i.e. at home, in school, at work), or limits socializing activities [*Dworkin & Sherman 2006*]. Moreover, if there are strong extraneous social and/or health influences or any other object loss like bereavement [*Lupton 1969, Pomp 1974, Lowental & Tau 1980*], unemployment, placing on the retired list, diagnosis of life-threatening illness (etc.), the individual's ability to accept dentures may also be seriously compromised [*Lowental & Tau 1980, Allen & McMillan 2003*]. The psychoemotional "strength" and supportive potential of family members, friends and other members of the social networks of patients also of high diagnostic and prognostic importance.

4.2.3. Evaluation of Orofacial Status (Physical Examination)

There are two major facets of physical examination such as extraoral examination and intraoral examination [*Laney & Gibilisco 1983*]. *Extraoral examination* should include the evaluation of facial contour, characteristics of abnormal swellings, lesions, deformities or other surface changes as well as the inspection of opening and closing movements [*Laney & Gibilisco 1983*]. Structures including bones, muscles and lymph nodes (if any) of paraoral region, lateral surfaces of the face, temporal and submandibular areas as well as the major salivary glands should be palpated. TMJ should also be palpated as the patient opens and closes his/her mouth [*Laney & Gibilisco 1983*] and mandibular deviations [*Dunteman & Swarm 1995*] as well as limitations of mouth opening (if any) should also be recognized [*de Laat et al. 1993, Dunteman & Swarm 1995*]. Posterior cervical musculature and anterior cervical infrahyoid muscles should also be examined, because the skull is maintained upon the vertebral column in a state of equilibrium by the posterior cervical musculature and by the anterior complex system of muscles (including masticatory muscles but also infrahyoid muscles) and skeletal elements (i.e. mandible and hyoid bone) [*Silverman 1961*]. The anatomic location, characteristics, as well as aggravating and relief giving factors of facial pain and/or any other facial symptom should also be evaluated [*Laney & Gibilisco 1983*]. Trigger zones (if any) referring to neuralgic pain as well as trigger points (see below) should also be recognized [*Tesserioli de Siqueira et al. 2004*].

Intraoral examination should include the inspection of the tonsillar area and all oral mucosal surfaces as well as the bimanual digital palpation of the sublingual tissues, the cheek and the lips. The pterygoid muscles and the bony structures should also be palpated intraorally [*Dunteman & Swarm 1995, Laney & Gibilisco 1983*]. Natural dentition, occlusion, the edentulous arch as well as the design and quality of dentures should also be evaluated carefully [*Laney & Gibilisco 1983, Brunello & Mandikos 1998*]. Loose retainers of fixed dentures (if any) should also be revealed [*Curtis et al. 2006*]. Intraorally available trigger points of the pterygoid muscles, suprahyoid musculature and temporal muscles should also be examined (see also *paragraph 4.2.4.* below). Intraoral trigger zones (if any) should also be recognized [*Tesserioli de Siqueira et al. 2004*].

4.2.4. Palpation of Trigger Points

Trigger points (TrP) are focal muscle areas of maximum tenderness (located within the muscle or its fascia [*Bell 1969, Schwartz 1955*]) typically found in taut muscle bands, which elicit severe local pain and/or aggravation of the referred pain with a characteristic pain referral pattern [*Dunteman & Swarm 1995, Sarlani et al. 2005/a*]. Usually, fascia gives sharply localized pain, while muscle gives diffuse pain that is referred [*Schwartz 1955*]. Trigger points in the *masseter and temporalis muscles* can refer pain to posterior teeth [*Sarlani et al. 2005/a*] and to the ear [*Dunteman & Swarm 1995*]. These TrPs may also cause tinnitus or vertigo occasionally [*Dunteman & Swarm 1995*]. Trigger points of *lateral pterygoid muscle* refer pain to maxillary sinus and may mimic sinusitis. Pain referral of these TrPs may also be coupled with autonomic reflex induced excessive nasal secretion occasionally [*Dunteman & Swarm 1995*], and they may also cause numbness or burning pain of the cheek occasionally [*Dunteman & Swarm 1995*]. Trigger points of *medial pterygoid muscle* may inhibit adjacent tensor-veli palatini openings of the Eustachian tube, which may simulate otitis with ear stuffiness (barohypoacusis) and pain [*Dunteman & Swarm 1995*]. Trigger points in the *sternocleidomastoid, digastric and trapezius muscles* often refer pain to jaws or temple [*Dunteman & Swarm 1995, Sarlani et al. 2005/a*].

4.2.5. X-Ray, MRI and PET

X-ray diagnostics include the evaluation of several 2-dimensional (2D) images including *intraoral radiographs, extraoral radiographs* and images of *orthopantomography* (OP). X-ray diagnostics also uses 3-dimensional (3D) images such as *computed tomography* (CT) [*Hazey et al. 2009*]. A number of technological advances in radiology have attempted to improve the standard of traditional (2D) and computed tomographic (3D) images [*Scarfe et al. 2006, Hazey et al. 2009*]. For enhance visualization of 2D images *magnification, gamma adjustment,* and *enhanced 2-dimensional imaging* [*Parks 2008, Hazey et al. 2009*] including *color enhancement, image reversal, histogram equalization* (accentuate a small area), *contrast enhancement* and several *measurement tools* [*Parks 2008, Hazey et al. 2009*] are the most important techniques. In the case of 3D computed tomography, a new and highly efficient method called *cone-beam computed tomography* (CBCT) was developed roughly ten years ago [*Mozzo et al. 1998*]. CBCT method reaches at least similar (or even higher) diagnostic value like other CT methods [*Scarfe et al. 2006, Hintze et al. 2007*]; but with the use of lower x-ray dose and at lower costs [*Berrington De Gonzalez & Darby 2004, Silva et al. 2008*].

X-ray diagnostics is highly efficient for the analysis of orofacial hard tissues including bone and teeth and related pathological conditions [*Scarfe et al. 2006, Nair & Nair 2007*]. Radiographic evidence of sialolithiasis and certain other pathological condition of the soft tissues like mineralization in the stylohyoid or stylomandibular ligament (Eagle's sy.) [*Correll & Wescott 1982*] may also be recognized; however, in such cases the diagnostic value of x-ray images is limited. Recently, 3D CT images of the cranium, mandible and dental surfaces can also be combined with computed three-dimensional movement recording (see also *paragraph 4.2.8.*), performing dynamic and precise simulation of condyle to fossa distances and occlusal contacts during mandibular function [*Palla et al. 2003, Terajima et al. 2008*].

Magnetic resonance imaging (MRI, fMRI) is a highly sensitive an noninvasive tool, especially suitable for the diagnosis of heterogeneous pathologies; because both soft tissues and bones as well as their changes during function (i.e. continuous moving images) may be analyzed [*Ogasawara et al. 2001, Larheim 2005*]. MRI is suitable to detect bone marrow and cortical bone abnormalities, osteoarthritis, sinovial proliferation, joint effusion (more fluid than seen in healthy), TMJ disc displacement, disc morphology and TMJ functioning [*de Laat et al. 1993, Larheim 2005*]. MRI may also be used to evaluate constriction or dilatation of blood vessels [*Ogasawara et al. 2001*], which could be highly important for the diagnosis of vascular orofacial pain symptoms.

Positron emission tomography (PET) is a highly sensitive tool for diagnosis of primary or metastatic malign tumors of the orofacial region, because actively growing malignant tumor cells take up much higher amount of nutritive (including positron emitting diagnostic radio-isotopes like ^{18}F, ^{11}C, ^{15}O, ^{13}N) from the environment than normal cells [*Rother 2001*]. Although this kind of tomography is rather expensive because of the use of positron-camera and the need of administered radioisotopes, in some cases it may be needed for proper somatic diagnosis (i.e. to verify or to exclude possible tumor behind the symptoms) [*Rother 2001, White & Pharoah 2008*].

4.2.6. Thermography

Thermography using highly sensitive sensors at 0.1 °C thermal accuracy seems to be a promising tool for diagnosis and differential diagnosis of orofacial pain [*Gratt et al. 1989, 1996, Gratt & Anbar 2005*] and other functional symptoms. Region of interest (ROI) can be considered as normal when thermal difference comparing to control (i.e. surrounding tissues or contralateral tissues) is less than ± 0.25 °C. Thermal difference of a ROI between ± 0,26 - 0.35 °C may be considered as "equivocal". ROI should be considered as "cold" when thermal difference is at least - 0,35 °C; whereas should be considered as "hot" when thermal difference is at least + 0.35 °C comparing to control [*Gratt et al.1996*].

In the case of *extraoral thermography,* normal finding of ROI may be indicative of the nervous origin of the symptom including central (psychological or neurological) processes, pre-trigeminal and trigeminal neuralgia as well as pain of dental pulp origin [*Gratt et al. 1996, McGimpsey et al. 2000*]. Cold value of ROI indicates local decrease of blood flow of deeper subcutaneous tissues because of arterial vasoconstriction [*Kemppainen et al. 2001, Lee et. al. 2007*] or obstruction. Cold value may also indicate facial angiooedema [*Ogasawara et al. 2001*]. Hot value of ROI may indicate *inflammatory processes* including TMJ arthropathy, maxillary sinusitis or bone related inflammations [*Gratt et al. 1996, McGimpsey et al. 2000, Ventä et al. 2001*]. Herpes labialis infection also induces hot values already in the prodromal phase [*Biagioni & Lamey 1995*]. Vascular pain with enhanced blood NO level may also be resulted in hot values [*Gratt & Anbar 2005*]. Local vasodilatation also induces hot values [*Lee et al. 2007*]. In the case of *intraoral thermography,* hot values ("hot spots") may appear in relation with increased secretory function of minor salivary glands [*Lamey et al. 2007*]. Pulpal blood flow of teeth may also be analyzed using intraoral thermography [*Porgel et al. 1989, Kells et al. 2000/a,b*]. Especially rewarming pattern of teeth following a controlled cold stimulus (i.e. 20 sec. cooling with an airstream at 20 ºC) seems to be promising, which may be used to test tooth vitality [*Porgel et al. 1989, Kells et al. 2000/a,b,*] and to recognize certain rare intrapulpal pathologies.

4.2.7. Diagnostic Tools for Allergic Reactions

Allergy may be diagnosed by allergen elimination test, skin tests, intraoral mucosa test and in vitro blood tests [*Borelli et al. 1988*]. For allergen elimination test removal of all dental restorations containing an expected allergen is needed [*Borelli et al. 1988, Garau et al. 2005, Issa et al. 2005*], therefore this method may be rather expensive, and may also lead to various complications [*Yontchev 1986, Yontchev et al. 1987*]. Advantage of this method is the high sensitivity, however it is not possible to discriminate between allergic and irritative reactions using this method [*Garau et al. 2005, Borelli et al. 1988*]. The strong placebo effect of this method should also be considered [*Osborne & Albino 1999*]; because misdiagnosis may occur because of transient (pseudo)recoveries which are frequently followed by recurrences in time [*Yontchev 1986, Yontchev et al. 1987*] (i.e. especially in the case of mucosal symptoms with major psychological component).

For skin tests, either series of small test peaces or standardized test solutions may be used. The most frequently used standardized test solutions contain metal salt solutions like nickel sulphate 5%, palladium chloride 1%, gold sodium thiosulfate 0,5%, cobalt chloride (1%), and ammonium tetrachloroplatinate 0,25% [*Garhammer et al 2001*]; but also other metal salts may be used. Similarly, acrylate/methacrylate allergens (diluted in petrolatum) including 2-hydroxyethyl methacrylate (2-HEMA; 2.0 %), methyl methacrylate (MMA; 2.0 %), ethylene glycol dimethacrylate (EGDMA; 2.0 %), diethyleneglycol diacrylate (DEGDA; 0.1 %), 1,6-hexanediol diacrylate (HDDA; 0.1 %), triethyleneglycol diacrylate (TREGDA; 0.1 %), triethyleneglycol dimethacrylate (TREGDMA; 2.0 %), 1,4-butanediol diacrylate (BUDA; 0.1 %), 2-hydroxy propyl acrylate (2-HPA), 2-hydroxypropyl metacrylate (2-HPMA; 2.0 %) and bis-phenol-diglycidyl-methacrylate (bis-GMA; 2.0 %) [*Goon et al. 2007, 2008*] are also frequently used for testing. Certainly, any other dental compounds available in standardized solution may also be tested [*Vamnes et al. 2004, Issa et al. 2005, Goon et al. 2007*]. Test pieces should be prepared exactly as if they would be used in the mouth [*Wöstmann 1996, Garhammer et al 2001*]. Dental alloys should be casted, sandblasted and polished before application [*Garhammer et al 2001*]. Alloy test pieces should also include areas covered by properly fused porcelain (or composite) when porcelain (or composite) fused to metal will be used for restoration. Similarly, acrylates and other composite materials should be polymerized and polished properly before use for such testing [*Wöstmann 1996*].

Test solution can be applied onto the skin (epicutan test, patch test) which is a standard method for delayed type (type IV) allergic reactions primarily responsible for denture related allergic symptoms [*Borelli et al. 1988, Hamann et al. 2005*]. Similarly, test solutions can also be applied into the skin (i.e. prick test, scarification test, intracutan test) which is primarily used for assessment of risk of immediate IgE mediated (type I) reactions [*Borelli et al. 1988, Hamann et al. 2005*]. Test pieces can be applied onto the skin only; and can be used for detection of delayed type (type IV reactions). Skin test using test pieces seems to be a method of rather low sensitivity [*Garhammer et al. 2001*]. Skin tests using test solutions are much more sensitive, however cross-reactions and irritative effect may lead to "pseudo-positive" results [*Wöstmann 1996, Garhammer et al. 2001*]. It should be also noted that, skin tests may lead to sensitization and/or serious anaphylactic reactions (especially if test solution is applied into the skin, see above) and there are also several potential test pitfalls for an inexperienced tester [*Storrs 1996, Mowad 2006*]. Therefore, skin tests should be carried out and assessed by the allergologist. It should be also considered that, data of skin tests cannot be simply related to mucosal reactions [*Spiechowicz et al. 1999*] because of the special morphological and immunological properties of the oral mucosa [*Garhammer et al. 2001, Novak et al. 2008, Fábián et al. 2009/b*] and because of the presence of saliva [*Fábián et al. 2007/a, 2008/a, 2009/b*].

For intraoral mucosa tests, test pieces prepared as described for skin tests (see above) can be used. Test pieces may be applied onto the surfaces of palatal or ridge mucosa with the help of individually prepared removable appliances (similar to removable orthodontic appliances or RPDs). For evaluation of buccal or labial mucosal reactions, test pieces may be fixed onto labial or buccal tooth surfaces (similarly to the method used for fixation of orthodontic brackets). Great advantage of the intraoral mucosa tests is that, their results are clearly refer to the individual's oral condition; however discrimination between allergic and irritative reactions is not possible using this method [*Borelli et al. 1988*]. Because of the presence of saliva [*Fábián et al. 2007/a, 2008/a, 2009/b*] and the phenomenon of oral mucosal allergen tolerance [*Novak et al. 2008, Fábián et al. 2009/b*] intraoral mucosal tests are rather safe, and can be carried out by the dentist in most cases. However, great care should be taken about patients with severe local reactions as well as with a history of urticaria, allergic type asthma bronchiale, angiooedema, anaphylactic shock or any other IgE mediated (type I) reactions. In such cases, even oral testing should be done under supervision of allergologist. Importantly, dentist dealing with such patients should be prepared for (and ready to use) first aid interventions against severe anaphylactic reactions. Mild symptoms such as pruritus or urticaria can be controlled by administration of 0.2 to 0.5 mL of 1:1000 epinephrine subcutaneously, with repeated doses as required at 3-min intervals for severe reactions. An intravenous infusion should be initiated to provide a route for administration of epinephrine (diluted 1:50.000), and volume expanders if intractable hypotension occurs [*Austen 1991*]. Laryngotomy may also be needed if laringeal angiooedema appear.

From the relatively large group of possible in vitro blood tests several methods seems to be especially important for dentist: (1) determination of allergen specific serum IgE level may refer to the risk of life dangerous IgE mediated (type I) reactions; (2) basophile granulocyte activation tests may refer either to risk of IgE mediated (type I) reaction or to pseudoallergic irritative reactions; (3) lymphocyte transformation test may refer to a delayed type (type IV) hypersensitivity [*Borelli et al. 1988*], which is primarily responsible for the majority of oral denture related allergic reactions; (4) leukocyte migration inhibitory tests also refer to delayed type (type IV) hypersensitivity. Although in vitro blood tests are rather expensive and there is also a need of a high-level laboratory background, these tests are of the best future perspective, especially because of their specificity and safety.

A relative risk of allergic reactions to dental alloys may also be assessed due to evaluation of oral corrosion and oral galvanic current. Oral corrosion is a release of metallic derivatives as a result of several chemical (or electrochemical) reactions of alloys being in touch with saliva, gingival crevicular fluid, immune cells and oral microbes [*Wirz et al. 1987, Schmalz et al. 1998, Pfeiffer & Schwickerath 1991, Garhammer et al. 2001, Geurtsen 2002, House et al. 2008*]. Corrosion may increase the risk of allergic reactions because of a relatively high amount of metallic derivatives released from alloys. Further, corrosion may also lead to mucosal toxic/irritative reactions of chemical origin, caused by the released metallic derivatives of intraorally used alloys [*Geurtsen 2002*]. There is some chairside method available for evaluation of corrosion processes in patient's mouth. Several compounds released by corrosion may be detected from the saliva [*Pfeiffer & Schwickerath 1991, Geurtsen 2002, Garhammer et al. 2004*], however there are relatively large differences in replicate samples [*Geurtsen 2002, Garhammer et al. 2004*]. Corrosion potential of intraoral dental alloys may also be measured with a high impedance voltmeter and a Ag/AgCl microreference electrode [*Sutow et al. 2006, 2007/a,b, 2008*].

Similarly to oral corrosion, occurrence of oral galvanic current may also increase the risk of allergic and toxic/irritative reactions in the mouth. For evaluation of galvanic current it should be considered that, there can be electric potential differences between several alloys placed into the mouth (and came into contact with saliva). Such potential differences may lead to the appearance of an electric potential of mV order of magnitude resulting in galvanic electric current being generally below 15 μA [*Sutow et al 2004*] (in some cases it may rise up to roughly 100 μA [*Sutow et al 2004*]). Notwithstanding that this current is rather low, but may exert significant biological effects on the oral mucosa resulting in gingival swelling, erythema, mucosal pain and lichenoid reactions [*Bánóczy et al. 1979, Schmalz and Garhammer 2002*]. Although, galvanic current induced symptoms should be clearly distinguished from "real" allergic reactions; appearance of galvanic currents may also indicate a risk of allergic (or toxic/irritative) reactions in sensitive patients because of the amount of ions released from the dental alloy surfaces. Although it is difficult to measure galvanic electric current directly; however, corrosion potential of several alloys present in a mouth can be measured chairside as mentioned above [*Sutow et al. 2006, 2007/a,b, 2008*]. Importantly, any differences between corrosion potentials of several alloys detected in the same mouth [*Sutow et al. 2008*] refer to a risk of oral galvanic current phenomena.

4.2.8. Tactile Sensation and Motor Ability Testing

Although tactile sensation and motor ability may appear as rather different things, they are strongly coupled to each other in some respects, because of the major role of muscle function in the oral tactile recognition [*Landt 1978, Müller & Hasse-Sander 1993, Jacobs et al. 1998*] and *vice versa* [*Munro 1975/a,b, Griffin et al. 1975, de Laat et al. 1985, van der Glas et al. 1985, 1988, Kossioni & Karkazis 1995*]. Notwithstanding that, there is no clear evaluation of the PDI-related diagnostic and prognostic value of the methods below; it is very likely that, all above tests are beneficial for the evaluation of sensory-motor function. However it should be emphasized that, both design and execution of such method may significantly influence the result [*Dahlström 1989, Kossioni & Karkazis 1995, Jacobs et al. 1998, Fábián et al. 2005, Fábián 2007*]. Therefore, experienced investigators as well as properly planned and standardized methods are needed for valid results. Frequently used methods to evaluate patient's tactile sensation and motor ability are evaluation of oral stereognosis, oral motor ability and occlusal thickness discriminative ability as well as testing of the reproducibility of closure and other masticatory movements. In certain cases, methods to detect subtle alterations of the neuromuscular regulation may also be used.

Oral stereognosis is the ability to recognize and discriminate form or shape in the oral cavity, which may be utilized to assess oral tactile perceptual abilities [*Jacobs et al. 1998*]. Oral stereognostic ability (OSA) decreases significantly with age [*Landt 1978, Jacobs et al. 1998, Ikebe et al. 2007*] with edentulousness [*Jacobs et al. 1998, Smith & McCord 2002*] but also because of some individual psychological factors [*Jacobs et al. 1998*]. An important role of oral stereognostic ability in accepting full dentures was expected in the literature [*Landt 1978, Smith & McCord 2002*]. Although there may be a lack of *general* correlation between oral stereognosis and PDI [*Eitner et al. 2007*], psychological stress induced insufficiency of oral stereognostic ability likely play a role in the appearance of complete denture related PDI. Oral stereognostic test is frequently performed in conjunction with an oral motor ability test (see below) in order to correlate the outcome of both tests [*Jacobs et al. 1998*].

Oral motor ability (OMA) provides an expression of the *complex oral sensorimotor function*, evaluating the ability to fit two test pieces (complementary in form) together [*Landt 1978, Müller & Hasse-Sander 1993, Jacobs et al. 1998*]. Oral motor ability also decreases with age [*Landt 1978, Müller & Hasse-Sander 1993*] and edentulousness, and it is also influenced by psychological factors similarly to stereognosis [*Jacobs et al. 1998*]. Similarly to oral stereognosis, oral motor function could also be expected as an important factor of accepting complete denture [*Michman & Langer 1975, Landt 1978, Müller & Hasse-Sander 1993*].

Thickness discrimination ability expresses the sensory perceptive ability in relation with occlusal interferences and/or small foreign bodies. It can be measured using occlusal registration foils or metal foils of different foil thickness [*Baba et al. 2005, Suganuma et al. 2007, Calderon et al. 2009*]. The minimal detectable thickness is roughly between 8 to 23 micrometers [*Calderon et al. 2009*], and may be decreased in the case of bruxers [*Suganuma et al. 2007*]. The sensitivity of thickness differences can be ranged between 8 to 14 micrometers and occlusal dysesthesia patients shows increased sensitivity comparing to control [*Baba et al. 2005*].

Closure reproducibility indicates the patient's ability to reproduce closure with the "same" first-occluding points of occlusal surfaces. For testing, occlusal sonographic registration [*Watt 1966/a,b*] and comparative evaluation of the evoked sound patterns of repeated closures *via* computer can be used [*Fábián et al. 2005, Fábián 2007*]. For such purposes, the "open-close-clench" cycle may be used advantageously. Although premised cycle is an artificial maneuver, it provides more consistent records than "free" chewing cycles [*Munro 1975/a*]. *Reproducibility of any other masticatory movements* may be evaluated *via* computed pantographic (three-dimensional) movement recording [*Fujita et al. 1983, Aoki et al. 1988/a, Koeck & Lückerath 1995, Terajima et al. 2008*]. The goal of this kind of analysis is rather similar to that of the previous one (i.e. closure reproducibility see above); however in this case the whole pattern of masticatory (and/or other) movements may be evaluated.

Subtle alterations of neuromuscular regulation may be recognized due to a detailed analysis of the masseteric EMG. Several methods may be used including the analysis of the *open-close-clench cycle* as well as the analysis of the *effect of chin tapping and/or tooth tapping during clenching*. In the case of a detailed analysis of *open-close-clench cycle* [*Munro 1975/a,b, Griffin et al. 1975*] especially increased latency time of inhibitory response (may refer to atypical facial pain [*Munro 1975/b*]), increased duration of muscle contraction before initial tooth contact (may refer to TMD or atypical facial pain [*Munro 1975/b*]), absence or incompleteness of the inhibitory response following tooth contact (may refer to TMD [*Munro 1975/b*]) and absence of the correlations of the phases of open-close-clench cycle (may also refer to TMD [*Griffin et al. 1975*]) are of particular interest. (Please consider that: ideally, there is a positive correlation of duration of muscle contraction before initial tooth contact to the duration of the inhibitory response, and a negative correlation of duration of muscle contraction before initial tooth contact to the latency time [*Griffin et al. 1975*].)

Effect of chin tapping during clenching on the EMG of masseter muscle [*Tallgren et al. 1987, Kossioni & Karkazis 1995*] may also be analyzed in order to recognize subtle alterations of neuromuscular regulation. In this case moderate taps (directed downwards or backwards) are applied on the centre of the chin under clenching at roughly 40 % of the maximum voluntary contraction [*Kossioni & Karkazis 1995*], using a reflex hammer and a custom acrylic chin template [*Kossioni & Karkazis 1995*]. Importantly, an absence or incompleteness of the "silent period" (inhibitory response) may refer to an adaptation period of an *inexperienced* patient to denture [*Kossioni & Karkazis 1995*] as well as to an improper neuromuscular adaptation ability to dentures. Similarly, appearance of double "silent periods" may also refer to improper neuromuscular adaptation [*Tallgren et al. 1987*]. Further, an abnormally lengthened inhibitory response ("silent period") may refer to TMD [*Bessette et al. 1971, Dahlström 1989*]. Besides chin tapping, *effect of tooth tapping during clenching* on masseteric EMG may also be used for recognizing subtle alterations of neuromuscular regulation. In this case moderate taps are applied on *vital* upper central or upper premolar tooth under clenching at roughly 5-10 % of maximum voluntary contraction [*de Laat et al. 1985, van der Glas et al. 1985*], using a light aluminum hammer mounted as a pendulum and with a glass (hard plastic) rod as tip [*de Laat et al. 1985, van der Glas et al. 1985, 1988*]. Importantly, a double wave inhibitory response appear in healthy control subjects; whereas there are single wave inhibitory responses in the case of myofascial pain patients and patients with bruxism [*de Laat et al. 1985*].

4.2.9. Taste and Retronasal Smell Reactivity

Primary taste recognition, concentration discriminative ability and *time need of proper evaluation* can be examined with a series of 5-10 ml samples representing tasteless, sweet, salty, sour and bitter taste substances presented in disposable plastic cups at room temperature [*Har-Zion et al. 2004*]. Measurement may be carried out via simple "mouth rinsing" with the solution. In this case the "denture in" and "denture out" conditions can be compared. Test solutions may also be applied in small amount onto specific taste sensitive areas of the tongue and palate [*Henkin & Christiansen 1976*] for more detailed analysis of taste sensation. (The taste sensitive area of the pharynx located near to the root of the tongue is not available for such testing [*Henkin & Christiansen 1976*]). Distilled water may serve as *tasteless* sample. For *primary taste* test solutions analytically pure chemicals (allowed for human use) dissolved in distilled water may be used as "dilution series" [*Beauchamp et al. 1998, Har-Zion et al. 2004, Hoehl et al. in press*] in the following concentrations [*Hoehl et al. in press*]: (1) *sucrose* in concentrations ranging from 0.34 g/L to 24.00 g/L (M_r 342.3 g/mol) as sweet stimuli; (2) *citric acid* in concentrations ranging from 0.13 g/L to 1.20 g/L (M_r 210.14 g/mol) as sour stimuli; (3) *NaCl* in concentrations ranging from 0,16 g/L to 4.00 g/L (M_r 58.44 g/mol) as salty stimuli; (4) *caffeine* in concentrations ranging from 0,06 g/L to 0.54 g/L (M_r 194.19 g/mol) as bitter stimuli [*Hoehl et al. in press*].

Existence and sensitivity of an *umami taste (glutamate taste) recognition* expected as a fifth primary taste [*Kurihara & Kashiwayanagi 1998*] may also be evaluated using *monosodium glutamate* (MSG) dilution series in concentrations ranging from 0.08 g/L to 2.00 g/L (M_r 187.13 g/mol) [*Hoehl et al. in press*]. Expected increasing effect of *monosodium glutamate* (MSG) on *primary* taste palatability may also be tested adding 0,01 M MSG to the other (sweet, salty, sour and bitter) primary taste test solutions [*Beauchamp et al. 1998*]. However, it should be considered that, these are still questions under debate whether umami taste exists as a primary taste or not; and whether increasing effect of MSG on palatability of foods is due to the alteration of any other *primary* taste sensations or not [*Yamaguchi 1987, Beauchamp et al. 1998, Kurihara & Kashiwayanagi 1998*].

Besides taste evaluation, *retro-nasal smell reactivity* and *discrimination ability* may also be evaluated chairside [*Har-Zion et al. 2004*] using chewing gums (or candy) of identical texture, color and hardness but with different flavor like mint, banana, orange etc. [*Har-Zion et al. 2004*]. In this case *time need of proper evaluation* may also be evaluated, however (especially when chewing gum is used) it should be considered that, in order to obtain a satisfactory intra-oral flavor (smell) stimulus, the chewing gum had to be manipulated for a certain period of time. This manipulation (chewing) of the chewing gum can be more difficult under "denture out" than under "denture in" conditions for certain patients, depending on the remaining teeth and type or quality of denture [*Har-Zion et al. 2004*].

Interestingly, retro-nasal smell recognition may also be investigated due to umami taste intensity evaluation, using visual (or numerical) analog scale by the patient. For such evaluation 10 ppm (µl/L) of *methyl-furyl-disulfide* ($C_{10}H_{10}S_2$) should be dissolved in a dilution series (see above) of *monosodium glutamate* (MSG) and the taste intensity of MSG series *with* and *without methyl-furyl-disulfide* should be compared [*Rolls et al. 1998*]. Methyl-furyl-disulfide has the odor present also in the odor of garlic and savory, and significantly enhances the umami taste (glutamate taste) due to retro-nasal *odor* effects [*Rolls et al. 1998*]. Therefore an increased umami taste perception in the presence of methyl-furyl-disulfide may indicate a properly functioning retro-nasal smell reactivity and discrimination ability.

4.2.10. Analysis of Saliva

Besides the important and simple measurement of salivary *secretory rate* [*Gemba et al. 1996*] which may refer to emotional changes, anxiety, depression, chronic stress (and other organic causes of dry mouth and ptyalismus) [*Gemba et al. 1996, Fábián et al. 2008/a,b*]; saliva can also be used as a highly effective diagnostic tool for both local and systemic conditions [*Fábián et al. 2008/a,b*]. However, importance of the type of collected saliva (i.e. ductal ⇔ whole; resting ⇔ stimulated) [*Fábián et al. 2008/a*] and specific intraoral locations (if any) of certain saliva collection techniques (i.e. vestibular ⇔ paralingual etc.) [*Harmon et al. 2008, Fábián et al. 2008/a*] should be considered for proper analysis. The method of stimulation (if any) should also be taken into account [*Fábián et al. 2003, Stokes & Davis 2007*]. Similarly, circadian rhythms of flow rate [*Dawes 1972, 1975*] and circadian rhythms of concentration of several constituents of saliva [*Dawes 1972, 1975, Brown et al. 2008*] should also be considered carefully [*Fábián et al. 2008/a*]. Further, evaluation of the level of *direct* blood contamination should also be carried out, especially before assessing molecules of blood origin [*Fábián et al. 2008/a,b*]. (For such purposes determination of the level of transferrin in saliva may be used advantageously [*Schwartz & Granger 2004, Granger et al. 2007/a*]).

There are numerous possible salivary parameters, which may be analyzed [*Fábián et al. 2008/a,b*]. For *general diagnostic purposes* serum free hormone levels (in the case of nonpeptide hormones), small peptide type neurotransmitters, DNA and mRNA as well as tumor markers, medication, other drugs and virus infections may be evaluated from saliva samples [*Fábián et al. 2008/a,b*]. Levels of *psychosocial stress markers* such as salivary cortisol [*Nejtek 2002, Krahwinkel et al. 2004, Dorn et al. 2007, Granger et al. 2007/b*], salivary amylase [*Chatterton Jr. et al. 1996, Nater et al. 2005, Granger et al. 2007/b*] and salivary chaperokine HSP70/HSPA [*Fábián et al. 2004/a, 2008/a,b*] may also be analyzed. *Stress reactivity* may also be evaluated using salivary stress parameters including the simple assay of salivary amylase level [*Nater et al. 2005, Kivlighan & Granger 2006*]. Salivary *microbiota* may also be evaluated [*Fábián et al. 2008/a,b*]. *Oral defense molecules* including cystatins histatins, lactoferrine, lysozyme, defensins, mucins (etc.) as well as molecules referring to *local and/or general immune surveillance* like salivary sIgA [*Kugler et al. 1992, Gruzelier et al. 1998*], several pro- and anti-inflammatory cytokines [Liskmann et al. 2006] and salivary chaperokine HSP70/HSPA [*Fábián et al. 2003*] may also be determined [*Fábián et al. 2008/a,b*].

Antioxidant capacity of saliva [*Ginsburg et al. 2004, Liksmann et al. 2007*] as well as the level of its synergism with polyphenols present in nutriments [*Ginsburg et al. 2004*] and on the surfaces of blood cells and oral microbes [*Ginsburg et al. 2004, Koren et al. in press/a,b*] may also be evaluated. Several metallic derivatives of intraoral alloys released due to *corrosion* (see *paragraph 4.2.7.*) may also be detected from the saliva [*Pfeiffer & Schwickerath 1991*] (although there are relatively large differences in replicate samples [*Garhammer et al. 2004*]). *Viscosity and wettability,* both of which refer to the "gluing" ability (i.e. adhesion, cohesion, surface tension [*Darvell & Clark 2000, Turner et al. 2008*]) and lubricating ability of saliva may also be measured [*Park et al. 2007, Stokes & Davis 2007, Zussman et al. 2007*]. *Buffering capacity* may also be analyzed [*de Lima et al. 2008*]. *Salivary pH* as a rather important determinant of the oral milieu and oral comfort feeling [*Fábián et al. 2008/a,b*] may also be measured [*Nikolopoulou & Tzortzopoulou 2007*] and/or monitored *continuously* (intraorally) daylong with a pH sensor connected with a radio-transmitter of data all of which are built in a removable denture [*Watanabe et al. 1999*]. This latter, exciting possibility may open promising diagnostic perspectives in the future for continuous control of several other salivary parameters as well.

4.2.11. Psychological and Pathopsychological Questionnaires

Expression Scale of *Psychological Screening Inventory* (PSI) was reported to be an efficient tool to *predict* psychogenic denture intolerance of complete denture patients [*Ismail et al. 1974*]. Further, *Global Severity Index* and *Positive Symptom Distress Index* of *Checklist-90-R* (SCL-90-R) and also cumulative value of *Center of Epidemiological Studies Depression Scale* (CES-D) could be used efficiently for *early differential diagnosis* and for *forensic verification* of diagnosis of complete denture related PDI [*Eitner et al. 2006*]. The *Beck Depression Inventory* (BDI) may also be used to assess depressive symptom severity of patients, and to recognize clinically meaningful depression behind their PDI symptoms [*Beck & Beamesderfer 1974, Beck et al. 1979*]. Similarly, anxiety level of patients may be measured with *Spielberger's State and Trait Anxiety Inventory* (STAI-S and STAI-T) [*Spielberger et al. 1970*]. Subjective well being may be measured with the *Marburg Questionnaire of well-being* [*Basler 1999*]. Patient's satisfaction with denture can be measured with *patient's satisfaction scales* [*Vervoorn et al. 1988, Fenlon & Sherriff 2008, Turker et al. 2009*]. Level of patient's oral health-related quality of life [*Giddon 1978*] (OHQOL or OHRQoL) can be measured using the *Oral Health Impact Profile* (OHIP) [*Slade & Spencer 1994*] or its short form [Slade 1997] as well as its complete denture specific short form [*Allen & Locker 2002*]. The single item *Perceived Oral Health Rating* may also be used [*Brunswick & Nikias 1975, Atchhison & Gift 1997*].

In the case of pain symptoms, pain beliefs may be recognized administrating the *Survey of Pain Attitudes* (SOPA), to recognize beliefs like "disability" (belief that one's pain is disabling), "harm" (belief that pain signifies damage and that activity should be avoided) and "control" (belief in one's personal control over pain) [*Strong et al. 1992, Jensen et al. 1994*]. Fear of Pain may be measured using the *Short form of Fear of Pain Questionnaire* (FPQ-SF) measuring four factors such as fear of severe-, minor-, injection- and dental-pain [*Asmundson et al. 2008*]. Pain coping strategies of the patient may be evaluated using the *Chronic Pain Coping Inventory* (CPCI) [*Jensen et al. 1995*] including eight factors such as "coping self statements", "guarding of walking/standing", "exercising/stretching", "task persistence", "seeking social support", "asking for assistance", "resting" and "structured relaxation" [*Jensen et al. 1995, Hadjistavropoulos et al. 1999*]. Other aspects of pain coping strategies may be evaluated using the *Coping Strategy Questionnaire* (CSQ) [*Rosenstiel & Keefe 1983, Keefe et al. 1989*] consist of subscales such as "praying", "ignoring pain sensation", "distancing from pain", "catastrophizing", "coping self statements" and "distraction" [*Rosenstiel & Keefe 1983, Keefe et al. 1989, Hadjistavropoulos et al. 1999*]. Pain induced affective distress may be measured with the *Pain Distress Inventory* including four factors namely "depression", "anger", "pain sensitivity" and "somatic anxiety" [*Osmann et al. 2003, 2005*]. Pain catastrophizing (a tendency to exaggerate the threat value of pain or potentially painful situations) may be evaluated by the *Catastrophizing Subscale* of *Coping Strategy Questionnaire* (CSQ, see above) [*Rosenstiel & Keefe 1983, Keefe et al. 1989, Swartzman et al. 1994*] or by the *Pain Catastrophizing Scale* (PCS) [*Sullivan et al. 1995*] measuring three factors such as "rumination", "magnification" and "helplessness" [*Sullivan et al. 1995, 1998, 2005, Osmann et al. 1997, 2000*].

Pain intensity may also be assessed using *visual analogue scale* (VAS) and/or *numerical analogue scale* (NAS). Such evaluations are usually carried out at the beginning, during and at the end of the therapy. Using NAS or VAS assessment, rating of *current* pain, as well as *usual* ("average") pain, *least* pain and *worst* pain in the past month (and/or week) are usually recommended [*Jensen et al. 1996, Turner et al. 2006*]. Obviously, not only intensity of pain, but also intensity of any other symptom may also be evaluated with VAS and NAS in a similar way. Importantly, not only VAS, and NAS but most premised pain related scales may also be used in relation with any other PDI symptoms, replacing the word "pain" with the word describing the other symptom at issue in the scales [*Reynolds 2000, Turner et al. 2006*]. (With other words: the pain related scales can be "re-worded" as necessary to apply to a certain symptom of interest [*Reynolds 2000, Turner et al. 2006*].) Besides these, some other questionnaires like *dental fear scales*, a scale for evaluation of *patient-dentist relationship* as well as scales for rating *exposure to stressful life events*, and *perceived stress* may also be used for certain diagnostic purposes (see also *paragraph 5.2.*).

4.2.12. Other Tools

Self-projective figure drawing tests [Silvermann et al. 1976, Tóth et al. 2006, Fábián et al. 2007] as well as the evaluation of patient's written free association (coupling) about mouth and/or teeth [Kaán et al. 2005, Fábián et al. 2004, 2007, Fejérdy et al. 2005] may also be helpful in some cases. In some cases anesthetic blockade may also be used for differentiation between somatic and psychogenic pain. (In general, psychogenic origin of pain should be considered when anesthetic blockade gives equivocal relief of pain [Gratt et al. 1989]). In certain cases of TMD related symptoms detailed three-dimensional analysis of mandibular movements [Fujita et al. 1983, Aoki et al. 1988/a, Koeck & Lückerath 1995] coupled with a detailed analysis of occlusal surfaces [Aoki et. al 1988/a,b, Koeck & Lückerath 1995] as well as arthroscopic investigation of the temporomandibular joint [Mairgünther & Dielert 1991, Zhang et al. 1999] may also be needed. Auscultation and/or audio-visual sound recording analysis [Sadowsky et al. 1985, Muhl et al. 1987] of TMJ sounds may also be useful. Sonographic audiospectral analysis of TMJ sounds may also be used occasionally [Ouellette 1974]. In some cases sleep electromyography and/or polysomnography (registration of sleep EMG coupled with registration of various other psychophysiological parameters) may also be needed to obtain sufficient, accurate and reliable data in relation with nocturnal parafunctions [Dahlström 1989, Lavigne et al. 1996, Glaros 2006].

4.3. STRATEGY OF DIAGNOSIS

4.3.1. Diagnosis Based on Definition

The essence of diagnosis based on definition is that, the symptom(s) should fit in the definition of denture intolerance (see *paragraph 2.2.2.*), which was defined in the present work as: *patient's refusal accepting or wearing* truly prepared (standard, properly made) *fixed* and/or *removable denture*(s) because of appearing *any kind of psychogenic* symptom(s) in relation to the *denture* or to the *treatment procedure* [*Fábián & Fábián 2000, Fábián et al. 2004/b, 2007/b*]. Since psychogenic symptoms may mimic a great variety of (most of) somatic symptoms; to assess that whether a symptom is of *psychogenic origin* or not, the next five characteristics of psychogenic symptoms [*Marxkors & Müller-Fahlbusch 1981*] can be considered as follows: (1) well-marked divergence between the symptoms and the clinical findings; (2) unsuccessful previous somatic treatments; (3) fluctuation of the symptoms; (4) conspicuous emotional involvement of the patient into the dental problem; (5) presumable relationship of the symptoms and the psychosocial history [*Marxkors & Müller-Fahlbusch 1981*]. Symptoms which meet at least four from the above five criteria are very likely to be of psychogenic origin [*Fábián et al. 2006*].

4.3.2. Diagnosis of Exclusion

It should be emphasized that, the diagnosis of PDI is also a diagnosis of exclusion [Fábián & Fábián 2000, 2007/b], therefore a careful and accurate dental examination is crucial [Brodine & Hartshorn 2004, Sarlani et al. 2005/a,b]. A detailed differential diagnosis considering possible disorders of the teeth, or oral- and maxillofacial tissues should also be carried out [Brodine & Hartshorn 2004, Sarlani et al. 2005/a,b] (see paragraphs 4.4.1., 4.4.2.). PDI may be expected only at those cases without any significant dental finding [Fábián & Fábián 2000, Fábián et al. 2004/b, 2007/b]. Following the careful dental examination, any other possible somatic causes behind the symptoms should also be excluded [Brodine & Hartshorn 2004, Sarlani et al. 2005/a,b]. For such purposes, exclusion of systemic diseases that may cause orofacial symptoms should also be carried out (see paragraphs 4.4.3., 4.4.4.) and medication induced symptoms should also be considered (see paragraph 4.4.5.). Further, referral to other professionals like maxillofacial surgeon, neurologist, psychiatrist, otorhinolaringologist, ophthalmologist, internist, rheumatologist (etc.) may also be needed, and especially recommended in the case of pain and other (pseudo)neurological symptoms [Sarlani et al. 2005/a.b]. It should be also considered that, the diagnosis may change later in the course of the disease as the clinical findings change and/or stabilize, therefore continuous monitoring and evaluation of the patient over time is essential [Sarlani et al. 2005/a.b].

4.4. DIFFERENTIAL DIAGNOSIS

4.4.1. Disorders of the Teeth and Periodontal Tissues

There are numerous possible somatic causes of tooth-located pain (and other symptoms) which make early diagnosis and differential diagnosis of tooth-located psychogenic pain (or other psychogenic symptoms) rather difficult [*Gratt et al. 1989, Golan 1997, Fábián 1999, Türp et al. 2009*]. Intrapulpal-, periapical and periodontal (periimplantal) inflammations of bacterial origin are the most frequent causes of tooth located symptoms [*Madléna et al. 2008, Hermann et al. 2009*], however other possibilities like cracked tooth [*Kahler 2008*], denticle, overhang, overload [*Dobó-Nagy et al. 2003*] and other mechanical trauma, abrasion, erosion as well as postoperative, postpreparative and postcementation pain and (hyper)sensitivity should also be considered carefully [*Brännström 1996, Kern et al. 1996, Türp et al. 2009*]. Long-term degenerative pulp reactions of abutment teeth should also be considered [*Zoellner et al. 1996*]. Odontalgia because of noninfectious vascular or neuropathic origin may also occur occasionally [*Baad-Hansen 2008*]. Unerupted and impacted teeth may also induce pain or other symptoms.

Besides premised primarily somatic causes of tooth-located symptoms, psychogenic pain (and/or other symptoms) centered on teeth, implants, or extraction sites may also occur certainly, causing huge diagnostic problem [*Gratt et al. 1996, Fábián 1999, Sarlani et al. 2005, Kromminga et al. 1991*] (see also *paragraph 3.2.2., 3.2.12.*). It should be also mentioned that, *locally asymptomatic* unerupted (especially impacted) teeth occasionally induce symptoms like fatigue, headache, dizziness, nausea, emotional tension and irritability

[*Eidelman 1979, 1982*]. Similarly, non-vital teeth and residual infections may also cause general health symptoms occasionally, like allergic or autoimmune reactions as well as fatigue, headache, dizziness, nausea, emotional tension, irritability [*Eidelman 1982*] even if they are asymptomatic locally.

4.4.2. Other Disorders of the Orofacial Region

There are numerous possible pathologies causing symptoms in the orofacial region. Many of them may cause difficulties and mistakes also in the diagnosis of PDI. Some (but far not all) of such disorders are listed below, to point out the importance of proper and careful clinical diagnosis and differential diagnosis of PDI cases. Before the diagnosis of PDI is established, various disorders of somatic origin should be considered. Oral infections [*Woda & Pionchon 2000*], especially *Candida*-associated denture-stomatitis [*Miyamoto & Ziccardi 1998, Vitkov et al. 1999, Taillandier et al. 2000, Hermann et al. 2001, Satoh 2004*] may be considered first. Similarly, local irritations of chemical, microbial or mechanical origin [*Woda & Pionchon 2000, de Baat 2006*] as well as appearance of electrical galvanic currents [*Bánóczy et al. 1979, Schmalz & Garhammer 2002, Sutow et al. 2004, Wartenberg et al. 2008*] may also be responsible for numerous denture related symptoms. Minor nerve trauma [*Woda & Pionchon 2000, de Baat 2006*] and sensory nerve impairment following preprosthetic dentoalveolar surgery [*Bataineh 2001, de Baat 2006*] as well as bone resorption to the mental foramen area and consequent nerve compression by the denture [*Sandler et al. 1995*] may also cause various symptoms. Similarly, sharp exostoses under denture base [*de Baat 2006*] should also be considered.

Maxillary sinusitis [*Gratt et al. 1996*], osteomyelitis [*Sandler et al. 1995*] osteonecrosis [*Woda & Pionchon 2000, Srinivasan et al. 2007, Kumar et al. 2008*] and any other local inflammation [*Woda & Pionchon 2000*] should also be considered. Bone fracture of jaws and mandible [*Sandler et al. 1995, Yassutaka et al. 2006*] as well as cysts of the bone and soft tissues [*Azevedo et al. 2008*] should also be excluded. Similarly, TMJ arthropathy [*Harris et al. 1993, Nuebler-Moritz et al. 1995, Gratt et al. 1996, Israel & Scrivani 2000*], sinovial chondromatosis of the TMJ [*Orden et al. 1989*] as well as any other severe TMJ pathologies should be excluded too. Certain other pathologies like Eagle's syndrome [*Correll & Wescott 1982, Sarlani et al. 2005/a*], pterygoid hamulus's bursitis [*Shankland 1996/a,b, Ramírez et al. 2006*], trigeminal and glossopharyngeal neuralgia [*Gratt et al. 1996, Israel & Scrivani 2000, Sarlani et al. 2005/a*] as well as salivary gland pathologies [*Sarlani et al. 2005/b, Márton et al. 2005, 2006*] and alterations of salivation [*Niedermeier 1991, Feinberg 1993, Márton et al. 2005, 2006, 2008*] should also be considered. Finally, orofacial tumors (see *paragraph 4.4.3.*) and non-topical organic and systemic diseases (see *paragraph 4.4.4.*) as well as medication induced orofacial symptoms (see *paragraphs 4.4.5.*) should also be excluded.

4.4.3. Tumors Behind Orofacial Symptoms

An important issue of differential diagnosis is the discrimination of psychogenic orofacial symptoms and symptoms of early stage (or not yet clearly detectable) tumors [*Castellanos & Lally 1982, Sandler et al. 1995, Wolowski 1995, Wong et al. 1998, Wertheimer-Hatch et al. 2000*]. In cases of *persistent and nontypical* psychosomatic *symptoms*, the somatic evaluation must be extended despite a lack of clear-cut organic findings [*Sandler et al. 1995, Wolowski 1995, Wong et al. 1998*]. Importantly, not only orofacial and/or pharyngeal [*Castellanos & Lally 1982, Wertheimer-Hatch et al. 2000, Gellrich et al. 2002*] but also any other neoplasms [*Sandler et al. 1995, Wong et al. 1998, Oneschuk et al. 2000, Israel & Scrivani 2000*] (i.e. tumors of the brain, peripheral nerves, blood cells, metastatic tumors etc.) should also be considered in these cases. Importantly, pain symptom that has worsened rapidly in a short period of time *may* indicate malignancy affecting almost any soft or hard tissue component of the surrounding oral and/or maxillofacial tissues [*Wong et al. 1998, Sarlani et al. 2005/b*]. In contrast, painless, slowly growing encapsulated submucosal firm or slightly fluctuant mass may refer to benign oral tumors [*Azevedo et al. 2008*]. In some cases tumors may be presenting as a "simple" asymptomatic swelling [*Azevedo et al. 2008*]. It is likely that, the relationships between patient's psychosocial history and the appearance of initial symptoms is much weaker in the case of tumors comparing to the psychosomatic symptoms [*Wolowski 1995*]; which aspect may also be considered for the differential diagnosis of unclear cases.

4.4.4. Non-Topical Organic and Systemic Diseases

There are numerous non-topical organic and systemic diseases that may cause complaints on the orofacial region [*Zumkley 1976, Sandler et al. 1995*]. Neurological disorders like migraine or cluster headache [*Drummond 1997, Israel & Scrivani 2000, Bernhardt et al. 2005, Sarlani et al. 2005/b*], chronic paroxysmal hemicrania [*Israel & Scrivani 2000, Sarlani et al. 2005*], giant cell arteritis [*Sarlani et al. 2005/b*] and other vascular pain of extracranial carotid arteries [*Sandler et al. 1995, Sarlani et al. 2005/b*] may cause orofacial pain. Alterations of peripheral and/or central sensory functions may also cause orofacial symptoms [*Grushka et al. 1987, Woda & Pionchon 2000, 2001*]. The clinical manifestation of Lyme disease [*Sandler et al. 1995, Heir 1997, Pertes 1998, Sarlani et al. 2005*] and multiple sclerosis [*Sarlani et al. 2005/b*] may also mimic various orofacial pain disorders. Several movement disorders of nervous origin [*Lobbezzo & Naeije 2007*] including orofacial dyskinesia and oromandibular dystonia [*Lobbezzo & Naeije 2007, Balasubramaniam & Ram 2008*] should also be considered. Cerebrovascular processes [*Israel & Scrivani 2000, Sarlani et al. 2005/b*] and seizure disorder (epilepsy) [*Károlyházy et al. 2003, 2005, Sarlani et al. 2005/b*] may also cause orofacial symptoms. Similarly, several psychiatric disorders (also those which are not closely related to PDI pathologies) may also be associated with chronic orofacial pain or other orofacial symptom [*Kaban & Belfer 1981, Pilling 1983, Israel & Scrivani 2000, Sarlani et al. 2005/a,b*].

Disease group of spondyloarthropathies including ankylosing spondylitis, spondyloarthritis and rheumatoid arthritis [*Sandler et al. 1995, Yamakawa et al. 2002,*

Hackard-Bouder et al. 2006, Herman et al. 2008, Fábián et al. 2009/a] as well as fibromyalgia [*Pertes 1998, Sarlani et al. 2005/a*] should also be considered. Similarly, autoimmune pathologies including polymyositis and dermatomyositis [*Márton et al. 2005*] as well as systemic sclerosis [*Scardina et al. 2002*] should be considered as well. Similarly, verifiable ("real") allergy [*Izumi 1982, Wirz et al. 2003, de Baat 2006*] behind certain symptoms should also be excluded. Paget's disease [*Sandler et al. 1995*], osteoporosis [*Baxter 1981, Woda & Pionchon 2000, 2001*] as well as changes of estrogen level [*Woda & Pionchon 2000, 2001*], menopausal symptoms [*Niedermeier et. al. 1979, Myers & Naylor 1989, Woda & Pionchon 2000, 2001*] and pregnancy [*Myers & Naylor 1989*] may also cause differential diagnostic difficulties. Diabetes mellitus [*Miyamoto & Ziccardi 1998, Vitkov et al. 1999*], nutritional deficiencies [*Touger-Decker 1998, Scala et al. 2003*] and certain eating disorders including anorexia nervosa [*Hellström 1977, Öhrn et al. 1999*] may also cause oral symptoms. Pathologies in distant structures, (including the neck, heart muscle, and thorax) can also be sources of referred orofacial pain symptoms [*Sandler et al. 1995, Israel & Scrivani 2000, Sarlani et al. 2005/a,b, de Baat 2006*] (and orofacial pain can be their presenting symptom [*Sandler et al. 1995, Sarlani et al. 2005/b, de Baat 2006*]).

4.4.5. Medication Induced Orofacial Symptoms

Several symptoms may also be induced by side-effects of medications. Oral contraceptives [*Pluvinage 1977, Myers & Naylor 1989*], anticholinergic drugs [*Feinberg 1993*], anxiolytics [*Friedlander et al. 2002, 2004*], antidepressants [*Friedlander et al. 2002, 2004*], antipsychotic drugs [*Magnusson et al. 1996, Friedlander et al. 2002*], hydantoines, calcium channel blockers, cyclosporines, bisphosphonates [*Cheng et al. 2005, Srinivasan et al. 2007, Kumar et al. 2008, Blazsek et al. in press*] and drugs of chemotherapy [*Oneschuk et al. 2000*], may be the most important medications, which may cause oral/orofacial symptoms. However, various other drugs may also be implicated in xerostomia [*Tredwin et al. 2005, Fábián et al. 2008/a*] in orofacial motor symptoms [*Clark 2006, Lobbezzo & Naeije 2007*], in taste alterations or in any other symptoms that are also frequently attributed to dentures [*Yontchev 1986, Yontchev et al. 1986*].

4.5. Referral to Other Professionals

Based on above data it is obvious that, referral for evaluation to other professionals may be a necessary component in both the diagnosis and management of PDI [*Wiens et al. 1983*]. Referral to maxillofacial surgeon, neurologist, otorhinolaryngologist, ophthalmologist, allergologist, rheumatologist, internist, and family doctor as well as to professionals of several dental specialties is frequently needed [*Pilling 1983, Wiens et al. 1983*]. To do this adequately, the referring dentist must know other professionals and have faith in their ability. There is also a great need of referral to psychiatrist certainly [*Kaban & Belfer 1981*], but unfortunately, many PDI patients often avoid this type of care until an emotional condition becomes so severe that hospitalization is necessary [*Pilling 1983*]. Since physical symptoms may arise as extensions of psychological defense mechanisms in the struggle to cope with an emotional conflict [*Wiens et al. 1983*]; PDI patients frequently recognize their symptom as "of obviously somatic origin" rather than to attempt resolution of the underlying psychological conflict [*Wiens et al. 1983*]. Consequently, they are not motivated for cooperating with the psychiatrist and being involved emotionally in the treatment. Therefore those psychiatrists who show a particular interest in such psychophysiological or psychosomatic problems will be more helpful and perceptive for this select group of PDI patients [*Wiens et al. 1983*] (comparing to those psychiatrists being frustrated because of the treatment-refusing behavior of such patients).

4.6. CONCLUSION

Since psychogenic symptoms may mimic a great variety of somatic symptoms; a clear-cut diagnosis and proper differential diagnosis of PDI could be rather difficult. Therefore it should be emphasized that, *the diagnosis of PDI is a presumptive one in many cases*. The diagnosis may change later in the course of the disease as the clinical findings change and/or stabilize, therefore continuous monitoring and evaluation of the patient over time is essential [*Sarlani et al. 2005/a.b*]. A detailed differential diagnosis considering possible disorders of the teeth, and/or oral- and maxillofacial tissues should also be carried out, and *any other possible somatic causes behind the symptoms should also be excluded*. For such purposes *referral to other professionals* like maxillofacial surgeon, neurologist, psychiatrist, otorhinolaringologist, ophthalmologist, internist, rheumatologist (etc.) may also be needed, and especially *recommended in the case of pain and other (pseudo)neurological symptoms* [*Sarlani et al. 2005/a.b*].

REFERENCES

[1]   Allen, PF. & Locker, D. A modified short version of the Oral Health Impact Profile for assessing health related quality of life in edentulous adults. *Int J Prosthodont*, 2002 15, 446-450.

[2]   Allen, PF. & McMillan, AS. A review of the functional and psychosocial outcomes of edentulousness treated with complete replacement dentures. *J Can Dent Assoc*, 2003 69, 662.

[3]   Aoki, H; Tamaki, K; Fujita, T; Fukase, A; Endo, Y; Yamamura, M; Watanabe, H. Role of advanced technology for studying coronal restorations and clinical assessment of mandibular function. *Bull Kanagawa Dent Coll*, 1988/a 16, 45-51.

[4]   Aoki, H; Tamaki, K; Fukase, A; Endo, Y; Fujita, T. Reevaluation of changing features in occlusal concepts. *Bull Kanagawa Dent Coll*, 1988/b 16, 59-61.

[5]   Asmundson, GJG; Bovell, CV; Carleton, RN; McWilliams, LA. The Fear of Pain Questionnaire - Short Form (FPQ-SF): Factor validity and psychometric properties. *Pain*, 2008 134, 51-58.

[6]   Atchison, KA. & Gift, HC. Perceived oral health in a diverse sample. *Adv Dent Res*, 1997 11, 272-280.

[7]   Austen, KF. Diseases of immediate type hypersensitivity. In: Wilson JD, Braunwald E, Isselbacher KJ, Petersdorf RG, Martin JB, Fauci AS, Root RK editors. *Harrison's Principles of Internal Medicine Vol. 2. (Twelfth Edition).* New York: McGraw-Hill; 1991; 1422-1428.

[8]   Azevedo, LR; Dos Santos, JN; De Lima, AAS; Machado, MAN; Grégio, AMT. Canalicular adenoma presenting as an asymptomatic swelling of the upper lip: A case report. *J Contemp Dent Pract*, 2008 9, 1.

[9]   Baad-Hansen, L. Atypical odontalgia - pathophysiology and clinical management. *J Oral Rehabil*, 2008 35, 1-11.

[10]   Baba, K; Aridome, K; Haketa, T; Kino, K; Ohyama, T. Sensory perceptive and discriminative abilities of patients with occlusal dysesthesia. *Nihon Hoteshu Shika Gakki Zasshi*, 2005 49, 599-607.

[11]   Balasubramaniam, R. & Ram, S. Orofacial movement disorders. *Oral Maxillofac Surg Clin North Am*, 2008 20, 273-285.

[12]   Bálint, M; Krause, M; Krause, WR; Kaán, B; Fejérdy, L; Gáspár, J; Fábián, TK. Modification of the photo-acoustic stimulation technique in the explorative therapy of oral psychosomatic patients. *Fogorv Szle*, 2003 96, 171-174.

[13]   Bánóczy, J; Roed-Petersen, B; Pindborg, JJ; Inovay, J. Clinical and hystologic studies on electrogalvanically induced oral white lesions. *Oral Surg Oral Med Oral Pathol*, 1979 48, 319-323.

[14]   Barsby, MJ. The use of hypnosis in the management of "gagging" and intolerance to dentures. *Br Dent J*, 1994 176, 97-102.

[15]   Basler, HD. Marburger Fragebogen zum habituellen Wohlbefinden. Untersuchung an Patienten mit chronischem Schmerz. *Schmerz*, 1999 13, 385-391.

[16]   Bataineh, AB. Sensory nerve impairment following mandibular third molar surgery. *J Oral Maxillofac Surg*, 2001 59, 1012-1017.

[17]   Baxter, JC. Relationship of osteoporosis to excessive residual ridge resorption. *J Prosthet Dent*, 1981 46, 123-125.

[18]   Beauchamp, GK; Bachmanov, A; Stein, LJ. Development and genetics of glutamate taste preference. *Ann NY Acad Sci*, 1998 855; 412-416.

[19]   Beck, AT; Beamesderfer, A. Assessment of depression: the depression inventory. In: Pichot P, editor. *Modern problems in pharmacopsychiatry. Vol. 7.* Basel, Switzerland: Karger; 1974; 151-169.

[20]   Beck, AT; Rush, AJ; Shaw, BF; Emery, G. *Cognitive therapy of depression.* New York: Guilford Press; 1979.

[21]   Bell, WH. Nonsurgical management of the pain-dysfunction syndrome. *JADA,* 1969 79, 161-170.

[22]   Bensing, J. Bridging the gap. The separate worlds of evidence-based medicine and patient-centered medicine. *Patient Education Counseling*, 2000 39, 17-25.

[23]   Bernhardt, O; Gesch, D; Schwahn, C; Mack, F; Meyer, G; John, U; Kocher, T. Risk factors for headache, including TMD signs and symptoms, and their impact on quality of life. Results of the study of Health in Pomerania (SHIP). *Quintessence Int*, 2005 36, 55-64.

[24]   Berrington De Gonzalez, A. & Darby, S. Risk of cancer from diagnostic X-rays: Estimates for the UK and 14 other countries. *Lancet*, 2004 363, 345-351.

[25] Bessette, R; Bishop, B; Mohl, N. Duration of masseteric silent period in patients with TMJ syndrome. *J Appl Physiol*, 1971 30, 864-869.

[26] Biagioni, PA. & Lamey, PJ. Electronic infrared thermography as a method of assessing herpes labialis infection. *Acta Derm Venereol*, 1995 75, 264-268.

[27] Blazsek, J; Dobó-Nagy, C; Blazsek, I; Varga, R; Vecsei, B; Fejérdy, P; Varga, G. Aminobisphosphonate stimulates bone regeneration and enforces consolidation of titanium implant. *Pathol Oncol Res*, in press; DOI: 10.1007/s12253-009-9156-y

[28] Borelli, S; Seifert, HU; Seifert, B. Sensibilisierung und allergische Reaktionen. In: hupfauf L (ed.) *Teilprothesen*. München: Urban & Schwarzenberg; 1988; 247-263.

[29] Brännström, M. Reducing the risk of sensitivity and pulpal complications after the placement of crowns and fixed partial dentures. *Quintessence Int*, 1996 27, 673-678.

[30] Brodine, AL. & Hartshorn, MA. Recognition and management of somatoform disorders. *J Prosthet Dent*, 2004 91, 268-273.

[31] Brown, GL; McGarvey, EL; Shirtcliff, EA; Keller, A; Granger, DA; Flavin, K. Salivary cortisol, dehydroepiandrosterone, and testosterone interrelationships in healthy young males: A pilot study with implications for studies of aggressive behavior. *Psychiatry Res*, 2008 159, 67-76.

[32] Brunello, DL. & Mandikos, MN. Construction faults, age gender, and relative medical health: factors associated with complaints in complete denture patients. *J Prosthet Dent*, 1998 79, 545-554.

[33] Brunswick, AF. & Nikias, M. Dentist ratings and adolescent's perception of oral health. *J Dent Res*, 1975 54, 836-843.

[34] Calderon, PS; Kogawa, EM; Corpas, LS. Lauris, JRP; Conti, PCR. The influence of gender and bruxism on human minimum interdental threshold ability. *J Appl Oral Sci*, 2009 17, 224-228.

[35] Castellanos, JL. & Lally, ET. Acinic cell tumor of the minor salivary glands. *J Oral Maxillofac Surg*, 1982 40, 428-431.

[36] Chatterton Jr., RT; Vogelsong, KM; Lu, YC; Ellman, AB; Hudgens, GA. Salivary alpha-amylase as a measure of endogenous adrenergic activity. *Clin Psychol*, 1996 16, 433-448.

[37] Cheng, A; Mavrokokki, A; Carter, G; Stein, B; Fazzalari, NL; Wilson, DF; Goss, AN. The dental implications of bisphosphonates and bone disease. *Aust Dent J*, 2005 50, S4-S13.

[38] Clark, GT. Medical management of oral motor disorders: dystonia, dyskinesia, and drug-induced dystonic extrapiramidal reactions. *J Calif Dent Assoc*, 2006 34, 657-667.

[39] Correll, RW. & Wescott, WB. Eagle's syndrome diagnosed after history of headache, dysphagia, otalgia, and limited neck movement. *JADA*, 1982 104, 491-492.

[40] Curtis, DA; Plesh, O; Sharma, A; Finzen, F. Complications associated with fixed partial dentures with a loose retainer. *J Prosthet Dent*, 2006 96, 245-251.

[41] Dahlsröm, L. Electromyographic studies of craniomandibular disorders: a review of the literature. *J Oral Rehabil*, 1989 16, 1-20.

[42] Darvell, BW. & Clark, RK. The physical mechanisms of complete denture retention. *Brit Dent J*, 2000 189, 248-252.

[43] Dawes, C. Circadian rhythms in human salivary flow rate and composition. *J Physiol*, 1972 220, 529-545.

[44] Dawes, C. Circadian rhythms in the flow rate and composition of unstimulated and stimulated human submandibular saliva. *J Physiol*, 1975 244, 535-548.

[45] de Baat, C. Pain in edentulous patients. *Ned Tijdschr Tandheelkd*, 2006 113, 463-468.

[46] de Laat, A; van der Glas, HW; Weytjens, JLF; van Steenberghe, D. The masseteric post-stimulus electromyographic-complex in people with dysfunction of the mandibular joint. *Arch Oral Biol*, 1985 30, 177-180.

[47] de Laat, A; Horvath, M; Bossuyt, M; Fossion, E; Baert, AL. Myogenous or arthrogenous limitation of mouth opening: Correlations between clinical findings, MRI, and clinical outcome. *J Orofac Pain*, 1993 7, 150-155.

[48] de Lima, DC; Nakata, GC; Balducci, I; Almeida, JD. Oral manifestations of diabetes mellitus in complete denture wearers. *J Prosthet Dent*, 2008 99, 60-65.

[49] Derra, C. Psychosomatische Diagnostik und Therapie des atypischen Gesichtsschmerzes. *ZWR*, 2002 111, 485-490.

[50] Dobó-Nagy, C; Fejérdy, P; Angyal, J; Harasztosi, L; Daróczi, L; Beke, D; Wesselink, PR. Measurement of periapical pressure created by occlusal loading. *Int Endodont J*, 2003 36, 700-704.

[51] Dorn, LD; Lucke, JF; Loucks, TL; Berga, SL. Salivary cortisol reflects serum cortisol: analysis of circadian profiles. *Ann Clin Biochem*, 2007 44. 281-284.

[52] Drummond, PD. Photophobia and autonomic responses to facial pain in migraine. *Brain*, 1997 120, 1857-1864.

[53] Duke, RL; Campbell, BH; Indressano, AT; Eaton, DJ; Marbella, AM; Myers, KB; Layde, PM. Dental status and quality of life in long-term head and neck cancer survivors. *Laryngoscope*, 2005 115, 678-683.

[54] Dunteman, E. & Swarm, R. Atypical facial "neuralgia". (Case reports). *Anesth Analg*, 1995 80, 188-190.

[55] Dworkin, SF. & Sherman J. Chronic orofacial pain: biobehavioral perspectives. In: Mostofsky DI, Forgione AG, Giddon, DB editors. *Behavioral dentistry*. Ames (Iowa): Blackwell Munksgaard; 2006; 99-113.

[56] Eidelman, D. "Fatigue or rest" and associated symptoms (headache, vertigo, blurred vision, nausea, tension and irritability) due to locally asymptomatic, unerupted, impacted teeth. *Med Hypothesis*, 1979 5, 339-346.

[57] Eidelman, D. Pathology in the lower half of the functional face - its significance in clinical medicine. *Med Hypothesis*, 1982 8, 149-154.

[58] Eitner, S; Wichmann, M; Heckmann, J; Holst, S. Pilot study on the psychologic evaluation of prosthesis incompatibility using the SCL-90-R scale and the CES-D scale. *Int J Prosthodont*, 2006 19, 482-490.

[59] Eitner, S; Wichmann, M; Schlegel, A; Holst, S. Clinical study on the correlation between psychogenic dental prosthesis incompatibility, oral stereognosis, and the psychogenic diagnostic tools SCL-90R and CES-D. *Int J Prosthodont*, 2007 20, 538-545.

[60] Emerson, WA, & Giddon, DR. Psychologic factors in adjustment to full denture prosthesis. *J Dent Res*, 1955 34, 683-684.

[61] Engel, G. The need for a new medical model: a challenge for biomedicine. *Science*, 1977 196, 129-136.

[62] Fábián G. Psychosomatic aspects of orthodontics. [Az orthodontia pszichoszomatikus vonatkozásai]. In: Fábián TK, Vértes G editors. *Psychosomatic dentistry* [*Fogorvosi pszichoszomatika*]. Budapest: Medicina; 2007; 137-146.

[63] Fábián, G; Fejérdy, L; Kaán, B; Fábián, Cs; Tóth, Zs; Fábián, TK. Background data about the high dental fear scores of Hungarian 8-15-year old primary school children. *Fogorv Szle*, 2004 97, 128-132.

[64] Fábián, G; Bálint, M; Fábián, TK. Psychology and psychosomatics of the orthodontic treatment. *Fogorv Szle*, 2005 98, 113-119.

[65] Fábián, G; Müller, O; Kovács, Sz; Nguyen, MT; Fábián, TK; Csermely, P; Fejérdy, P. Attitude towards death. Does influence dental fear? *Ann NY Acad Sci*, 2007 1113, 339-349.

[66] Fábián, TK. Treatment possibilities of denture intolerance. Use of photo-acoustic stimulation and hypnotherapy in a difficult clinical case. [Adalékok a protézis intolerancia gyógyításához. Fény-hang kezeléssel kombinált hipnoterápia alkalmazásának szokatlan módja egy eset kapcsán.] *Hipno Info*,1999 38, 81-88.

[67] Fábián, TK. & Fábián, G. Dental stress. In: Fink G, editor in chef. *Encyclopedia of Stress. Vol. 1*. San Diego: Academic Press; 2000; 657-659.

[68] Fábián, TK; Gáspár, J; Fejérdy, L; Kaán, B; Bálint, M; Csermely, P; Fejérdy, P. Hsp70 is present in human saliva. *Med Sci Monitor*, 2003 9, BR62-65.

[69] Fábián, TK; Tóth, Zs; Fejérdy, L; Kaán, B; Csermely, P; Fejérdy, P. Photo-acoustic stimulation increases the amount of 70 kDa heat shock protein (Hsp70) in human whole saliva. A pilot study. *Int J Psychophysiol*, 2004/a 52, 211-216.

[70] Fábián, TK; Kaán, B; Fejérdy, L; Tóth, Zs; Fejérdy, P. Effectiveness of psychotherapy in the treatment of denture intolerance. Evaluation of 25 cases. *Fogorv Szle*, 2004/b 97, 163-168.

[71] Fábián, TK; Mierzwińska-Nastalska, E; Fejérdy, P. Photo-acoustic stimulation. A suitable method in the treatment of psychogenic denture intolerance. *Protet Stomatol*, 2006 56, 335-340.

[72] Fábián, TK; Fejérdy, P; Nguyen, MT; Sőti, Cs; Csermely, P. Potential immunological functions of salivary Hsp70 in mucosal and periodontal defense mechanisms. *Arch Immunol Ther Exp*, 2007/a 55, 91-98.

[73] Fábián, TK; Fábián, G; Fejérdy, P. Dental Stress. In: Fink G, editor in chef. *Encyclopedia of Stress. 2-nd enlarged edition, Vol. 1*. Oxford: Academic Press; 2007/b; 733-736.

[74] Fábián, TK; Fejérdy, P; Csermely, P. Chemical biology of saliva in health and disease. In: Begley T, editor in chief. *Wiley encyclopedia of chemical biology*. Hoboken: John Wiley & sons; 2008/a. DOI: 10.1002/9780470048672.wecb643

[75] Fábián, TK; Fejérdy, P; Csermely, P. Salivary genomics, transcriptomics and proteomics: The emerging concept of the oral ecosystem and their use in the early diagnosis of cancer and other diseases. *Current Genomics*, 2008/b 9, 11-21.

[76] Fábián, TK; Csermely, P; Fábián, G; Fejérdy P. Spondyloarthropathies and bone resorption. Possible role of Hsp70. *Acta Physiol Hungarica*, 2009/a 96, 149-155.

[77] Fábián, TK; Gótai, L; Beck, A; Fábián, G; Fejérdy, P. The role of molecular chaperones (HSPAs/HSP70s) in oral health and oral inflammatory diseases: A review. *Eur J Inflammation*, 2009/b 7, 53-61.

[78] Feinberg, M. The problems of anticholinergic adverse effects in older patients. *Drugs Aging*, 1993 3, 335-348.

[79] Fejérdy, L; Kaán, B; Fábián, G; Tóth, Zs; Fábián, TK. Background data about the high dental fear scores of Hungarian secondary school students. *Fogorv Szle*, 2005 98, 9-13.

[80] Fenlon, MR. & Sherriff, M. An investigation of factors influencing patients' satisfaction with new complete dentures using structural equation modeling. *J Dentistry*, 2008 36, 427-434.

[81] Freeman, R. The determinants of dental health attitudes and behaviors. *Brit Dent J*, 1999 187, 15-18.

[82] Friedlander, AH; Friedlander, IK; Marder, SR. Bipolar I disorder. Psychopathology, medical management and dental implications. *JADA*, 2002 133, 1209-1217.

[83] Friedlander, AH; Marder, SR; Sung, EC. Panic disorder. Psychopathology, medical management and dental implications. *JADA*, 2004 135, 771-778.

[84] Fujita, T; Aoki, H; Shimizu, T; Kikuta, D; Kawagoe, Y; Watanabe, H; Yamamura, M; Ukiya, M. Background information on the measuring system for mandibular motion. *Bull Kanagawa Dent Coll*, 1983 11, 69-78.

[85] Gale, EN. & Carlsson, SG. Look carefully; a short note on symptom substitution. *Behav Res Ther*, 1976 14, 77.

[86] Garau, V; Masala, MG; Cortis, MC; Pittau, R. Contact stomatitis due to palladium in dental alloys: A clinical report. *J Prosthet Dent*, 2005 93, 318-320.

[87] Garhammer, P; Schmalz, G; Hiller, KA; Reitinger, T; Stolz, W. Patients with local adverse effects from dental alloys: frequency, complaints, symptoms, allergy. *Clin Oral Invest*, 2001 5, 240-249.

[88] Garhammer, P; Hiller, KA; Reitinger, T; Schmalz, G. Metal content of saliva of patients with and without metal restorations. *Clin Oral Invest*, 2004 8, 238-242.

[89] Gellrich, NC; Schramm, A; Böckmann, R; Kugler, J. Follow-up in patients with oral cancer. *J Oral Maxillofac Surg*, 2002 60, 380-386.

[90] Gemba, H; Teranaka, A; Takemura, K. Influences of emotion upon parotid secretion in human. *Neurosci Lett*, 1996 211, 159-162.

[91] Geurtsen, W. Biocompatibility of dental casting alloys. *Crit Rev Oral biol Med*, 2002 13, 71-84.

[92] Giddon, DB. The mouth and the quality of life. *NY J Dentistry*, 1978 48, 3-10.

[93] Ginsburg, I; Sadovnic, M; Oron, M; Kohen, R. Novel chemiluminescence-inducing cocktails, part II: measurement of the anti-oxidant capacity of vitamins, thiols, body fluids, alcoholic beverages and edible oils. *Inflammopharmacology*, 2004 12, 305-320.

[94] Glaros, AG. Bruxism. In: Mostofsky DI, Forgione AG, Giddon, DB editors. *Behavioral dentistry*. Ames (Iowa): Blackwell Munksgaard; 2006; 127-137.

[95] Golan, HP. The use of hypnosis in the treatment of psychogenic oral pain. *Am J Clin Hypn*, 1997 40, 89-96.

[96] Goon, ATJ; Bruze, M; Zimerson, E; Goh, CL; Isakson, M. Contact allergy to acrylates/methacrylates in the acrylate and nail acrylics series in southern Sweden: simultaneous positive patch test reaction patterns and possible screening allergens. *Contact Dematitis*, 2007 57, 21-27.

[97] Goon, ATJ; Bruze, M; Zimerson, E; Goh, CL; Koh, DSQ; Isakson, M. Screening for acrylate/methacrylate allergy in the baseline series: our experience in Sweden and Singapore . *Contact Dematitis*, 2008 59, 307-313.

[98] Granger, DA; Cicchetti, D; Rogosch, FA; Hibel, LC; Teisl, M; Flores, E. Blood contamination in children's saliva: Prevalence, stability, and impact on the measurement of salivary cortisol, testosterone, and dehydroepiandrosterone. *Psychoneuroendocinology*, 2007 32, 724-733.

[99] Granger, DA; Kivlighan, KT; Fortunato, C; Harmon, AG; Hibel, LC; Schwartz, EB; Whembolua, GL. Integration of salivary biomarkers into developmental and behaviorally-oriented research: Problems and solutions for collecting specimens. *Physiol Behav*, 2007/b 92, 583-590.

[100] Gratt, BM. & Anbar, M. A pilot study of nitric oxide blood levels in patients with chronic orofacial pain. *Oral Surg Oral Med Oral Pathol Oral Radiol Endod*, 2005 100, 441-448.

[101] Gratt, BM; Sickless, EA; Graff-Radford, SB; Solberg, WK. Electronic thermography in the diagnosis of atypical odontalgia: a pilot study. *Oral Surg Oral Med Oral Pathol*, 1989 68, 472-481.

[102] Gratt, BM; Graff-Radford, SB; Shetty, V; Solberg, WK; Sickles, EA. A 6-year clinical assessment of electrical facial thermography. *Dentomaxillofac Radiol*, 1996 25, 247-255.

[103] Green, CS. & Laskin, DM. Temporomandibular disorders: Moving from a dentally based to a medically based model. *J Dent Res*, 2000 79, 1736-1739.

[104] Griffin, CJ, Watson, JE; Marshall, WG: Electromyographic analysis of the effects of treatment in patients with the temporomandibular joint syndrome. In: Griffin CJ, Harris R editors. *The temporomandibular joint syndrome. The masticatory apparatus of man in normal and abnormal function.* (Monographs in oral science, Vol. 4.) Basel - München - Paris - London - New York - Sydney: Karger; 1975; 188-200.

[105] Grushka, M; Sessle, BJ; Howley, TP. Psychophysical assessment of tactile, pain and thermal sensory functions in burning mouth syndrome. *Pain*, 1987 28, 169-184.

[106] Gruzelier, J; Clow, A; Evans, P; Lazar, I; Walker, L. Mind-body influences on immunity: Lateralized control, stress, individual difference predictors and prophylaxis. *Ann NY Acad Sci*, 1998 851, 487-494.

[107] Hacquard-Bouder, C; Ittah, M; Breban, M. Animal models of HLA-B27-associated diseases: new outcomes. *Joint Bone Spine*, 2006 73, 132-138.

[108] Hadjistavropoulos, HD; MacLeod, FK; Asmundson, GJG. Validation of the Chronic Pain Coping Inventory. *Pain*, 1999 80, 471-481.

[109] Hamann, CP; Depaola, LG; Rodgers, PA. Occupation-related allergies in dentistry. *JADA*, 2005 136, 500-510.

[110] Harmon, AG; Towe-Goodman, NR; Fortunato, CK; Granger, DA. Differences in saliva collection location and disparities in baseline and diurnal rhythms of alpha amylase: A preliminary note of caution. *Hormones Behavior*, 2008 54, 592-596.

[111] Harris, M; Feinmann, C; Wise, M; Treasure, F. Temporomandibular joint and orofacial pain: clinical and medicolegal management problems. *Brit Dent J*, 1993 174, 129-136.

[112] Har-Zion, G; Brin, I; Steiner, J. Psychophysiological testing of taste and flavour reactivity in young patients undergoing treatment with removable orthodontic appliances. *Eur J Orthodontics*, 2004 26, 73-78.

[113] Hazey III, MA; Ngan, P; Reed, H; Razmus, T; Crout, R; Kao, E. Comparison of computer-generated, enhanced and conventional 2-dimensional radiographic imaging. *AM J Orthod Dentofacial Orthop*, 2009 135, 463-467.

[114] Heir, GM. Differentiation of orofacial pain related to Lyme disease from other dental and facial pain disorders. *Dent Clin North Am*, 1997 41, 243-258.

[115] Hellström, I. Oral complications in anorexia nervosa. *Scand J Dent Res*, 1977 85, 71-86.

[116] Henkin, RI. & Christiansen, RL. Taste localization on the tongue, palate, and pharinx of normal man. *J Appl Physiol*, 1967 22, 316-320.

[117] Herman, S; Krönke, G; Schett, G. Molecular mechanisms of inflammatory bone damage: emerging targets for therapy. *Trends Mol Med*, 2008 14, 245-253.

[118] Hermann, P; Berek, Zs; Nagy, G; Kamotsay, K; Rozgonyi, F. Pathogenesis, microbiological and clinical aspects of oral candidiasis (candidosis). *Acta Microbiol Immunol Hungarica*, 2001 48, 479-495.

[119] Hermann, P. Gera, I; Borbély J; Fejérdy, P; Madléna, M. Periodontal health of an adult population in Hungary: findings of a national survey. *J Clin Periodontol*, 2009 36, 449-457.

[120] Hintze, H; Wiese, M; Wenzel, A. Cone beam CT and conventional tomography for the detection of morphological temporomandibular joint changes. *Dentomaxillofacial Radiol*, 2007 36, 192-197.

[121] Hoehl, K; Schoenberger, GU; Busch-Stockfisch, M. Water quality and taste sensitivity for basic tastes and metallic sensation. *Food Quality Preference*, in press. DOI: 10.1016/j.foodqual.2009.06.007

[122] House, K; Sernetz, F; Dymock, D; Sandy, JR; Ireland, AJ. Corrosion of orthodontic appliances - should we care? *Am J Orthod Dentofacial Orthop*, 2008 133, 584-592.

[123] Ikebe, K; Amemiya, M; Morii, K; Matsuda, K; Furuya-Yoshinaka, M; Nokubi, T. Comparison of oral stereognosis in relation to age end the use of complete dentures. *J Oral Rehabil*, 2007 34, 345-350.

[124] Ismail, Y; Zullo, T; Kruper, D. The use of the psychological screening inventory as a predictor of problem denture patients. J Dent Res, 1974 54 (spec. issue. A), L128.

[125] Israel, HA. & Scrivani, SJ. The interdisciplinary approach to oral, facial and head pain. *JADA*, 2000 131, 919-926.

[126] Issa, Y; Duxbury, AJ; Macfarlane, TV; Brunton, PA. Oral lichenoid lesions related to dental restorative materials. *Brit Dent J*, 2005 198, 361-366.

[127] Izumi, AK. Allergic contact gingivostomatitis due to gold. *Arch Dermatol Res*, 1982 272, 387-391.

[128] Jacobs, R; Serhal, CB; van Steenberge, D. Oral stereognosis: a review of the literature. *Clin Oral Invest*, 1998 2, 3-10.

[129] Jensen, MP; Turner, JA; Romano, JM; Lawler, BK. Relationship of pain-specific beliefs to chronic pain adjustment. *Pain*, 1994 57, 301-309.

[130] Jensen, MP; Turner, JA; Romano, JM; Strom, SE. The chronic pain coping inventory: development and preliminary validation. *Pain*, 1995 60, 203-216.

[131] Jensen, MP; Turner, LR; Turner, JA; Romano, JM. The use of multiple-item scales for pain intensity measurement in chronic pain patients. *Pain*, 1996 67, 35-40.

[132] Kaán, B; Fejérdy, L; Tóth, Zs; Fábián, G; Korchmáros, R; Fábián, TK. Lexicological parameters of free association (coupling) about teeth of Hungarian primary school children. An initial study. *Fogorv Szle*, 2005 98, 239-244.

[133] Kaban, LB. & Belfer, ML. Temporomandibular joint dysfunction: an occasional manifestation of serious psychopathology. *J Oral Surg*, 1981 39, 742-746.

[134] Kahler, W. The cracked tooth conundrum: terminology, classification, diagnosis, and management. *Am J Dent*, 2008 21, 275-282.

[135] Károlyházy, K; Kovács, E; Kivovics, P; Fejérdy, P; Arányi, Z. Dental status and oral health of patients with epilepsy: an epidemiologic study. *Epilepsia*, 2003 44, 1103-1108.

[136] Károlyházy, K; Kivovics, P; Fejérdy, P; Arányi, Z. Prosthodontic status and recommended care of patients with epilepsy. *J Prosthet Dent*, 2005 93, 177-182.

[137] Keefe, FJ; Brown, GK; Wallston, KA; Caldwell, DS. Coping with rheumatoid arthritis pain: catastrophizing as a maladaptive strategy. *Pain*, 1989 37, 51-56.

[138] Kells, BE; Kennedy, JG; Biagioni, PA; Lamey, PJ. Computerized infrared thermographic imaging and pulpal blood flow: Part 1. A protocol for thermal imaging of human teeth. *Int Endod J*, 2000/a 33, 442-447.

[139] Kells, BE; Kennedy, JG; Biagioni, PA; Lamey, PJ. Computerized infrared thermographic imaging and pulpal blood flow: Part 2. Rewarming of healthy human teeth following a controlled cold stimulus. *Int Endod J*, 2000/b 33, 448-462.

[140] Kemppainen, P; Forster, C; Handwerker, HO. The importance of stimulus site and intensity in differences of pain-induced vascular reflexes in human orofacial regions. *Pain*, 2001 91, 331-338.

[141] Kern, M; Kleimeier, B; Schaller, HG; Strub, JR. Clinical comparison of postoperative sensitivity for a glass ionomer and a zinc phosphate luting cement. *J Prosthet Dent*, 1996 75, 159-162.

[142] Kivlighan, KT. & Granger, DA. Salivary α-amylase response to competition: Relation to gender, previous experience, and attitudes. *Psychoneuroendocrinology*, 2006 31, 703-714.

[143] Koeck, B. & Lückerath, W. Instrumentelle Funktionsdiagnostik. In: Koeck B, editor. *Funktionsstörungen des Kauorgans.* München - Wien - Baltimore: Urban & Schwarzenberg; 1995; *115*-149.

[144] Koren, E; Kohen, R., Ginsburg, I. A cobalt-based tetrazolium salts reduction test to assay polyphenols. *J Agric Food Chem*, in press/a. DOI: 10.1021/jf9006449

[145] Koren, E; Kohen, R; Ovadia, H; Ginsburg, I. Bacteria coated by polyphenols acquire potent oxidant-scaveging capacities. *Exp Biol Med*, in press/b. DOI: 10.3181/0901-RM-22

[146] Kossioni AE. & Karzakis, HC. Variation in the masseteric silent period in older dentate humans and in denture wearers. *Arch Oral Biol*, 1995 40, 1143-1150.

[147] Krahwinkel, T; Nastali, S; Azrak, B; Willershausen, B. The effect of examination stress conditions on the cortisol content of saliva - a study of students from clinical semesters. *Eur J Med Res*, 2004 28, 256-260.

[148] Kreyer, G. Psychosomatics of the orofacial system. *Wien Med Wochenschr*, 2000 150, 213-216.

[149] Kromminga, R; Habel, G; Müller-Fahlbusch, H. Failure of dental implants following psychosomatic disturbances in the stomatognathic system - a clinical-catamnestic study. *Dtsch Stomatol*, 1991 41, 233-236.

[150] Kugler, J; Hess, M; Haake, D. Secretion of salivary immunoglobulin A in relation to age, saliva flow, mood states, secretion of albumin, cortisol, and catecholamines in saliva. *J Clin Immunol*, 1992 12, 45-49.

[151] Kumar, SKS; Meru, MC; Sedghizadeh, PP. Osteonecrosis of the jaws secondary to bisphosphonate therapy: A case series. *J Contemp Dent Practice*, 2008 9, 1.

[152] Kurihara, K. & Kashiwayanagi M. Introductory remarks on umami taste. *Ann NY Acad Sci*, 1998 855, 393-397.

[153] Lamey, PJ; Biagioni, PA; AlHashimi, I. The feasibility of using infrared thermography to evaluate minor salivary gland function in euhydrated, dehydrated and rehydrated subjects. *J Oral Pathol Med*, 2007 36, 127-131.

[154] Landt, H. Adaptationsprobleme bei der oralen prothetischen Rehabilitation des alternden Menschen. In: Körber E, editor. *Die zahnärztlich-protetische Versorgung des älternden Menschen*. München, Wien: Carl Hanser Verlag; 1978; 69-92.

[155] Laney, WR. & Gibilisco, JA. History, laboratory data and physical examination. In: Laney WR, Gibilisco JA editors. *Diagnosis and treatment in prosthodontics*. Philadelphia: Lea & Febiger; 1983; 26-72.

[156] Larheim, TA. Role of magnetic resonance imaging in the clinical diagnosis of the temporomandibular joint. *Cells Tissues Organs*, 2005 180, 6-21.

[157] Lavigne, GJ; Rompé, PH; Montplaisir, JY. Sleep bruxism: Validity of clinical research diagnostic criteria in a controlled polysomnographic study. *J Dent Res*, 1996 75, 546-552.

[158] Lee, JG; Kim, SG; Lim, KJ; Choi, KC. Thermographic assessment of inferior alveolar nerve injury in patients with dentofacial deformity. *J Oral Maxillofac Surg*, 2007 65, 74-78.

[159] Lesse, S. Atypical facial pain syndromes of psychogenic origin. Complications of their misdiagnosis. *J Nerv Ment Dis*, 1956 124, 346-351.

[160] Liskmann, S; Vihalemm, T; Salum, O; Zilmer, K; Fischer, K; Zilmer, M. Correlations between clinical parameters and interleukin-6 and interleukin-10 levels in saliva from totally edentulous patients with peri-implant disease. *Int J Oral Maxillofac Implants*, 2006 21, 543-550.

[161] Liskmann, S; Vihalemm, T; Salum, O; Zilmer, K; Fischer, K; Zilmer, M. Characterization of the antioxidant profile of human saliva in peri-implant health and disease. *Clin Oral Impl Res*, 2007 18, 27-33.

[162] Lobbezoo, F. & Naeije, M. Dental implications of some common movement disorders: A concise review. *Arch Oral Biol*, 2007 52, 395-398.

[163] Lowenthal, U. & Tau, S. Effects of ethnic origin, age, and bereavement on complete denture patients. *J Prosthet Dent*, 1980 44, 133-136.

[164] Lupton, DE. Psychological aspects of temporomandibular joint dysfunction. *JADA*, 1969 79, 131-136.

[165] Macfarlane, TV; Blinkhorn, AS; Davies, RM; Worthington, HV. Association between local mechanical factors and orofacial pain: survey in the community. *J Dentistry*, 2003 31, 535-542.

[166] Madléna, M; Hermann, P; Jáhn, M; Fejérdy, P. Caries prevalence and tooth loss in Hungarian adult population: results of a national survey. *BMC Public Health*, 2008 8, 364.

[167] Magnusson, A; Opjordsmoen, S; Dietrichs, E. Drug-induced dystonia misinterpreted as hysteria. *Tidsskr Nor Laegeforen*, 1996 116, 844-845.

[168] Mairgünther, R. & Dielert, E. Temporomandibular joint examination under general anesthesia - a case report. *Dtsch Stomatol*, 1991 41, 393-395.

[169] Márton, K; Hermann, P; Dankó, K; Fejérdy, P; Madléna, M; Nagy, G. Evaluation of oral manifestations and masticatory force in patients with polymyositis and dermatomyositis. *J Oral Pathol Med*, 2005 34, 164-169.

[170] Márton, K; Boros, I; Varga, G; Zelles, T; Fejérdy, P; Zeher, M; Nagy, G. Evaluation of palatal saliva flow rate and oral manifestations in patients with Sjögren's syndrome. *Oral Dis*, 2006 12, 480-486.

[171] Márton, K; Madléna, M; Bánóczy, J; Varga, G; Fejérdy, P; Sreebny, LM; Nagy, G. Unstimulated whole saliva flow rate in relation to sicca symptoms in Hungary. *Oral Dis*, 2008 14, 472-477.

[172] Marxkors, R. & Müller-Fahlbusch, H. Zur Diagnose psychosomatischer Störungen in der zahnärztlich-prothetischen Praxis. *Deutsch Zahnärztl Z*, 1981 36, 787-790.

[173] McGimpsey, JG; Vaidya, A, Biagioni, PA; Lamey, PJ. Role of thermography in the assessment of infraorbital nerve injury after malar fractures. *Brit J Oral Maxillofac Surg*, 2000 38, 581-584.

[174] Michman, J. & Langer, A. Postinsertion changes in complete dentures. *J Prosthet Dent*, 1975 34, 125-134.

[175] Miyachi, H; Wake, H; Tamaki, K; Mitsuhashi, A; Ikeda, T; Inoue, K; Tanaka, S; Tanaka, K; Miyaoka, H. Detecting mental disorders in dental patients with occlusion-related problems. *Psychiatry Clin Neurosci*, 2007 61, 313-319.

[176] Miyamoto, SA. & Ziccardi, VB. Burning mouth syndrome. *Mt Sinai J Med*, 1998 65, 343-347.

[177] Mowad, CM. Patch testing: pitfalls and performance. *Curr Opin Allergy Clin Immunol*, 2006 6, 340-344.

[178] Mozzo, P; Procacci, C; Tacconi, A; Tinazzi Martini, P; Bergamo Andreis, IA. A new volumetric CT machine for dental imaging based on the cone-beam technique: preliminary results. *Eur Radiol*, 1998 8, 1558-1564.

[179] Muhl, ZF; Sadowsky, C; Sakols, EI. Timing of temporomandibular joint sounds in orthodontic patients. *J Dent Res*, 1987 66, 1389-1392.

[180] Munro, RR. Electromyography of the muscles of mastication. In: Griffin CJ, Harris R editors. *The temporomandibular joint syndrome. The masticatory apparatus of man in normal and abnormal function.* (Monographs in oral science, Vol. 4.) Basel - München - Paris - London - New York - Sydney: Karger; 1975/a; 87-116.

[181] Munro, RR. Electromyography of the masseter and anterior temporalis muscles in the open-close-clench cycle in temporomandibular joint dysfunction. In: Griffin CJ, Harris R editors. *The temporomandibular joint syndrome. The masticatory apparatus of man in normal and abnormal function.* (Monographs in oral science, Vol. 4.) Basel - München - Paris - London - New York - Sydney: Karger; 1975/b; 117-125.

[182] Müller, F. & Hasse-Sander, I. Experimental studies of adaptation to complete dentures related to ageing. *Gerodontology*, 1993 10, 23-27.

[183] Müller-Fahlbusch, H. & Sone, K. Präprotetische Psychagogik. *Deutsch Zahnärztl Z*, 1982 37, 703-707.

[184] Myers, A. & Naylor, GD. Glossodynia as an oral manifestation of sex hormone alterations. *Ear Nose Throat J*, 1989 68, 786, 789-790.

[185] Nair, MK. & Nair, UP. Digital and advanced imaging in endodontics: A review. *J Endod*, 2007 33, 1-6.

[186] Nakaminami, T; Omae, T; Akanishi, M; Maruyama, T. Psychosomatic aspects of the patients with stomatognathic dysfunction. 2. *Nihon Hotetsu Shika Gakkai Zasshi*, 1989 33, 395-400.

[187] Nater, UM; Rohlender, N; Gaab, J; Berger, S; Jud, A; Kirschbaum, C; Ehlert, U. Human salivary alpha amylase reactivity in a psychosocial stress paradigm. *Int J Psychophysiol.* 2005 55, 333-342.

[188] Nejtek, VA. High and low emotion events influence emotional stress perceptions and are associated with salivary cortisol response changes in a consecutive stress paradigm. *Psychoneuroendocrinology*, 2002 27, 337- 352.

[189] Niedermeier, W. Physiology and pathophysiology of the minor salivary glands. *Dtsch Z Mund Kiefer Gesichtschir*, 1991 15, 6-15.

[190] Niedermeier, W; Becker, H, Christ, F; Habermann, PG. Effect of menopausal syndromes on symptoms of denture intolerance. *Schweiz Mschr Zahnheilk*, 1979 89, 1011-1018.

[191] Nikolopoulou, F. & Tzortzopoulou E. Salivary pH in edentulous patients before and after wearing conventional dentures and implant overdentures: a clinical study. *Implant Dent*, 2007 16, 397-403.

[192] Novak, N; Haberstok, J; Bieber, T; Allam, JP. The immune privilege of the oral mucosa. *Trends Mol Med*, 2008 14, 191-198.

[193] Ogasawara, T; Kitagawa, Y; Ogawa, T; Yamada, T; Kawamura, Y; Sano, K. MR imaging and thermography of facial angiooedema: A case report. *Oral Surg Oral Med Oral Pathol Oral Radiol Endod*, 2001 92, 473-476.

[194] Oneschuk, D; Hanson, J, Bruera, E. A survey of mouth pain and dryness in patients with advanced cancer. *Support Care Cancer*, 2000 8, 372-376.

[195] Orden, A; Laskin, DM; Lew, D. Chronic preauricular swelling. *J Oral Maxillofac Surg*, 1989 47, 390-397.

[196] Osborne, JW. & Albino, JE. Psychological and medical effects of mercury intake from dental amalgam. A status report for the American Journal of Dentistry. *Am J Dent*, 1999 12, 151-156.

[197] Osman, A; Barrios, FX; Kopper, BA; Hauptmann, W; Jones, J; O'Neill, E. Factor structure, reliability, and validity of the Pain Catastrophizing Scale. *J Behav Med*, 1997 20, 589-605.

[198] Osman, A; Barrios, FX; Gutierrez, P; Kopper, BA; Merrifield, T; Grittmann, L. The Pain Catastrophizing Scale: Further psychometric evaluation with adult samples. *J Behav Med*, 2000 23, 351- 365.

[199] Osman, A; Barrios, FX; Gutierrez, PM; Kopper, BA; Butler, A; Bagge, CL. The Pain Distress Inventory: development and initial psychometric properties. *J Clin Psychol*, 2003 59, 767-785.

[200] Osman, A; Barrios, FX; Gutierrez, PM. Reliability and construct validity of the pain distress inventory. *J Behav Med*, 2005 28, 169-180.

[201] Ouellette, PL. TMJ sound prints: electronic auscultation and sonographic audiospectral analysis of the temporomandibular joint. *JADA*, 1974 89, 623-628.

[202] Öhrn, R; Enzell, K, Angmar-Månsson, B. Oral status of 81 subjects with eating disorders. *Eur J Oral Sci*, 1999 107, 157-163.

[203] Palla, S; Gallo, LM; Gössi, D. Dynamic stereometry of the temporomandibular joint. *Orthod Craniofac Res*, 2003 6 (suppl.1), 37-47.

[204] Park, MS; Chung, JW; Kim, YK; Chung, SC; Kho, HS. Viscosity and wettability of animal mucin solutions and human saliva. *Oral Diseases*, 2007 13, 181-186.

[205] Parks, ET. Digital radiographic imaging. Is the dental practice ready? *JADA*, 2008 139, 477-481.

[206] Pertes, RA. Differential diagnosis of orofacial pain. *Mt Sinai J Med*, 1998 65, 348-354.

[207] Pfeiffer, P. & Schwickerath, H. Nickel solubility and metallic taste. *ZWR*, 1991 100, 762-770.

[208] Pilling, LF. Psychiatric aspects of diagnosis and treatment. In: Laney WR, Gibilisco JA editors. *Diagnosis and treatment in prosthodontics*. Philadelphia: Lea & Febiger; 1983; 129-140.

[209] Pluvinage, RJ. Headaches, migraine and oral contraception. *Contracept Fertil Sex (Paris)*, 1977 5, 113-117.

[210] Pomp, AM. Psychotherapy for the myofascial pain-dysfunction syndrome: a study of factors coinciding with symptom remission. *JADA*, 1974 89, 629-632.

[211] Porgel, MA; Yen, CK; Taylor, RC. Studies in tooth crown temperature gradients with the use of infrared thermography. *Oral Surg Oral Med Oral Pathol*, 1989 67, 583-587.

[212] Ramírez, LM; Ballesteros, LE; Sandoval, GP. Hamular bursitis and its possible craniofacial referred symptomatology: Two case reports. *Med Oral Patol Oral Cir Bucal*, 2006 11, E329-333.

[213] Reynolds, F. Relationships between catastrophic thoughts, perceived control and distress during menopausal hot flushes: exploring the correlates of a questionnaire measure. *Maturitas*, 2000 36, 113-122.

[214] Rolls, ET; Critchley, HD; Browning, A; Hernadi, I. The neurophysiology of taste and olfaction in primates, and umami flavor. *Ann NY Acad Sci*, 1998 855, 426-437.

[215] Rosentiel, AK. & Keefe, FJ. The use of coping strategies in chronic low back pain patients: relationship to patient characteristics and current adjustment. *Pain*, 1983 17, 33-44.

[216] Ross, GL; Bentley, HJ; Greene Jr., GW. The psychosomatic concept in dentistry. *Psychosom Med*, 1953 15, 168-173.

[217] Rother, UJ. *Moderne bildgebende Diagnostic in der Zahn-, Mund-, und Kieferheilkunde*. München: Urban & Fisher; 2001; 171,

[218] Sadowsky, C; Muhl, ZF; Sakols, EI; Sommerville, JM. Temporomandibular joint sounds related to orthodontic therapy. *J Dent Res*, 1985 64, 1392-1395.

[219] Salé, H. & Isberg, A. Delayed temporomandibular joint pain and dysfunction induced whiplash trauma. A controlled prospective study. *JADA*, 2007 138, 1084-1091.

[220] Sandler, NA; Ziccardi, V; Ochs, M. Differential diagnosis of jaw pain in the elderly. *JADA*, 1995 126, 1263-1272.

[221] Sarlani, E; Balciunas, BA; Grace, EG. Orofacial pain - Part I. Assessment and management of musculoskeletal and neuropathic causes. *AACN Clin Issues*, 2005/a 16, 333-346.

[222] Sarlani, E; Balciunas, BA; Grace, EG. Orofacial pain - Part II. Assessment and management of vascular, neurovascular, idiopathic, secondary, and psychogenic causes. *AACN Clin Issues*, 2005/b 16, 347-358.

[223] Satoh, T. Clinical and fundamental investigations on recurrent glossodynia. *Nippon Ishinkin Gakkai Zasshi*, 2004 45, 233-237.

[224] Scala, A; Checchi, L; Montevecchi, M; Marini, I. Giamberardino, MA. Update on burning mouth syndrome: overview and patient management. *Crit Rev Oral Biol Med*, 2003 14, 275-291.

[225] Scardina, GA; Mazzulo, M; Messina, P. Early diagnosis of progressive systemic sclerosis: the role of orofacial phenomena. *Minerva Stomatol*, 2002 51, 311-317.

[226] Scarfe, WC; Farman, AG; Sukovic, P. Clinical applications of cone-beam computed tomography in dental practice. *JCDA*, 2006 72, 75-80.

[227] Schmalz, G. & Garhammer, P. Biological interactions of dental cast alloys with oral tissues. *Dent Mater*, 2002 18, 396-406.

[228] Schmalz, G; Langer, H; Schweikl, H. Cytotoxicity of dental alloy extracts and corresponding metal salt solution. *J Dent Res*, 1998 77, 1772-1778.

[229] Schwartz, LL. Pain associated with the temporomandibular joint. *JADA*, 1955 51, 394-397.

[230] Schwartz, E. & Granger, DA. Transferrin enzyme immunoassay for quantitative monitoring of blood contamination in saliva. *Clinical Chemistry*, 2004 50, 654-656.

[231] Shankland 2nd, WE. Pterygoid hamulus bursitis: One cause of craniofacial pain. *J Prosthet Dent*, 1996/a 75, 205-210.

[232] Shankland 2nd, WE. Bursitis of the hamular process. Part II: Diagnosis, treatment and report of three case studies. *Cranio*, 1996/b 14, 306-311.

[233] Silva, MAG; Wolf, U; Heincke, F; Bumann, A; Visser, H; Hirsch, E. Cone-beam computed tomography for routine orthodontic treatment planning: A radiation dose evaluation. *Am J Orthod Dentofac Orthop*, 2008 133, 640.e1-640.e5.

[234] Silverman, SI. *Oral physiology*. St Louis: Mosby; 1961; 362.

[235] Silverman, S; Silverman, SI; Silverman, B; Garfinkel, L. Self-image and its relation to denture acceptance. *J Prosthet Dent*, 1976 35, 131-141.

[236] Slade, GD. Derivation and validation of a short form oral health impact profile. *Comm Dent Oral Epidemiol*, 1997 25, 284-290.

[237] Slade, GD. & Spencer, AJ. Development and evaluation of the Oral Health Impact Profile. *Community Dent Health*, 1994 11, 3-11.

[238] Smith, PW. & McCord, JF. Oral stereognostic ability in edentulous and dentate individuals. *Eur J Prosthodont Restor Dent*, 2002 10, 53-56.

[239] Spiechowicz, E; Glantz, PO; Axell, T; Grochowski, P. A long-term follow-up of allergy to nickel among fixed prostheses wearers. *Eur J Prosthodont Restor Dent*, 1999 7, 41-44.

[240] Spielberger, CD; Gorsuch, RL; Lushene, RE. *Manual for the State-Trait Anxiety Inventory*. Palo Alto, CA: Consulting Psychologist Press; 1970.

[241] Srinivasan, D; Shetty, S; Ashworth, D; Gew, N; Millar, B. Orofacial pain - a presenting symptom of bisphosphonate associated osteonecrosis of the jaws. *Brit Dent J*, 2007 203, 91-92.

[242] Stokes, JR. & Davies, GA. Viscoelasticity of human whole saliva collected after acid and mechanical stimulation. *Biorheology*, 2007 44, 141-160.

[243] Storrs, FJ. Technical and ethical problems associated with patch testing. *Clin Rev Allergy Immunol*, 1996 14, 185-198.

[244] Strong, J; Ashton, R; Chant, D. The measurement of attitudes towards and beliefs about pain. *Pain*, 1992 48, 227-236.

[245] Suganuma, T; Ono, Y; Shinya, A; Furuya, R. The effect of bruxism on periodontal sensation in the molar region: A pilot study. *J Prosthet Dent*, 2007 98, 30-35.

[246] Sullivan, MJL; Bishop, SR; Pivik, J. The pain catastrophizing scale: development and validation. *Psychol Assess*, 1995 7, 524-532.

[247] Sullivan, MJL; Stanish, W; Waite, H; Sullivan, M; Tripp, DA. Catastrophizing, pain, and disability in patients with soft-tissue injuries. *Pain*, 1998 77, 253-260.

[248] Sullivan, MJL; Lynch, ME; Clark, AJ. Dimensions of catastrophic thinking associated with pain experience and disability in patients with neuropathic pain conditions. *Pain*, 2005 113, 310-315.

[249] Sutow, EJ; Maillet, WA; Taylor, JC; Hall, GC. In vivo galvanic currents of intermittently contacting dental amalgam and other metallic restorations. *Dental Materials*, 2004 20, 823-831.

[250] Sutow, EJ; Maillet, WA; Hall, GC. Corrosion potential variation of aged dental amalgam restorations over time. *Dental Materials*, 2006 22, 325-329.

[251] Sutow, EJ; Maillet, JP; Maillet, WA; Hall, GC; Millar, M. Corrosion potential recovery of dental amalgam restorations following prophylaxis. *Dental Materials*, 2007/a 23, 840-843.

[252] Sutow, EJ; Maillet, WA; Taylor, JC; Hall, GC; Millar, M. Time-dependent corrosion potential of newly-placed admixed dental amalgam restorations. *Dental Materials*, 2007/b 23, 644-647.

[253] Sutow, EJ; Taylor, JC; Maillet, WA; Hall, GC; Millar, M. Existence of an electrically insulating layer in amalgam-containing galvanic couples. *Dental Materials*, 2008 24, 874-879.

[254] Swartzman, LC; Gwadry, FG; Shapiro, AP; Teasell, RW. The factor structure of the Coping Strategies Questionnaire. *Pain*, 1994 57, 311-316.

[255] Taillandier, J; Esnault, Y; Alemanni, M. A comparison of fluconazole oral suspension and amphotericin B oral suspension in older patients with oropharingeal candidosis. Multicentre Study Group. *Age Aging*, 2000 29, 117-123.

[256] Tallgren, A; McCall Jr., WD; Mansour, NN; Ash Jr., MM. Follow-up study of silent periods in complete denture wearers. *J Oral Rehabil*, 1987 14, 345-353.

[257] Terajima, M; Endo, M; Aoki, Y; Yuuda, K; Hayasaki, H; Goto, TK; Tokumori, K; Nakasima, A. Four-dimensional analysis of stomatognathic function. *Am J Orthod Dentofacial Orthop*, 2008 134, 276-287.

[258] Tesserioli de Siqueria, SRD; Nóbrega, JCM; Valle, LBS; Teixeira, MJ; Tesserioli de Siqueria, JT. Idiopathic trigeminal neuralgia: Clinical aspects and dental procedures. *Oral Surg Oral Med Oral Pathol Oral Radiol Endod*, 2004 98, 311-315.

[259] Tickle, M; Craven, R; Worthington, HV. A comparison of the subjective oral health status of older adults from deprived and affluent communities. *Community Dent Oral Epidemiol*, 1997 25, 217-222.

[260] Tóth, Zs; Fejérdy, L; Fábián, Cs; Kaán, B; Müller, O; Fábián, TK. Initial analysis of tooth drawings of 8-18 years old schoolchildren from normal population. *Fogorv Szle*, 2006 99, 47-52.

[261] Touger-Decker, R. Oral manifestations of nutrient deficiencies. *Mt Sinai J Med*, 1998 65, 355-361.

[262] Tredwin, CJ; Scully, C; Bagan-Sebastian, JV. Drug-induced disorders of teeth. *J Dent Res*, 2005 84, 596-602.

[263] Turker, SB; Sener, ID; Özkan, YK. Satisfaction of the complete denture wearers related to various factors. *Arch Gerontol Geriatr*, 2009 49, e126-e129.

[264] Turner, JA; Mancl, L; Aaron, LA. Short- and long-term efficacy of brief cognitive-behavioral therapy for patients with chronic temporomandibular disorder pain: A randomized controlled trial. *Pain*, 2006 121, 181-194.

[265] Turner, M; Jahangiri, L; Ship, JA. Hyposalivation, xerostomia and the complete denture. A systematic review. *JADA*, 2008 139, 146-150.

[266] Türp, JC; Hugger, A; Löst, C; Nilges, P; Schindler, HJ; Staehle, HJ. Vorschlag einer Klassifikation der Odontalgien. *Schmerz*, 2009 23, 448-460.

[267] Vamnes, JS; Lygre, GB; Grönningsæter, AG, Gjerdet, NR. Four years of clinical experience with an adverse reaction unit for dental biomaterials. *Community Dent Oral Epidemiol*, 2004 32, 150-157.

[268] van der Glas, HW; de Laat, A; van Steenberghe, D. Oral pressure mediate a series of inhibitory and excitatory periods in the masseteric poststimulus EMG complex following tapping of a tooth in man. *Brain Res*, 1985 337, 117-125.

[269] van der Glas, HW; de Laat, A; Carels, C; van Steenberghe, D. Interactive periodontal and acoustic influences on the masseteric post-stimulus electromyographic complex in man. *Brain Res*, 1988 444, 284-294.

[270] Ventä, I; Hyrkäs, T; Paakkari, I; Ylipaavalniemi, P. Thermographic imaging of postoperative inflammation modified by anti-inflammatory pretreatment. *J Oral Maxillofac Surg*, 2001 59, 145-150.

[271] Vervoorn, JM; Duinkerke, ASH; Luteijn, F; Van de Poel, ACM. Assessment of denture satisfaction. *Community Dent Oral Epidemiol*, 1988 16, 364-367.

[272] Vitkov, L; Weitgasser, R; Lungstein, A; Noack, MJ; Fuchs, K; Krautgartner, WD. Glycaemic disorders in denture stomatitis. *J Oral Pathol Med*, 1999 28, 406-409.

[273] Wartenberg, M; Wirtz, N; Grob, A; Niedermeier, W; Hescheler, J. Direct current electrical fields induce apoptosis in oral mucosa cancer cells by NADPH Oxidase-Derived reactive oxygen species. *Bioelectromagnetics*, 2008 29, 47-54.

[274] Watanabe, T; Kobayashi, K; Suzuki, T; Oizumi, M; Clark, GT. A preliminary report on continuous recording of salivary pH using telemetry in an edentulous patient. *Int J Prosthodont*, 1999 12, 313-317.

[275] Watt, DM. Clinical application of gnathosonics. *J Prosthet Dent*, 1966/a 16, 83-95.

[276] Watt, DM. Gnathosonics - A study of sounds produced by the masticatory mechanism. *J Prosthet Dent*, 1966/b 16, 73-82.

[277] Wertheimer-Hatch, L; Hatch (III), GF; Hatch, KF; Davis, GB; Blanchard, DK; Foster Jr., RS; Skandalakis, JE. Tumors of the oral cavity and pharinx. *World J Surg*, 2000 24, 395-400.

[278] White, SC. & Pharoah, MJ. The evolution and application of dental maxillofacial imaging modalities. *Dent Clin North Am*, 2008 52, 689-705.

[279] Wiens, JP; Milliner, EK; Maruta, T; Gibilisco, JA. Management of craniofacial pain. In: Laney WR, Gibilisco JA editors. *Diagnosis and treatment in prosthodontics.* Philadelphia: Lea & Febiger; 1983; 141-156.

[280] Wirz, J; Jäger, K; Schmidli, F. Klinische Korrosion. *Schweiz Monatschr Zahnmed*, 1987 97, 1151-1156.

[281] Wirz, J; Schmidli, F; Petrini, MG. Metal intolerance. A frequent condition, but difficult to diagnose. *Schweiz Monatschr Zahnmed*, 2003 113, 284-295.

[282] Woda, A. & Pionchon, P. A unified concept of idiopathic orofacial pain: pathophysiologic features. *J Orofac Pain*, 2000 14, 196-212.

[283] Woda, A. & Pionchon, P. Orofacial idiopathic pain: clinical signs, causes and mechanisms. *Rev Neurol Paris*, 2001 157, 265-283.

[284] Wolowski, A. Symptoms six months before the appearance of a malignant or psychosomatic illness. *J Facial Somato Prosthetics*, 1995, 23-28.

[285] Wong, JK; Wood, RE; McLean, M. Pain preceding recurrent head and neck cancer. *J Orofac Pain*, 1998 12, 52-59.

[286] Wöstmann, B. Psychogene Zahnersatzunverträglichkeit. In: Sergl HG, editor. *Psychologie und Psychosomatik in der Zahnheilkunde*. München - Wien - Baltimore: Urban & Schwarzenberg; 1996; 187-213.

[287] Yamaguchi, S. Fundamental properties of umami in human taste sensation. In: Kawamura Y, Kare MR editors. *Umami: A basic taste*. New York: Marcel Dekker; 1987; 41-73.

[288] Yamakawa, M; Ansai, T; Kasai, S; Ohmaru, T; Takeuchi, H; Kawaguchi, T; Takehara, T. Dentition status and temporomandibular joint disorders in patients with rheumatoid arthritis. *Cranio*, 2002 20, 165-171.

[289] Yassutaka Faria Yaedú, R; Regina Fisher Rubira-Bullen, I; Sant'Ana E. Spontaneous fracture of genial tubercles: case report. *Quintessence Int*, 2006 37, 737-739.

[290] Yontchev, EA; Studies of individuals with orofacial discomfort complaints. An investigation of a group of patients who related their sufferings to effects of dental materials and constructions. *Swed Dent J Suppl*, 1986 38, 1-45.

[291] Yontchev, E; Hedegård, B; Carlsson, GE. Reported symptoms, diseases, and medication of patients with orofacial discomfort complaints. *Int J Oral Maxillofac Surg*, 1986 15, 687-695.

[292] Yontchev, E; Hedegård, B; Carlsson, GE. Outcome of treatment of patients with orofacial discomfort complaints. *Int J Oral Maxillofac Surg*, 1987 16, 312-318.

[293] Zhang, ZK; Ma, XC; Gao, S; Gu, ZY; Fu, KY. Studies on contributing factors in temporomandibular disorders. *Chin J Dent Res*, 1999 2, 7-20.

[294] Zoellner, A; Herzberg, S; Gaengler, P. Histobacteriology and pulp reactions to long-term dental restorations. *J Marmara Univ Dent Fac*, 1996 2, 483-490.

[295] Zumkley, H. The patient's intolerance of dentures from the internal medicine viewpoint. *Dtsch Zahnärztl Z*, 1976 31, 8-9.

[296] Zusmann, E; Yarin, AL; Nagler, RM. Age- and flow-dependency of salivary viscoelasticity. *J Dent Res*, 2007 86, 281-285.

Chapter 5

PREVENTION OF PSYCHOGENIC DENTURE INTOLERANCE

ABSTRACT

Prevention is likely to be the most important tool for the management of psychogenic denture intolerance related problems at a social level; therefore, prevention of PDI is clearly a scope of *every* dentist's duties. Besides high quality preparative dental skills and technical background, cornerstones of prevention are screening of risk patients, proper treatment planning, proper communication with the patient, screening of the patient-nurse-dentist interrelationships, as well as prevention of dental fear, prevention of treatment-induced pain and prevention of relapse. It is also crucial for the prevention that patients must be made aware of their responsibilities in achieving a satisfactory outcome. It is also a matter of considerable significance that the clinician carefully weighs the option of nontreatment in certain cases. Dental team members should also be able to accept a patient from the bottom of hart as well as to understand and accept own emotions for a proper and successful treatment and for the avoidance of treatment failure. Therefore, *dentists and other team members should become a mature, well-disposed and good person on behalf of the patients as well as on behalf of their own interest.* Maintenance of the mental health of dental team is also crucial for the prevention of PDI. Lack of attention to all above aspects may invite treatment failure and may lead to the occurrence of PDI.

5.1. INTRODUCTION

Prevention is likely to be the most important tool for the management of psychogenic denture intolerance related problems at a social level; therefore, prevention of PDI is clearly a scope of *every* dentist's duties. Besides high quality preparative dental skills and technical background, cornerstones of prevention are screening of risk patients, proper treatment planning, proper communication with the patient, screening of the patient-nurse-dentist interrelationships [*Fábián & Fábián 2000/a, Fejérdy & Orosz 2007*], as well as prevention of dental fear, prevention of treatment induced pain and prevention of relapse [*Fábián & Fábián 2000/a, Fábián et al. 2007*]. Maintenance of the mental health of dental team is also crucial for the prevention of PDI [*Fejérdy et al. 2004*]. The most important knowledge in relation with premised fundamental parts of prevention will be introduced in details below.

5.2. SCREENING OF RISK PATIENTS

Screening of risk patient is primarily based on the collection of a detailed patient's history (see *paragraph 4.2.1.*) as well as on careful evaluation of medical- psychosocial and orofacial status (see *paragraphs 4.2.2., 4.2.3.*). Dissatisfaction with the existing denture may also indicate a risk of PDI [*Levin & Landesman 1976, Kawai et al. in press*]. Semi-structured interview [*Levin & Landesman 1976, Kaban & Belfer 1981*], as well as certain psychological and pathopsychological questionnaires (see *paragraph 4.2.11.*) may also be used for screening purposes efficiently. Patients with *high dental fear* and with *previous disturbances of patient-dentist relationship* may also be considered as risk patients, because dental fear and disturbances of patient-dentist relationship may lead to significant psychological stress that may turn into PDI symptoms. Accordingly, patients with high level of perceived stress may also be considered as risk patients.

Although some patients may deny suffering from dental fear but express it behaviorally [*Fox et al. 1989*]; in most cases patients with increased dental fear could be recognized using the *Dental Anxiety Scale* (DAS) [*Corah 1969*], the *Dental Fear Survey* (DFS) [*Kleinknecht et al. 1973, 1984*] or the single-item *Dental Anxiety Question* (DAQ) [*Neverlien 1990*]. Risk patients in relation with dental fear may also be recognized using the "*Expectation Scale*" [*Fábián et al. 2003, 2007*]. Fear of pain may be measured using the *Short form of Fear of Pain Questionnaire* (FPQ-SF) measuring four factors such as fear of severe-, minor-, injection- and dental-pain [*Asmundson et al. 2008*]. Previous disturbances of the patient-dentist relationship may be recognized using the *Getz's Dental Beliefs Survey* (DBS) [*Milgrom et al. 1985*]. Exposure to stressful life events during the preceding period may be measured using the *Social Readjustment Rating Scale* (SRRS) [*Holmes & Rahe 1967*]. Similarly, patients' perception of stress may be measured using the *Perceived Stress Scale* (PSS) [*Cohen et al. 1983*]. Shortest form (*Form C*) of *Cattell's 16 PF questionnaire* may also be used to predict the appearance of PDI [*Cattell et al. 1970, Reeve et al. 1984*] (See also *paragraph 4.2.11.* for another psychological screening tools.)

5.3. PROPER TREATMENT PLANING

Lack of attention to all facets of treatment planning may invite treatment failure; therefore, assessment of both *mental* (psychosocial) as well as *physical* (biomedical) conditions should be evaluated carefully [*Laney 1983, Bensing 2000, Green & Laskin 2000*]. Therefore, patient's *subjective* need as well as the *normatively determined* need for replacement of missing teeth should be evaluated carefully before any prosthodontic treatment [*Elias & Sheiham 1998, Heft et al. 2003, Mazurat & Mazurat 2003, Graham et al. 2006*]. Importantly, the success of a prosthetic treatment strongly depends on the patients' perception of the value of such replacement [*Mazurat & Mazurat 2003*]. It should be also considered that, patients are rather focused on social meaning of the mouth than to physical function of the teeth when defining subjective need for replacement of missing teeth [*Graham et al. 2006*]. Although occlusion of a complete dental arch is preferable *normatively* in most cases, many people are really satisfied with less than 28 natural (± wisdom) teeth [*Rosenoer & Sheiham 1995, Elias & Sheiham 1998, Jones et al. 2003, Ekanayake & Perera 2005, Cunha-Cruz et al. 2007*]. In fact, there is a discrepancy between the normative need and perceived need even for complete denture services in edentulous [*Allen & McMillan 2003*]. Therefore, prompt replacement of absent teeth *without a subjective need* of patients may lead to an overtreatment and discomfort [*Witter et al. 1994, 1999, Mazurat & Mazurat 2003*] especially when RPDs are used because of financial (or other) reasons [*Witter et al. 1994, 1999, Mazurat & Mazurat 2003, Bae et al. 2006*].

It should be also considered that aesthetics seems to be more important than other functions for a great majority of individuals [*Elias & Sheiham 1998, Shor et al. 2005, Zlatarić & Celebić 2008*]; therefore there can be a lack of *subjective* need for replacement of missing posterior (particularly molar) teeth [*Witter et al. 1994, Elias & Sheiham 1998, Mazurat & Mazurat 2003*] especially if only a few teeth are absent [*Zitzmann et al. 2007*]. Although there is a slightly more satisfaction with more than four functional occluding pairs (supporting units, occlusal units) of molars and/or premolars [*Rosenoer & Sheiham 1995*] and perceived oral health rating gradually worsen with increase of number of missing posterior teeth [*Cunha-Cruz et al. 2007*]; patients are usually more concerned about missing anterior teeth and having anterior rather than posterior teeth replaced [*Elias & Sheiham 1998, Mazurat & Mazurat 2003*]. Consequently, there is a relatively large number of those patients not wearing their free end RPDs replacing absent molars [*Elias & Sheiham 1998, Witter et al. 1994, 1999, Mazurat & Mazurat 2003*]. On the other hand, patients with *less* than 20 teeth present (consequently at least one but may be more anterior or premolar teeth are also missing) are significantly more dissatisfied with their appearance than those with complete dentures [*Lester et al. 1998*]; which clearly indicate the subjective need for dentures in this group (even if only RPDs can be managed financially).

Although aesthetics seems to be more important than other functions for a great majority of individuals [*Elias & Sheiham 1998, Shor et al. 2005, Zlatarić & Celebić 2008*], expectations and wishes of patient related to *chewing* [*Mazurat & Mazurat 2003, Szentpétery et al. 2005, Zlatarić & Celebić 2008, Roumanas 2009*] must also not be underestimated [*Fábián & Fábián 2000/a, Mazurat & Mazurat 2003, Fábián et al. 2007, Zlatarić & Celebić 2008*]. Although chewing ability can be acceptable for patients functioning from second premolar to second premolar (i.e. when all molars missing) [*Mazurat & Mazurat 2003*]; more advanced loss of teeth may induce strong difficulties of chewing. In such cases improvement of *mastication* may be a highly important wish of patients certainly [*Mazurat & Mazurat 2003*]. Patients' expectations related to *speech* may also influence satisfaction with dentures strongly [*Zlatarić & Celebić 2008, Roumanas 2009*]. Similarly, numerous other expectations and wishes of patients related to the denture and/or dental treatment may also appear [*Levin & Landesman 1976, Fábián & Fábián 2000/a, Fábián et al. 2007, Roumanas 2009*]. Importantly, executable and acceptable wishes and expectations of patient should be fulfilled [*Fábián & Fábián 2000/a, Mazurat & Mazurat 2003, Fábián et al. 2007*]. If inexecutable and/or unacceptable wishes and expectations also appear, the clinician should carefully weigh the option of nontreatment [*Levin & Landesman 1976, Stein 1983, Fábián & Fábián 2000/a, Fábián et al. 2007*].

Besides premised subjective need and *conscious wishes* [*Fábián & Fábián 2000/a, Smith & McCord 2004, Fábián et al. 2007*] related to denture function, *unconscious* wishes of patients related to both dental treatment and denture (as well as to dentist) should also be considered [*Fábián & Fábián 2000/a, Fábián et al. 2007, Fejérdy & Orosz 2007*]. In contrast to conscious wishes, understanding unconscious wishes (e.g. to look younger, to stop the appearance of aging, to be loved by the dentist etc.) may be more challenging but is similarly important for preventing the manifestation of PDI symptoms [*Fábián & Fábián 2000/a, Fábián et al. 2007, Fejérdy & Orosz 2007*]. It may occur that, the patient's conscious and/or unconscious wishes related to the dental treatment and/or dentures and/or dentist may not harmonize with the reality and possibilities of a prosthetic treatment. It is a matter of considerable significance that the clinician carefully weighs the option of nontreatment in such cases [*Stein 1983, Fábián & Fábián 2000/a, Fábián et al. 2007, Fejérdy & Orosz 2007*].

It should be also considered that, fixed dentures are usually preferable to a removable one for most patient [*Szentpétery et al. 2005*]. Therefore *properly planned* fixed dentures supported either by natural abutment teeth or by *properly inserted* [*Bartling et al. 1999*] dental implants may decrease the risk of triggering psychogenic symptoms (comparing to the estimated risk of similar cases treated with *RPDs*). However, *financial means* [*Ringland et al. 2004, Roumanas 2009*] and *compliance* of the patient as well as the amount of *stress* and possible *complications* induced by preparation of teeth [*Cronström et al. 1998, Goodacre et al. 2003/a*] and/or implant-surgical interventions [*Kaptein et al. 1998, Bartling et al. 1999, Walton 2000, Goodacre et al. 2003/b*] should also be considered very carefully. Because of the high success rate of endosseus dental implants [*Nedir et al. 2004, Comfort et al. 2005, Goené et al. 2005, Schwartz-Arad et al. 2007*], *strategic extraction* of *compromised* tooth/teeth and their replacement with implant supported fixed dentures should be considered [*Barone et al. 2006, Schwartz-Arad et al. 2007, Kao 2008*], especially because compromised teeth may significantly worsen the perceived oral health [*Cunha-Cruz et al. 2007*].

Fixed dentures are especially preferable in instances in which a space created by the loss of a single tooth or perhaps two adjacent teeth is bounded by clinically adequate abutments [*Laney 1983*]. Besides bridges, use of implant supported single crown(s) may also be a proper solution in such cases [*Nedir et al. 2004, Schwartz-Arad et al. 2007, Kao 2008*]. If the edentulous areas are longer, multiple abutments are usually necessary to support fixed restorations [*Laney 1983*]; however, the increased length of the span may invite symptoms in sensitive patients. Implant supported fixed prostheses may also be a proper solution also in such cases [*Goené et al. 2005, Schwartz-Arad et al. 2007, Kao 2008*]. It should be also considered that, the farther the pontics deviate from the straight line through the abutments, the longer is the operative lever arm that may also invite problems due to tipping forces [*Laney 1983*, see also *Appendix*]. In cases of increased estimated tipping forces, either insertion of implants or orthodontic movement of the abutment tooth/teeth or use of an RPD may be preferable. In the absence of sufficient number (and/or quality) of abutment teeth (and/or implants) RPDs should be used. Combinations of RPDs and fixed dentures may also be used advantageously in such cases. In cases with only a *few remaining teeth* (and/or implants), RPDs may be used. In such cases, especially *rotary movements* (especially *two-*

directional rotary movements around intermediary abutment tooth interrupting long edentulous areas) may be difficult to control [*Laney 1983*]. (For few more details about treatment planning of partial dentures, see also *Appendix*)

Use of oral implants should also be considered for treatment planning of *edentulous patients*. Use of oral implants as a support/retainer of complete dentures significantly improve oral health related quality of life [*Kaptein et al. 1998, Heydecke et al. 2003, Doundoulakis et al. 2003, Stellingsma et al. 2003*] as well as functional status of the masticatory system [*Lundqvist 1993, Bergendal & Magnusson 2000, Doundoulakis et al. 2003*] including function of the temporomandibular joint [*Bergendal & Magnusson 2000*], biting force [*Lundqvist 1993, Fontijn-Tekamp et al. 1998, 2000*], chewing ability [*Lundqvist 1993, Kaptein et al. 1998, Bergendal & Magnusson 2000, Doundoulakis et al. 2003*] and speech function [*Lundqvist 1993, Kaptein et al. 1998*] of edentulous patients. Similarly, use of implant supported/retained prostheses (instead of full dentures) also improve joint- muscle- mucosal- and cutaneous mechanoreceptor based [*Klineberg & Murray 1999, Jacobs & Van Steenberghe 2006*] psychophysiological discriminatory ability [*Klineberg & Murray 1999, Jacobs & Van Steenberghe 2006*], as well as oral stereognostic ability [*Lundqvist 1993, Klineberg & Murray 1999, Jacobs & Van Steenberghe 2006*] and oral motor ability [*Lundqvist 1993*] of *edentulous* patients. Osseoperception of edentulous arch may also be improved significantly with dental implants [*Lundqvist 1993, Jacobs & Van Steenberghe 2006, Batista et al. 2008*] due to a significant change of bone related somatosensory inputs to the brain and neuroplasticity based compensatory changes of several sensory and motor brain areas [*Yan et al. 2008*].

Although mean tactile threshold of implant supported/retained *overdentures* are still less comparing to the natural dentition [*Trulsson 2006, Batista et al. 2008*]; tactile threshold of implant supported *fixed prostheses* occluding with either implant supported fixed prostheses or natural dentition is comparable to (statistically not different from) that of natural dentition [*Batista et al. 2008*]. (Notwithstanding that, the highly sensitive sensory-motor function of human periodontal mechanoreceptors [*Jacobs & Van Steenberghe 2006, Trulsson 2006*] are lost.) Besides improving masticatory and sensory functions, implant supported *fixed* dentures [*De Bruyn et al. 2008*] significantly improve self-esteem and self-image of edentulous patients as well [*Trulsson et al. 2002*]; leading to a self-image may be labeled as "becoming the person I once was" [*Trulsson et al. 2002*]. Based on the numerous advantages mentioned above it is likely that, *properly planned* insertion [*Bartling et al. 1999*] and use of dental implants may prevent triggering numerous psychosomatic symptoms in many *edentulous* patients. However, financial means [*Roumanas 2009*] and compliance of the patient as well as the amount of stress induced by the implant-surgical intervention [*Walton & MacEntee 2005*] including post surgical pain [*Kaptein et al. 1998, Stellingsma et al. 2003, Cannizzaro et al. 2007*] and other symptoms (even if they are mostly transient [*Bartling et al. 1999, Walton 2000, Cannizzaro et al. 2007*]) should also be considered carefully before implant treatment. Implant treatment seems to be especially reasonable for edentulous patients with persistent functional problems due to severely resorbed mandible [*Fueki et al. 2007*], with poor chewing ability [*Walton & MacEntee 2005*] and with poor speech ability [*Walton & MacEntee 2005*] as well as for patients discarding of a mandibular (or rarely maxillary) denture [*Kotkin et al. 1998*] and/or having pain complaints related to dentures [*Kotkin et al. 1998, Walton &*

MacEntee 2005]. (But only in the absence of psychological causes behind premised symptoms.)

Besides above, there are some other aspects of prosthodontic treatment that should also be considered for proper treatment planning. Possibilities to *correct patients' existing malocclusion* (if any) should be considered before prosthodontic treatment. Occlusal early contacts [*Biondi & Picardi 1993, Learreta et al. 2007*], alterations of horizontal maxillomandibular relationship [*Biondi & Picardi 1993*] and improper vertical dimension [*Piquero et al. 1999*] should be corrected with the new denture(s). Possibilities to *decrease the risk of an inflammatory response* in the pulp following tooth preparation should also be considered; and time need of careful preparation technique, making well fitting provisional crowns/bridges, applying chemical defense of the stump, and proper methodology for the cementation of both provisorical and permanent restorations [Kern et al. 1996, Brännström 1996] should also be taken into account. Time need of *proper shaping of occlusal contacts* for both provisional and permanent dentures (avoiding the "prophylactic" removal of occlusal contacts as a "pain preventive measure" [Creech et al. 1984]) as well as time need of *accurate precise shaping of marginal closure and gingival site* for both provisorical and permanent dentures should also be considered for planning.

Importantly, planning of a *time-schedule ensuring enough time* to carry out a high quality, precise, "*lege artis*" dental treatment is one of the most important point to prevent triggering psychogenic symptoms. Timing of the start of prosthetic treatment and the insertion of dentures may also be of particular importance [*Müller-Fahlbusch & Sone 1982*], because heavy psychosocial and/or psychoemotional stress condition as well as the active phases of psychiatric disorders significantly increase the risk of PDI [*Müller-Fahlbusch & Sohne 1982*]. Therefore, starting of prosthetic treatment or insertion of dentures under any heavy psychological stress conditions and/or active phases of psychiatric disorders should be avoided [*Müller-Fahlbusch & Sone 1982*]; and the prosthetic treatment or insertion of denture should be delayed [*Müller-Fahlbusch & Sone 1982*].

5.4. COMMUNICATION WITH THE PATIENT

Communication with patient is a key factor of the prevention of PDI [*Pomp 1974, Müller-Fahlbusch & Sone 1982, Fejérdy et al. 2004*]. There are three major facets of proper and efficient patient-dentist communication including (1) good interpersonal relationship and mutual trust, (2) exchange of information, and (3) making treatment related decisions [*Laney 1983, Ong et al. 1995, Kulich 2000, Lechner & Roessler 2001, Fejérdy et al. 2004; Fejérdy & Orosz 2007*]. *A good interpersonal relationship* and *mutual trust* can be created due to friendliness, genuineness, readiness to help, empathy, respect, warmth, as well as eliciting feelings, paraphrasing and reflecting [*Laney 1983, Kulich 2000, Lechner & Roessler 2001, Fejérdy et al. 2004*]. Silence as well as humor may also be very useful in certain cases. Genuineness and congruence of any nonverbal communication is also highly important for creating a good interpersonal relationship and mutual trust [*Laney 1983, Kulich 2000, Fejérdy et al. 2004, Fejérdy & Orosz 2007*]. Simple basic techniques such as verbal following (to show he/she is listening to what the other say) [*Deneen et al. 1973*] and verbal reflection (to restate the essential feelings and contents of the message) [*Deneen et al. 1973*] as well as greeting the patient and using the patient's name [*Wanless & Holloway 1994*] should also not be forgotten.

Exchange of information consists of information giving and information seeking [*Bensing 1991, Ong et al. 1995*], and to meet their needs, both dentists and patients alternate between information giving and information seeking [*Ong et al. 1995*]. Patients need to know that what is the cause of their disorder as well as what are the treatment possibilities and possible treatment outcomes [*Lechner & Roessler 2001, Fejérdy & Orosz 2007*]. Clear information about treatment procedures and their conditions should also be presented for patients [*Lechner & Roessler 2001, Fejérdy & Orosz 2007*]; and patients' level of understanding should be raised until they clearly understand how the proposed treatment will meet their needs [*Shigli et al. 2008*]. Patients also need to know if the dentist accepts him/her and takes him/her seriously [*Kulich 2000*]. Dentist need information to establish the right diagnosis and treatment plan. For such purposes, listening to what the patient saying but also to what he/she is unable to say is crucial [*Kulich 2000, Fejérdy & Orosz 2007*].

Treatment related decisions-making should be based on mutuality, because not only the dentist but also the patient is responsible for his/her own health [*Laney 1983, Freeman 1999, Kulich 2000, Lechner & Roessler 2001, Ma et al. 2008*]. The dentist should give up to hiding behind the facade of a professional authority and should share the problem and problem solving with the patient [*Freeman 1999/a,b, Kulich 2000, Lechner & Roessler 2001*]. However, if the dentist has unresolved issues regarding power and control, dependency and insecurity, self-esteem, prejudice, or other similar issues [*Cohen 1994*] such a "shared" decision-making could be rather untoward. Therefore, dentist's skills should include both an understanding of the patient as well as an understanding of oneself [*Groves 1978, Cohen 1994, Kulich 2000, Fejérdy & Orosz 2007*].

5.5. PREVENTION OF DENTAL FEAR

Prevention (or at least a reduction) of dental fear should be integrated into dental treatment of every patients regularly, and especially into the treatment of patients with increased dental fear values [*Kreyer 1989, Benson 2000, Hermes et al. 2006*]. Especially because traumatizing dental events may trigger PDI symptoms [*Müller-Fahlbusch & Sone 1982*]. The most common reasons of dental fear are bad (painful or fearful) dental experiences [*Moore & Birn 1990, Gáspár et al. 2004, Fábián et al. 2004, Fejérdy et al. 2005, Kaán et al. 2005*], lack of control over the social situation in the dental chair [*Moore & Birn 1990*], lack of control over personal emotional reactions [*Moore & Birn 1990*], feeling of powerlessness during treatment [*Moore & Birn 1990*] and social learning processes with a negative image of dentists [*Moore & Birn 1990*]. Dental fear may also be rooted in (and/or coupled with) other fear types like fear of unknown, fear of intrusion, fear of actual pain (or its anticipation), fear of loss of control and fear of betrayal (lack of trust) [*Chapman & Kirby-turner 1999*]. Fear of death may also have significant impact on dental fear, especially in the case of higher dental fear values [*Fábián et al. 2007*]. There is also an important role of the parents (especially of mother [*Kaán et al. 2005*]) in how the children see dental events

[*Fábián et al. 2003, Kaán et al. 2005*]. Dislike of dentist's behavior and treatment error may also induce high dental fear [*Gáspár et al. 2004*]. Time pressure during dental treatment may also increase dental fear of the patient [*Gáspár et al. 2003/a, Markovics et al. 2005*]. Patients with severe systemic disease [*Facco et al. 2008*], and patients who are divorced [*Fejérdy et al. 2003*], less educated [*Peretz & Mersel 2000*], or attend a given dental office for the first time [*Peretz & Mersel 2000*] are more likely to experience higher dental fear; therefore such patients may merit special considerations [*Peretz & Mersel 2000*]. Living in a foreign language environment (i.e. minorities, migrant employees, guest employees, foreign students or tourists etc.) may also increase the level of dental fear [*Domoto et al. 1991, Markovics et al. 2005*].

The most important method for reduction of dental fear is *communication*. Great care should be taken to avoid fear producing terms or phrases describing the dental treatment or the dental instruments. It is also highly important that, to make only those promises that can be backed [*Botto 2006*]. It is also important that, to give the perception of being in control to the patient [*Botto 2006*]. For such purposes, the "*tell-show-do*" technique [*Addelston 1959*] may be used efficiently. This method includes describing in simple terms what is about to occur ("*tell*"); than allowing the patient to see, feel, explore and manipulate the tools or instruments ("*show*"); and than the starting of the procedure ("*do*") [*Addelston 1959, Allen 2006*]. Online support groups [*White & Dorman 2001, Winzelberg et al. 2002, Eysenbach et al. 2004, Coulson 2005*] may also be used to improve patients' perception of being in control, and for consequent prevention of dental fear [*Coulson & Buchanan 2008*].

Methods for *distraction* to refocus patient's attention away from the potentially painful/fearful stimulus or procedure may also be used, advantageously [*Allen 2006, Botto 2006*]. Offering of brief brakes during treatment is the simplest method for such purposes [*Allen 2006*]. Another simple forms of distraction include jiggling of the patients' cheek or asking them to hold their legs up in the air during a critical procedure (i.e. administrating of local anesthesia, or making impression) [*Botto 2006*]. Music expressing positive emotions [*Suda et al. 2008*] may also be used for distraction during the dental treatment [*Vinard & Ravier-rosenblaum 1989, Botto 2006*]. Fear inducing effect of the noise environment during dental treatments (especially the noise of high-speed turbine [*Vinard & Ravier-rosenblaum 1989*]) may also be decreased easily due to the use of music. Audiovisual methods like video games [*Allen 2006*], two-dimensional DVD-glasses and three-dimensional virtual reality technology [*Askay et al. 2009*] may also be used.

Mind-body therapies (see *paragraph 6.4.*) including hypnosis [*Gokli et al. 1994, Fábián & Fábián 1998, Fábián 1995/a,b, 1996/a,b, Staats & Krause 1995, Schmierer 1997, Benson 2000, Hermes et al. 2003, Eitner et al. 2006, Fábián et al. 2009/a*], self-hypnosis [*Taylor 1995, Shaw & Niven 1996*], photo-acoustic stimulation [*Fábián & Fábián 2000/b, Fábián & Vértes 2007, Fábián et al. 2005, 2009/a*] relaxation [*Tóth & Fábián 2006, Fábián 2007, Botto 2006*] and *several biofeedback methods* [*Litt et al. 1993, Botto 2006*] are also suitable for distraction during the dental treatment (see also *paragraph 6.4.*). *Breathing exercises* leading to slow normal breathing may also be used advantageously [*Botto 2006*]. In some cases *pharmacological methods* including premedication with anxiolytics [*Lu 1994*], relative analgesia (inhalation of nitrous oxide - oxygen mixture) [*Roberts 1979, Crawford 1990*], conscious sedation (intravenously administered benzodiazepines) and occasionally general anaesthesia [*Murray 1993, Matharu & Ashley 2006*] as well as *psychotherapeutic approaches* (see *paragraph 6.3.*) may also be used to reduce dental fear.

5.6. PREVENTION OF TREATMENT IDUCED PAIN

Similarly, to fearful treatment, painful dental treatment may also trigger PDI, especially when patient was emotionally traumatized [*Müller-Fahlbusch & Sone 1982*]. Patients with higher pain catastrophizing scores report heightened pain during [*Sullivan & Neish 1997, 1998*] and following (dental)surgery [*Pavli et al. 2005*], and increased anxiety, dental fear and emotional distress in relation with the dental treatment [*Sullivan & Neish 1997*]. Therefore, pain catastrophizing behavior of patients (if any) should be considered before, during, and also after the treatment. The use of highly efficient anaesthesia (including postoperative anaesthesia) and the use of psychological stress reducing interventions *before* treatment (i.e. cognitive or behavior therapy), *during* treatment (i.e. relaxation, hypnosis etc.) and *after* treatment (i.e. post hypnotic suggestions, self-hypnosis etc.) is also crucial for such patients. Despite local anaesthesia that have made painless dentistry a reality, psychological methods for alleviation of pain (and/or fear of pain) are still needed for sensitive patients [*Benson 2000*].

Procedural pain can be decreased efficiently using several mind-body methods (see *paragraph 6.4.*) especially hypnosis [*Staats & Krause 1995, Schmierer 1997, Fábián & Fábián 1998, Fábián 1995/a,b, Benson 2000, Fábián et al. 2009/a, Gáspár et al. 2003/b*] or self-hypnosis [*Jenkins 1995*]. Since decrease of dental fear and anxiety may significantly improve analgesic effects [*Fábián 1996/b, Fábián & Fábián 1998, Fábián et al. 2009*]; methods used for prevention of dental fear (see *paragraph 5.5.*) are also suitable for the prevention of treatment-induced pain. Pre-operative treatment and/or post-operative treatment of the teeth (or other oral tissues) with certain physiotherapies (i.e. low level laser or pulsed electromagnetic field therapy) may also be useful [*Fábián et al. 2009/b*] to decrease tissue damage [*Godoy et al. 2007*] and to reduce post operative pain [*Kreisler et al. 2004, Koszowski et al. 2006, Marković & Todorović 2006*]. Administration of non-steroid anti-inflammatory drugs (NSAIDs) before and/or after dental treatment may also be useful in certain cases.

5.7. PATIENT-NURSE-DENTIST INTERRELATIONSHIPS

Psychological factors in patient-nurse-dentist interrelationships are major determinants of treatment outcome [*Green & Laskin 1974, Pomp 1974, Laskin & Block 1986, Fábián & Fábián 2000/a, Fábián et al. 2007, Fejérdy & Orosz 2007*]. The importance of patient involvement in the development of the denture should be also emphasized in this relation [*Freeman 1999/a,b, Lechner & Roessler 2001, Ma et al. 2008*]. Patients must be made aware of their responsibilities in achieving a satisfactory outcome [*Freeman 1999/a,b, Lechner & Roessler 2001, Ma et al. 2008*]. Similarly, dentist should involve also the nurse into certain aspects of decision-making and patient care. Four major facets of patient-nurse-dentist relationships should also be considered, such as the *real relationship* and the *boundaries of relationship* as well as the *regression* and the *transference* phenomena.

The *real relationship* is an equal and unique relationship between persons [*Freeman 1999/b*]. This is a genuine and realistic interaction in which the uniqueness of the dentist is complemented by the uniqueness of the patient and the uniqueness of the nurse [*Freeman 1999/b*]. The real relationship between the patient and the dentist (and/or nurse) should be protected by *boundaries* [*Reid et al. 2007*]. Acceptance of gifts, dinner invitations or unconventional payments for treatment (i.e. exchanging dental services for housepainting service, or for a discount on an automobile purchase etc.) put the dentist and/or the nurse at high risk of violating boundaries with patients [*Reid et al. 2007*]. Consequently, conflicts of interest may appear, which may erode their ability to make objective decisions on behalf of the patient [*Reid et al. 2007*]. Importantly, relation between the dentist and the nurse should also be protected by similar boundaries [*Fábián & Fábián 2000/a, Fábián et al. 2007, Fejérdy & Orosz 2007*].

Regression simply describes the psychological state of the patients (and/or nurse and/or dentist) as they change from being in an emotionally controlled to a less well-controlled emotional state, which is associated with a change in relationship status [*Freeman 1999/b*]. Because of regression, the relationship may show a typical pattern of interaction between a parent and child [*Freeman 1999/b*] or any other pattern of emotionally deep-rooted relationships. Regression is frequently coupled with transference phenomena. Within the *transference* patients (and/or nurse, and/or dentist) will re-experience emotions and psycho-emotional patterns of previous relations (primarily from the childhood) [*Freeman 1999/b*]. The transference is particularly important because the dentist (as a "major target" of transference) may, therefore, be perceived emotionally as a "caring parent" or as a "powerful" or "threatening" person (or "any other" important person) [*Freeman 1999/b, Fábián & Fábián 2000/a, Fábián et al. 2007, Fejérdy & Orosz 2007*]; which may lead to patient's (and/or nurse's) behavior appearing as inadequate and disturbing from the viewpoint of the dentist.

5.8. PREVENTION OF RELAPSE

Prevention of relapse is primarily based on inducing and maintenance of long run changes of patients' health related behavior in respect of somatic (dental and medical) as well as mental health. It should be considered that, a structural plan for patient education has a better chance for success than one based only on intuition. Therefore, a clear identification and establishment of the educational needs of patients is crucial [*Wentz 1972*]. Subsequently, identification of possible/available motivation stimuli and concrete goal setting should be carried out [*Wentz 1972*]. Next goals of education plan should be achieved due to motivation and learning reinforcement [*Wentz 1972*]. Finally, results should be evaluated and controlled regularly [*Wentz 1972*]. Importantly, whatever structural plane is to be used, it must incorporate some means of providing information other than in an advice-giving format [*Freeman 1999*].

Information must be presented in such a way that patients feel its importance, and in a way that they can "take ownership" of it [*Freeman 1999*]. Importantly, patients can take such "ownership" (more precisely: "co-ownership") of the health-education interaction (and in doing so acknowledge their readiness to change) *only* within an *equality of the dentist-patient relationship* [*Freeman 1999*]. Depending on their personality, somatic condition, family/social background and symptoms, various methods may be offered for the patients. Most preferable *home practice* of several *mind-body methods* (see *paragraph 6.4.*), *diet- and medicinal herb therapy* (see *chapter 7.*) as well as *CAM methods* (see *chapter 8.*) may be offered. *Online support groups* [*White & Dorman 2001, Winzelberg et al. 2002, Eysenbach et al. 2004, Coulson 2005, Coulson & Buchanan 2007*] as well as *patients' clubs* could be another promising possibility for prevention of relapse of PDI patients. Although prevention of relapse is primarily based on the patients' self-reliance, patient should be told to return for care if symptoms recur and cannot be quickly controlled by the previously used (home practice) procedures [*Laskin & Block 1986*].

5.9. MENTAL HEALTH OF THE DENTAL TEAM

It should be emphasized that, many dentists (an other members of the dental team) have a working situation with rather hard work conditions and occupational stress [*Kreyer 1992, Newton & Gibbons 1996, Hjalmers et al. 2003*]. Further, dentist's profession is coupled with a difficult psychoemotional challenge as well [*Kreyer 1992*]. The active inhibition of dentist's emotional expression (especially when dealing with problem patients) may also lead to increased working stress and risk for a variety of health problems [*Berry & Pennebaker 1993*]. No wonder that, irritability, nervousness, bruxism, tremor, sweating, tenseness, articular pain (especially spinal pain), certain cardiovascular symptoms (i.e. functional irregularities), tiredness and poor concentration are frequently noticed by dentists being under working load [*Kreyer 1992*].

Although premised conditions not necessarily induce physical or mental difficulties in a short run [*Ozawa et al. 1989*], dentists may suffer from many physical and mental troubles linked to the working situation in longer run [*Kreyer 1992, Newton & Gibbons 1996, Hjalmers et al. 2003*]. Accordingly, a rather high prevalence of fatigue (70 %), and back-neck- or shoulder pain (76 %) were reported among female unpromoted general dental practitioners; from which 83 % and 95 % of the symptoms were likely related to the dental profession respectively [*Hjalmers et al. 2003*]. Thus, it is obvious that, dentists (and any member of the dental team) should take great care about their mental and physical health.

There is an obvious role of *disadvantageous body posture* of dentists and dental nurses during dental treatment. Body posture may be improved by several body exercises (see *paragraphs 8.5., 8.6.*), and by offering of brief brakes during the workday which may be utilized advantageously for practicing brief relaxation exercises (see *paragraph 6.4.1.*) and/or brief breathing exercises (see *paragraph 8.4.*). The *stress inducing effect of the noise environment* on dentist and dental nurse and the consequent sympathetic activation should also be considered [*Vinard & Ravier-Rosenblaum 1989*]. From this point of view, especially the noise of high-speed *turbine*, and the *telephone ringing* should be considered as highly disturbing and stress inducing during treatment [*Vinard & Ravier-rosenblaum 1989*]. Stress inducing effect of such noises can be significantly reduced by using turbines of high quality and decreasing the sound intensity of telephone ring as well as with the use of harmonious background music during the treatment [*Vinard & Ravier-rosenblaum 1989*].

It should be also considered that, facial muscles react to *psychoemotional stress* with more pronounced *increase of tension* comparing to other muscles of the body [*Heggendorn et al. 1979*]. Further, *consciously controlled face expressions* are more strongly expressed in the left side of the face leading to a rather asymmetric load of the facial muscles [*Baumann et al. 2005*] (especially in the case of women, because of the higher emotional sensitivity of their facial muscles [*Baumann et al. 2005*]). Therefore, member of the dental team (especially the dentist) can be of higher *risk of orofacial dysfunction*; and may pay a high price of "keep smiling" when their facial expressions are shaped by either stress or "marketing aspects" rather than the acceptance of patient and kindness of hart.

Consequently, dental team members should be able to accept a patient from the bottom of hart as well as to understand and accept own emotions. Thus, *dentists and other team members should become a mature, well-disposed and good person on behalf of the patients as well as on behalf of their own interest*. For such purposes several psychotherapeutic approaches (see *paragraph 6.3.*) as well as several mind-body methods (see *paragraph 6.4.*) are available and may be useful for dentists as well. Besides intrapersonal problems, *interpersonal problems of team members* should also be managed [*Kreyer 1992*]. In this respect, the most important is to *recognize, verbalize and discuss the appearing problem*. Recognition of interpersonal problems may be facilitated by anonym questionnaires [*Fejérdy et al. 2004*]. Verbalization and discussion can also be facilitated due to organizing regular formal team meetings as well as *informal* team meetings [*Fejérdy et al. 2004*].

5.10. CONCLUSION

Cornerstones of prevention are screening of risk patients, proper treatment planning, proper communication with the patient, screening of the patient-nurse-dentist interrelationships, as well as prevention of dental fear, prevention of treatment induced pain and prevention of relapse [*Fábián & Fábián 2000/a, Fábián et al. 2007, Fejérdy & Orosz 2007*]. It is crucial also for the prevention that, patients must be made aware of their responsibilities in achieving a satisfactory outcome. It is also a matter of considerable significance that the clinician carefully weigh the option of nontreatment in certain cases [*Levin & Landesman 1976, Stein 1983, Fábián & Fábián 2000/a, Fábián et al. 2007*]. Dental team members should also be able to accept a patient from the bottom of hart as well as to understand and accept own emotions for a proper and successful treatment and to avoid treatment failure. Therefore, *dentists and other team members should become a mature, well-disposed and good person on behalf of the patients as well as on behalf of their own interest*. Maintenance of the mental health of dental team is also crucial for the prevention of PDI [*Fejérdy et al. 2004*]. Lack of attention to all above facets of prevention may invite treatment failure and may lead to the occurrence of PDI.

REFERENCES

[1]   Addelston, H. Child patient training. *CDS Review*, 1959 38, 27-29.

[2]   Allen, KD. Management of children's disruptive behavior during dental treatment. In: Mostofsky DI, Forgione AG, Giddon, DB editors. *Behavioral dentistry*. Ames (Iowa): Blackwell Munksgaard; 2006; 175-187.

[3]   Allen, PF. & McMillan, AS. A review of the functional and psychosocial outcomes of edentulousness treated with complete replacement dentures. *J Can Dent Assoc*, 2003 69, 662.

[4]   Askay, SW; Patterson, DR; Sharar, SR. Virtual reality hypnosis. *Contemp Hypnosis*, 2009 26, 40-47.

[5]   Asmundson, GJG; Bovell, CV; Carleton, RN; McWilliams, LA. The Fear of Pain Questionnaire - Short Form (FPQ-SF): Factor validity and psychometric properties. *Pain*, 2008 134, 51-58.

[6]   Bae, KH; Kim, C; Paik, DI; Kim, JB. A comparison of oral health related quality of life between complete and partial removable denture-wearing older adults in Korea. *J Oral Rehabil*. 2006 33, 317-322.

[7]   Barone, A; Rispoli, L; Vozza, I; Quaranta, A; Covani, U. Immediate restoration of single implants placed immediately after tooth extraction. *J Periodontol*, 2006 77, 1914-1920.

[8]   Bartling, R; Freeman, K; Kraut, RA. The incidence of altered sensation of the mental nerve after mandibular implant placement. *J Oral Maxillofac Surg*, 1999 57, 1408-1410.

[9]   Batista, M; Bonachella, W; Soares, J. Progressive recovery of osseoperception as a function of the combination of implant-supported prostheses. *Clin Oral Impl Res*, 2008 19, 565-569.

[10]   Baumann, K; Kessler, H; Linden, M. Die Messung von Emotionen. *Verhaltenstherapie und Verhaltensmedizin*, 2005 26, 169-197.

[11]   Bensing, JM. Doctor-patient communication and quality of care. An observation study into affective and instrumental behavior in general practice. *Social Sci Med*, 1991 32, 1301-1310.

[12]   Bensing, J. Bridging the gap. The separate worlds of evidence-based medicine and patient-centered medicine. *Patient Education Counseling*, 2000 39, 17-25.

[13]   Benson, PE. Suggestion can help. *Ann R Australas Coll Dent Surg*, 2000 15, 284-285.

[14]   Bergendal, T. & Magnusson, T. Changes in signs and symptoms of temporomandibular disorders following treatment with implant supported fixed prostheses: a prospective 3-year follow up. *Int J Prosthodont*, 2000 13, 392-398.

[15]   Berry, DS. & Pennebaker, JW. Nonverbal and verbal emotional expressions and health. *Psychother Psychosom*, 1993 59, 11-19.

[16]   Biondi, M. & Picardi, A. Temporomandibular joint pain-dysfunction syndrome and bruxism: etiopathogenesis and treatment from a psychosomatic integrative viewpoint. *Psychother Psychosom*, 1993 59, 84-98.

[17]   Botto, RW. Chairside techniques for reducing dental fear. In: Mostofsky DI, Forgione AG, Giddon DB editors. *Behavioral dentistry*. Ames (Iowa): Blackwell Munksgaard; 2006; 115-125.

[18] Brännström, M. Reducing the risk of sensitivity and pulpal complications after the placement of crowns and fixed partial dentures. *Quintessence Int*, 1996 27, 673-678.

[19] Cannizzaro, G; Leone, M; Esposito, M. Immediate functional loading of implants placed with flapless surgery in the edentulous maxilla: 1-year follow-up of a single cohort study. *Int J Oral Maxillofac Implants*. 2007 22, 87-95.

[20] Cattell, RB; Eber, HW; Tatsuoka, M. *Handbook for the 16 PF Questionnaire*. Champaign, Illinois: Institute of Personality and Ability Testing; 1970.

[21] Chapman, HR. & Kirby-Turner, NC. Dental fear in children - a proposed model. *Brit Dent J*, 1999 187, 408-412.

[22] Cohen, PA. Recognizing and managing the difficult patient. *CDS Review*, 1994, 11-16.

[23] Cohen, S; Kamarck, T; Mermelstein, R. A global measure of perceived stress. *J Health Soc Behav*, 1983 24, 385-396.

[24] Comfort, MB; Chu, FC; Chai, J; Wat, PY; Chow, TW. A 5-year prospective study on small diameter screw-shaped oral implants. *J Oral Rehabil*, 2005 32, 341-345.

[25] Corah, NL. Development of a Dental Anxiety Scale. *J Dent Res*, 1969 48, 596.

[26] Coulson, NS. Receiving social support online: an analysis of a computer -mediated support group for individuals living with irritable bowel syndrome. *CyberPsychol Behav*, 2005 8, 580-584.

[27] Coulson, NS. & Buchanan, H. Self-reported efficacy of an online dental anxiety support group: a pilot study. *Community Dent Oral Epidemiol*, 2008 36, 43-46.

[28] Crawford, AN. The use of nitrous oxide-oxygen inhalation sedation with local anaesthesia as an alternative to general anaesthesia for dental extractions in children. *Brit Dent J*, 1990 168, 395-398.

[29] Creech 3rd, JL; Walton, RE; Kaltenbach, R. Effect of occlusal relief on endodontic pain. *JADA*, 1984 109, 64-67.

[30] Cronström, R; Owall, B; René, N. Treatment injuries in dentistry - cases from one year in the Swedish Patient Insurance Scheme. *Int Dent J*, 1998 48, 187-195.

[31] Cunha-Cruz, J; Hujoel, PP; Kressin, NR. Oral health-related quality of life of periodontal patients. *J Periodont Res*, 2007 42, 169-176.

[32] De Bruyn, H; Van de Velde, T; Collaert, B. Immediate functional loading of TiOblast dental implants in full-arch edentulous mandibles: a 3-year prospective study. *Clin Oral Impl Res*, 2008 19, 717-723.

[33] Deneen, LJ; Heid, DW; Smith, AA. Effective interpersonal and management skills in dentistry. *JADA*, 1973 87, 878-880.

[34] Domoto, P; Weinstein, P; Kamo, Y; Wohlers, K; Fiset, L; Tanaka, A. Dental fear of Japanese residents in the United States. *Anesth Prog*, 1991 38, 90-95.

[35] Doundoulakis, JH; Eckert, SE; Lindquist, CC; Jeffcoat, MK. The implant supported overdenture as an alternative to the complete mandibular denture. *JADA*, 2003 134, 1455-1458.

[36] Eitner, S; Schultze-Mosgau, S; Heckmann, J; Wichmann, M; Holst, S. Changes in neurophysiologic parameters in a patient with dental anxiety by hypnosis during surgical treatment. *J Oral Rehabil*, 2006 33, 496-500.

[37] Ekanayake, L. & Perera, I. Perceived need for dental care among dentate older individuals in Sri Lanka. *Spec Care Dentist*, 2005 25, 199-205.

[38] Elias, AC. & Sheiham, A. The relationship between satisfaction with mouth and number and position of teeth. *J Oral Rehabil*, 1998 25, 649-661.

[39] Eysenbach, G; Powell, J; Englesakis, M; Rizo, C; Stern, A. Health related virtual communities and electronic support groups: systemic review of the effects of online peer-to-peer interactions. *BMJ*, 2004 328, 1166-1171.

[40] Facco, E; Zanette, G; Manani, G. Italian version of Corah's Dental anxiety Scale: Normative data in patients undergoing oral surgery and relationship with the ASA physical status classification. *Anesth Prog*, 2008 55, 109-115.

[41] Fábián, G; Fejérdy, L; Fábián, Cs; Kaán, B; Gáspár, J; Fábián, TK. Dental fear scores of 8-15 years old primary school children in Hungary. *Fogorv Szle*, 2003 96, 129-133.

[42] Fábián, G; Fejérdy, L; Kaán, B; Fábián, Cs; Tóth, Zs; Fábián, TK. Background data about the high dental fear scores of Hungarian 8-15-year old primary school children. *Fogorv Szle*, 2004 97, 128-132.

[43] Fábián, G; Müller, O; Kovács, Sz; Nguyen, MT; Fábián, TK; Csermely, P; Fejérdy, P. Attitude toward death: Does it influence dental fear? *Ann NY Acad Sci*, 2007 1113, 339-349.

[44] Fábián, TK. Hypnosis in dentistry. I. Comparative evaluation of 45 cases of hypnosis. *Fogorv Szle*, 1995/a 88, 111-115.

[45] Fábián, TK. Hypnosis in dentistry. II. Amnesia, analgesia, loss of time perception: spontaneous manifestations during use of hypnosis in dentistry. *Fogorv Szle*, 1995/b 88, 237-242.

[46] Fábián, TK. Hypnotic desensitization as a supplemental method in dental care of patients with panic disorder. Report of a case. *Fogorv Szle*, 1996/a 89, 57-62.

[47] Fábián TK. Anxiety as a dynamic factor of dental hypnosis. *Fogorv Szle*, 1996/b 89, 153-157.

[48] Fábián, TK. Relaxation techniques [Relaxációs módszerek]. In: Fábián TK, Vértes G editors. *Psychosomatic dentistry* [*Fogorvosi pszichoszomatika*]. Budapest: Medicina; 2007; 185-192.

[49] Fábián, TK. & Fábián, G. Stress of life, stress of death: Anxiety in dentistry from the viewpoint of hypnotherapy. *Ann NY Acad Sci*, 1998 851, 495-500.

[50] Fábián, TK. & Fábián, G. Dental stress. In: Fink G, editor in chief. *Encyclopedia of stress. (vol. 1.)*. San Diego: Academic Press; 2000/a; 567-659.

[51] Fábián, TK. & Fábián, G. The use of photo-acoustic stimulation in dental practice. *Fogorv Szle*, 2000/b 93, 195-201.

[52] Fábián, TK. & Vértes, G. Photo-acoustic stimulation [Fény-hang stimuláció]. In: Fábián TK, Vértes G editors. *Psychosomatic dentistry* [*Fogorvosi pszichoszomatika*]. Budapest: Medicina; 2007; 192-200.

[53] Fábián, TK; Krause, WR; Krause, M; Fejérdy, P. Photo-acoustic stimulation and hypnotherapy in the treatment of oral psychosomatic disorders. *Hypnos*, 2005 32, 198-202.

[54] Fábián, TK; Fábián, G; Fejérdy, P. Dental stress. In: Fink G, editor in chief. *Encyclopedia of stress. Second edition. (vol. 1.)* .Oxford: Academic Press; 2007; 733-736.

[55] Fábián, TK; Gótai, L; Krause, WR; Fejérdy, P. Zahnärztliche Hypnoseforschung an der Semmelweis Universität Budapest. *Deutsche Z Zahnärztl Hypn*, 2009/a 8, 9-14.

[56] Fábián, TK; Gótai, L; Beck, A; Fábián, G; Fejérdy, P. The role of molecular chaperones (HSPAs/HSP70s) in oral health and oral inflammatory diseases: A review. *Eur J Inflammation*, 2009/b 7, 53-61.

[57] Fejérdy, L; Fábián, Cs; Kaán, B; Fábián, G; Gáspár, J; Fábián, TK. Epidemiological study of dental fear scores in several Hungarian sub-populations. *Fogorv Szle*, 2003 96, 277-281.

[58] Fejérdy, L; Kaán, B; Fábián, G; Tóth, Zs; Fábián, TK. Background data about the high dental fear scores of Hungarian secondary school students. *Fogorv Szle*, 2005 98, 9-13.

[59] Fejérdy, P. & Orosz, M. Personality of the dentist and patient-assistant-dentist interrelationships [A fogorvos személyisége, a beteg-asszisztens-fogorvos kapcsolatrendszer] In: Vértes G, Fábián TK editors. *Psychosomatic dentistry [Fogorvosi Pszichoszomatika]* Budapest: Medicina; 2007; 22-31.

[60] Fejérdy, P; Fábián, TK; Krause, WR. Mentalhygienische Aufgaben von Krankenschwestern in der Zahnmedizin. Kommunikation mit den Patienten und dem Zahnarzt. *Deutsche Z Zahnärztl Hypn*, 2004 3, 32-34.

[61] Fontijn-Tekamp, FA; Slagter, AP; van 't Hof, MA; Geertman, ME; Kalk, W. Bite forces with mandibular implant-retained overdentures. *J Dent Res,* 1998 77, 1832-1839.

[62] Fontijn-Tekamp, FA; Slagter, AP; van 't Hof; MA; Kalk, W; Jansen, JA. Pain and instability during biting with mandibular implant-retained overdentures. *Clin Oral Impl Res*, 2000 12, 46-51.

[63] Fox, E; O'Boyle, C; Barry, H; McCreary, C. Repressing coping style and anxiety in stressful dental surgery. *Br J Med Psychol*, 1989 62, 371-380.

[64] Freeman, R. Strategies for motivating the non-compliant patient. *Brit Dent J*, 1999/a 187, 307-312.

[65] Freeman, R. A psychodynamic understanding of the dentist-patient interaction. *Brit Dent J*, 1999/b 186, 503-505.

[66] Fueki, K; Kimoto, K; Ogawa, T; Garrett, NR. Effect of implant-supported or retained dentures on masticatory performance: a systemic review. *J Prosthet Dent*, 2007 98, 470-477.

[67] Gáspár, J; Fejérdy, L; Kaán, B; Tóth, Zs; Fábián, TK. The Hungarian version of Getz's Dental Beliefs Survey (DBS), First data about the Hungarian population. *Fogorv Szle*, 2003/a 96, 261-167.

[68] Gáspár, J; Linninger, M; Kaán, M; Bálint, M; Fejérdy, L; Fábián, TK. The effectivity of standardized direct suggestions under dental hypnotic conditions. *Fogorv Szle*, 2003/b 96, 205-210.

[69] Gáspár, J; Tóth, Zs; Fejérdy, L; Kaán, B; Fábián TK. Some background data about the high dental anxiety values of the Hungarian population. *Fogorv Szle*, 2004 97, 85-89.

[70] Godoy, BM; Arana-Chavez, VE; Núñez, SC; Ribeiro, MS. Effects of low-power red laser on dentine-pulp interface after cavity preparation. An ultrastructural study. *Arch Oral Biol*, 2007 52, 899-903.

[71] Goené, R; Bianchesi, C; Hüerzeler, M; Del Lupo, R; Testori, T; Davarpanah, M; Jalbout, Z. Performance of short implants in partial restorations: 3-year follow-up of Osseotite implants. *Implant Dent*, 2005 14, 274-280.

[72] Gokli, MA; Wood, J; Mourino, AP; Farrington, FH; Best, AM. Hypnosis as an adjunct to the administration of local anesthetic in pediatric patients. *J Dent Child*, 1994 61, 272-273.

[73] Goodacre, CJ; Bernal, G; Rungcharassaeng, K; Kan, YKK. Clinical complications in fixed prosthodontics. *J Prosthet Dent*, 2003/a 90, 31-41.

[74] Goodacre, CJ; Bernal, G; Rungcharassaeng, K; Kan, YKK. Clinical complications with implant and implant prostheses. *J Prosthet Dent*, 2003/b 90, 121-132.

[75] Graham, R; Mihaylov, S; Jepson, N; Allen, PF; Bond, S. Determining "need" for a removable partial denture: a qualitative study of factors that influence dentist provision and patient use. *Brit Dent J*, 2006 200, 155-158,

[76] Green, CS. & Laskin, DM. Long-term evaluation of conservative treatment for myofascial pain-dysfunction syndrome. *JADA*, 1974 89, 1365-1368.

[77] Green, CS. & Laskin, DM. Temporomandibular disorders: Moving from a dentally based model to a medically based model. *J Dent Res*, 2000 79, 1736-1739.

[78] Groves, JE. Taking care of the hateful patient. *New Engl J Med*, 1978 298, 883-887.

[79] Heft, MW; Gilbert, GH; Shelton, BJ; Duncan, RP. Relationship of dental status, sociodemographic status, and oral symptoms to perceived need for dental care. *Community Dent Oral Epidemiol*, 2003 31, 351-360.

[80] Heggendorn, H; Voght, HP; Graber, G. Experimentelle Untersuchungen über die orale Hyperaktivität bei psychischer belastung, im besonderen bei Aggression. *Schweiz Mschr Zahnheilk*, 1979 89, 1148-1161.

[81] Hermes, D; Hakim, SG; Trübger, D; Sieg, P. Tape Recorded Hypnosis. Eine effiziente Therapieoption zur Verbesserung des Behandlungskomforts in der Oral- und Mund-Kiefer-Gesichtschirurgie. *Quintessenz*, 2003 54, 911-919.

[82] Hermes, D; Saka, B; Bahlmann, L; Matthes, M. Behandlungsangst in der Mund-, Kiefer- und Gesichtschirurgie. *Mund Kiefer GesichtsChir*, 2006 10, 307-313.

[83] Heydecke, G; Locker, D; Awad, MA; Lund, JP; Feine, JS. Oral and general health-related quality of life with conventional and implant dentures. *Community Dent Oral Epidemiol*, 2003 31, 161-168.

[84] Hjalmers, K; Söderfeldt, B; Axtelius, B. Psychosomatic symptoms among female unpromoted general practice dentists. *Swed Dent J*, 2003 27, 35-41.

[85] Holmes, TH. & Rahe, RH. The Social Readjustment Rating Scale. *J Psychosom Res*, 1967 11, 213.

[86] Jacobs, R. & Van Steenberghe, D. From osseoperception to implant-mediated sensory-motor interactions and related clinical implications. *J Oral Rehabil*, 2006 33, 282-292.

[87] Jenkins, M. Teaching patients to block post-operative pain by self-hypnosis. *Eur J Clin Hypn*, 1995 2, 54-55.

[88] Jones, JA; Orner, MB; Spiro, A(3rd); Kressin, NR. Tooth loss and dentures: patients' perspectives. *Int Dent J*, 2003 53 (5 Suppl.), 327-334.

[89] Kaán, B; Fejérdy, L; Tóth, Zs; Fábián, G; Korchmáros, R; Fábián, TK. Lexicological parameters of free association (coupling) about teeth of Hungarian primary school children. An initial study. *Fogorv Szle*, 2005 98, 239-244.

[90] Kaban, LB. & Belfer, ML. Temporomandibular joint dysfunction: an occasional manifestation of serious psychopathology. *J Oral Surg*, 1981 39, 742-746.

[91]   Kaptein, MLA; Hoogstraten, J; Putter de, C; Lange de, GL; Blijdorp, PA. Dental implants in the atrophic maxilla: measurements of patients' satisfaction and treatment experience. *Clin Oral Impl Res*, 1998 9, 321-326.

[92]   Kao, RT. Strategic extraction: A paradigm shift that is changing our profession *J Periodontol*, 2008 79, 971-977.

[93]   Kawai, Y; Matsumaru, Y; Kanno, K; Kawase, M; Shu, K; Izawa, T; Gunji, A; Kobayashi, K. The use of existing denture-satisfaction ratings for a diagnostic test to indicate prognosis with newly delivered complete dentures. *J Prosthodontic Res*, in press, DOI: 10.1016/j.jpor.2009.05.002

[94]   Kern, M; Kleimeier, B; Schaller, HG; Strub, JR. Clinical comparison of postoperative sensitivity for a glass ionomer and a zinc phosphate luting cement. *J Prosthet Dent*, 1996 75, 159-162.

[95]   Kleinknecht, RA; Klepac, RK; Alexander, LD. Origins and characteristics of fear of dentistry. *J Am Dent Assoc*, 1973 86, 842-848.

[96]   Kleinknecht, RA; Thorndike, RM; McGlynn, FD; Harkavy, J. Factor analysis of the Dental Fear Survey with cross-validation. *J Am Dent Assoc*, 1984 108, 59-61.

[97]   Klineberg, I. & Murray, G. Osseoperception: Sensory function and proprioception. *Adv Dent Res*, 1999 13, 120-129.

[98]   Koszowski, R; Smieszek-Wilczewska, J; Dawiec, G. Comparison of analgesic effect of magnetic and laser stimulation before oral surgery procedures. *Wiad Lek*, 2006 59, 630-633.

[99]   Kotkin, H; Slabbert, JC; Becker, PJ; Carr, L. Perceptions of complete dentures by prospective implant patients. *Int J Prosthodont*, 1998 11, 240-245.

[100] Kreisler, MB; Haj, HA; Noroozi, N; Willershausen, B. Efficacy of low level laser therapy in reducing postoperative pain after endodontic surgery - a randomized double blind clinical study. *Int J Oral Maxillofac Surg*, 2004 33, 38-41.

[101] Kreyer, G. Advances in dental psychology. *Z Stomatol*, 1989 86, 123-130.

[102] Kreyer, G. Zur Inzidenz und Wertigkeit von psychischen, somatischen und psychosomatischen Belastungsfaktoren bei österreichischen Zahnbehandlern. *Z Stomatol*, 1992 89, 319-331.

[103] Kulich, KR. *Interpersonal skills in the dentist-patient relationship. (Ph.D. thesis).* Göteborg: Göteborg University; 2000; 9-15.

[104] Laney, WR. Considerations in treatment planning. In: Laney WR, Gibilisco JA editors. *Diagnosis and treatment in prosthodontics.* Philadelphia: Lea & Febiger; 1983; 157-181.

[105] Laskin, DM. & Block, S. Diagnosis and treatment of myofacial pain-dysfunction (MPD) syndrome. *J Prosthet Dent*, 1986 56, 75-85

[106] Learreta, JA; Beas J; Bono, AE; Durst A. Muscular activity disorders in relation to intentional occlusal interferences. *Cranio*, 2007 25, 193-199.

[107] Lechner, SK. & Roessler, D. Strategies for complete denture success: beyond techniqual excellence. *Compend Contin Educ Dent*, 2001 22, 553-559.

[108] Lester, V; Ashley, FP; Gibbons, DE. The relationship between socio-dental indices of handicap, felt need for dental treatment and dental state in a group of frail and functionally dependent older adults. *Community Dent Oral Epidemiol*, 1998 26, 155-159.

[109] Levin, B. & Landesmann, HM. A practical questionnaire for predicting denture success of failure. *J Prosthet Dent*, 1976 35, 124-130.

[110] Litt, MD; NYE, C; Shafer, D. Coping with oral surgery by self-efficacy enhancement and perceptions of control. *J Dent Res*, 1993 72, 1237-1243.

[111] Lu, DP. The use of hypnosis for smooth sedation induction and reduction of postoperative violent emergencies from anesthesia in pediatric dental patients. *J Dentistry Children*, 1994, 182-185.

[112] Lundqvist, S. Speech and other oral functions. Clinical and experimental studies with special reference to maxillary rehabilitation on osseointegrated implants. *Swed Dent J Suppl*, 1993 91, 1-39.

[113] Ma, H; Sun, HQ, Ji, P. How to deal with esthetically overcritical patients who need complete dentures: A case report. *J Contemp Dent Pract*, 2008 9, 22-27.

[114] Marković, AB. & Todorović, L. Postoperative analgesia after lower third molar surgery: contribution of the use of long-acting local anesthetics, low-power laser, and diclofenac. *Oral Surg Oral Med Oral Pathol Oral Radiol Endod*, 2006 102, e4-e8.

[115] Markovics, E; Markovics, P; Fábián, G; Vértes, G; Fábián, TK; Fejérdy, P. Dental fear scores of 12-19-year-old school children of the Hungarian minority in Transylvania. *Fogorv Szle*, 2005 98, 165-169.

[116] Matharu, LL. & Ashley, PF. What is the evidence for pediatric dental sedation? *J Dentistry*, 2007 35, 2-20.

[117] Mazurat, NM. & Mazurat, RD. Discuss before fabricating: Communicating the realities of partial denture therapy. Part I: Patient expectations. *J Can Dent Assoc*, 2003 69, 90-94.

[118] Milgrom, P; Weinstein, P; Kleinknecht, RA; Getz, T. Treating fearful dental patients: a clinical handbook. Reston (Virginia): Reston Publishing Company; 1985; 138-142.

[119] Moore, R. & Birn, H. Phenomenon of dental fear. *Tandlaegebladet*, 1990 94, 34-41.

[120] Murray, JJ. General anesthesia and children's dental health: Present trends and future needs. *Anesth Pain Conrol Dent*, 1993 2, 209-216.

[121] Müller-Fahlbusch, H. & Sone, K. Präprotetische Psychagogik. *Deutsch Zahnärztl Z*, 1982 37, 703-707.

[122] Nedir, R; Bischof, M; Briaux, JM; Beyer, S; Szmukler-Moncler, S; Bernard, JP. A 7-year life table analysis from a prospective study on ITI implants with special emphasis on the use of short implants. Results from a private practice. *Clin Oral Implant Res*, 2004 15, 150-157.

[123] Neverlien, PO. Assessment of a single-item dental anxiety question. *Acta Odontol Scand*, 1990 48, 365-369.

[124] Newton, JT. & Gibbons, DE. Stress in dental practice: a qualitative comparison of dentists working within the NHS and those working within an independent capitation scheme. *Brit Dent J*, 1996 180, 329-334.

[125] Ong, LML; De Haes, JCJM; Hoos, AM; Lammes, FB. Doctor-patient communication: A review of the literature. *Social Sci Med*, 1995 40, 903-918.

[126] Ozawa, M; Yamaguchi, M; Kawano, J. Psychological aspects of dental students in the course clinical prosthetics. *Nihon Hoteshu Shika Gakkai Zassi*, 1989 33, 1099-1105.

[127] Pavlin, DJ; Sullivan, MJ; Freund, PR; Roesen, K. Catastrophizing: a risk factor for postsurgical pain. *Clin J Pain*, 2005 21, 83-90.

[128] Peretz, B. & Mersel, A. Non-Institutionalized elderly dental patients in Israel: socia-demographics, health concerns, and dental anxiety. *Spec Care Dentist*, 2000 20, 61-65.

[129] Piquero, K; Ando, T; Sakurai, K. Buccal mucosa ridging and tongue indentation: incidence and associated factors. *Bull Tokyo Dent Coll*, 1999 40, 71-78.

[130] Pomp, AM. Psychotherapy for the myofascial pain-dysfunction syndrome: a study of factors coinciding with symptom remission. *JADA*, 1974 89, 629-632.

[131] Reeve, PE; Watson, CJ; Stafford, GD. The role of personality in the management of complete denture patients. *Brit Dent J*, 1984 156, 356-362.

[132] Reid, KI; Mueller, PS; Barnes, SA. Attitudes of general dentists regarding the acceptance of gifts and unconventional payment from patients. *JADA*, 2007 138, 1127-1133.

[133] Ringland, C; Taylor, L; Bell, J; Lim, K. Demographic and socio-economic factors associated with dental health among older people in NSW. *Aust N Z J Public Health*, 2004 28, 53-61.

[134] Roberts, GJ. Relative analgesia. - An introduction. *Dental update*, 1979 6, 271-284.

[135] Rosenoer, LM. & Sheiham, A. Dental impacts on daily life and satisfaction with teeth in relation to dental status in adults. *J Oral Rehabil*, 1995 22, 469-480.

[136] Roumanas, ED. The social solution - denture esthetics, phonetics, and function. *J Prosthodont*, 2009 18, 112-115.

[137] Schmierer, H. *Einführung in die zahnärztliche Hypnose.* Berlin: Quintesenz; 1997; 236-269.

[138] Schwartz-Arad, D; Laviv, A; Levin, L. Survival of immediately provisionalized dental implants placed immediately into fresh extraction sockets. *J Periodontol*, 2007 78, 219-223.

[139] Shaw, AJ. & Niven, N. Theoretical concepts and practical applications of hypnosis in the treatment of children and adolescents with dental fear and anxiety. *Brit Dent J*, 1996 180, 11-16.

[140] Shigli, K; Shivappa Angadi, G; Hedge, P; Hebbal, M. Patients' knowledge and understanding of the implications of wearing dentures. Report of a survey conducted at a dental institute in the south of India. *Prim Dent Care*, 2008 15, 85-89.

[141] Shor, A; Shor, K; Goto, Y. The edentulous patient and body image - achieving greater patient satisfaction. *Pract Proced Aesthet Dent*, 2005 17, 289-295.

[142] Smith, PW. & McCOrd, JF. What do patients expect from complete dentures? *J Dentistry*, 2004 32, 3-7.

[143] Staats, J. & Krause, WR. *Hypnotherapie in der zahnärztlichen Praxis.* Heidelberg: Hüthig; 1995; 77-124.

[144] Stein, RS. Mutual protective complex of dental restorations. In: Laney WR, Gibilisco JA editors. *Diagnosis and treatment of prosthodontics.* Philadelphia: Lea & Febiger; 1983; 306-326.

[145] Stellingsma, K; Bouma, J; Stegenga, B; Meijer, HJA; Raghoebar, GM. Satisfaction and psychological aspects of patients with an extremely resorbed mandible treated with implant-retained overdentures. *Clin Oral Impl Res*, 2003 14, 166-172.

[146] Suda, M; Morimoto, K; Obata, A; Koizumi, H; Maki, A. Emotional responses to music: towards scientific perspectives on music therapy. *NeuroReport*, 2008 19, 75-78.

[147] Sullivan, MJ. & Neish, NR. Psychological predictors of pain during dental hygiene treatment. *Probe*, 1997 31, 123-126, 135.

[148] Sullivan, MJ. & Neish, NR. Catastrophizing, anxiety and pain during dental hygiene treatment. *Community Dent Oral Epidemiol*, 1998 26, 344-349.

[149] Szentpétery, AG; John, MT; Slaze, GD; Setz, JM. Problems reported by patients before and after prosthodontic treatment. *Int J Prosthodont*, 2005 18, 124-131.

[150] Taylor, D. Extracting patients' fears of dentistry with hypnosis. *Eur J Clin Hypn*, 1995 2, 17-19.

[151] Tóth, Zs. & Fábián, TK. Relaxation techniques in dentistry. *Fogorv Szle*, 2006 99, 15-20.

[152] Trulsson, M. Sensory-motor function of human periodontal mechanoreceptors. *J Oral Rehabil*, 2006 33, 262-273.

[153] Trulsson, U; Engstrand, P; Berggren, U; Nannmark, U; Brånemark, PI. Edentulousness and oral rehabilitation: experiences from the patients' perspective. *Eur J Oral Sci*, 2002 110, 417-424.

[154] Vinard, H. & Ravier-Rosenblaum, C. The psychosomatic effects of the sonic environment in the dental office. *Rev Odontostomatol (Paris)*, 1989 18, 101-108.

[155] Walton, JN. Altered sensation associated with implants in the anterior mandible: a prospective study. *J Prosthet Dent*, 2000 83, 443-449.

[156] Walton, JN. & MacEntee, MI. Choosing or refusing oral implants: a prospective study of edentulous volunteers for a clinical trial. *Int J Prosthodont*, 2005 18, 483-488.

[157] Wanless, MB. & Holloway, PJ. An analysis of audio-recordings of general dental practitioners' consultations with adolescent patients. *Brit Dent J*, 1994 177, 94-98.

[158] Wentz FM. Patient motivation: a new challenge to the dental profession for effective control of plaque. *JADA*, 1972 85, 887-891.

[159] White, M. & Dorman, SM. Receiving social support online: implications for health education. *Health Educ Res*, 2001 16, 693-707.

[160] Winzelberg, AJ; Classen, C; Alpers, GW; Roberts, H; Koopman, C; Adams, RE; Ernst, H; Dev, P; Barr Taylo, C. Evaluation of an internet support group for women with primary breast cancer. *Cancer*, 2002 97, 1164-1173.

[161] Witter, DJ; De Haan, AF; Käyser, AF; Van Rossum, GM. A 6-year follow up study of oral function in shortened dental arches. Part II: Craniomandibular dysfunction and oral comfort. *J Oral Rehabil*, 1994 21, 353-366.

[162] Witter, DJ; van Palenstein Helderman, WH; Creugers, NH; Käyser, AF. The shortened dental arch concept and its implications for oral health care. *Community Dent Oral Epidemiol*, 1999 27, 249-258.

[163] Yan, C; Ye, L; Zhen, J; Ke, L; Gang, L. Neuroplasticity of edentulous patients with implant-supported full dentures. *Eur J Oral Sci*, 2008 116, 387-393.

[164] Zitzmann, NU; Hagmann, E; Weiger, R. What is the prevalence of various types of prosthetic dental restorations in Europe? *Clin Oral Implant Res*, 2007 18 (Suppl. 3), 20-33.

[165] Zlataric, DK. & Celebic, A. Factors related to patients' general satisfaction with removable partial dentures: a stepwise multiple regression analysis. *Int J Prosthodont*, 2008 21, 86-88.

Chapter 6

PSYCHOSOMATIC DENTAL THERAPY

ABSTRACT

Majority of psychogenic denture intolerance patients refuse to accept psychological background of their symptoms; therefore, a simple referral to psychiatrist and/or psychotherapist would not solve the problem in most cases. Consequently, an initial psychosomatic therapy is needed. The most important goals of initial psychosomatic therapy are avoidance of further useless invasive dental treatment as well as obtaining decrease (recovery) of symptoms and motivation of patients to participate in a definitive psychosomatic therapy. Gradual escalation of therapy and avoidance of irreversible forms of treatment are "cornerstones" of the initial psychosomatic therapy; which utilizes several placebo and/or palliative methods combined with supportive communication techniques. Administration of any mind-body therapies as "basic therapeutics" for psychosomatic disorders is also an important goal. Definitive psychosomatic therapy should be offered for patients being refractory to the initial psychosomatic therapy, and for patients responding to it but without a stable treatment outcome. *Psychosomatic dental therapy* induce changes towards an over-all improvement of psychological abilities, social functioning, and stress resistance; which may lead to an improvement of psychosomatic symptoms. Appearance of certain "mental wellness" may also occur. Autonomic and hormonal changes, including decrease of sympathetic activity, blood pressure, HPA axis hormones and catecholamine levels and advantageous changes of heart rate variability (HRV) also may occur; which may support the treatment of stress related orofacial symptoms. General improvement of musculoskeletal functions as well as improvement of pain tolerance may also occur as a result of the psychosomatic treatment. Further, psychosomatic therapies may upregulate immune system and increase immune surveillance. Immunomodulatory effects may also occur, indicating that, exaggerated immunological reactions such as allergy or autoimmune conditions may also be balanced due to the therapy. Salivation problems and pseudoneurological symptoms may also be treated efficiently in many cases.

6.1. INTRODUCTION

Majority of psychogenic denture intolerance patients refuse to accept psychological background of their symptoms [*Ross et al 1953, Fábián et al. 2005/a, Schwichtenberg & Doering 2008*], and instead of psychiatrists or psychotherapists, first they visit dentist and insist on the somatic origin of their symptoms [*Ross et al. 1953, Fábián et al. 2005/a*]. Therefore, a simple referral to psychiatrist and/or psychotherapist would not solve the problem in most cases. Consequently, an initial psychosomatic therapy is needed prior to definitive therapy, which is a scope of dental profession's duty [*Moulton et al. 1957, Pomp 1974*]. The most important goals of initial psychosomatic therapy are avoidance of further useless invasive dental treatment [*Brodine & Hartshorn 2004, Sarlani et al. 2005/b, Reewes & Merrill 2007, Baad-Hansen 2008*] as well as obtaining decrease (recovery) of symptoms and motivation of patients to participate in a definitive psychosomatic therapy (which is the highest level care of psychogenic denture intolerance patients).

Gradual escalation of therapy and avoidance of irreversible forms of treatment are "cornerstones" of the initial psychosomatic therapy [*Laskin & Block 1986*]; which utilizes several placebo and/or palliative methods (i.e. physiotherapies, medication, medicinal herb therapy, diet therapy, CAM therapy etc.) combined with supportive communication techniques. Administration of any mind-body therapies (which are the "basic therapeutics" for psychosomatic disorders [*Iversen 1989, Binder & Bider 1989, Krause 1994*]) is also an important goal of initial therapy. In contrast to initial therapy, definitive psychosomatic therapy should be carried out by *specialized dental professionals* as members of a specialized *psychosomatic team* including *experienced dentists and other medical and psychotherapeutical professionals*. Definitive psychosomatic therapy should be offered for patients being refractory to the initial psychosomatic therapy, and for patients responding to it but without a stable treatment outcome in a long run (i.e. patients with frequent relapses). Fundamentals of the complex process of dental psychosomatic therapy will be discussed in details below.

6.2. STRATEGY OF PSYCHOSOMATIC THERAPY

6.2.1. Initial Psychosomatic Therapy

As already indicated above, most of oral psychosomatic patients (especially PDI patients) refuse to accept psychological background of their symptoms [*Ross et al 1953, Fábián et al. 2005/a, Schwichtenberg & Doering 2008*]. Instead of psychiatrists or psychotherapists, first they visit dentist and insist on the somatic origin of their symptoms [*Ross et al. 1953, Fábián et al. 2005/a*]. In a dental psychosomatic unit, at least three-fourth (76,1 %) of the patients would surely need psychotherapy [*Schwichtenberg & Doering 2008*] but only 37,8 % of the patients would really begin a psychotherapeutic treatment [*Schwichtenberg & Doering 2008*]. Those, who do not begin definitive psychotherapy (the majority of such patients), are apt to continue doing "dentist shopping" (i.e. frequent and useless change of dentist) [*Schwichtenberg & Doering 2008*], with futile attempts at somatic therapies and/or surgical interventions [*Kreyer 2000*].

These data clearly indicate that, a simple referral to psychiatrist and/or psychotherapist would not solve the problem of the majority of PDI patients. Therefore, an initial psychosomatic therapy (IPT) is needed prior to definitive therapy, which is a scope of dental profession's duty [*Moulton et al. 1957, Pomp 1974*]. Initial psychosomatic therapy (IPT) is a scope of *every dentist's* duties currently, because of the absence of an extended network of specialized dental professionals. However, management of oral psychosomatic patients in *specialized dental groups* appears to be a meaningful perspective for the future [*Dahlström et al. 1997, Green & Laskin 2000, Schwichtenberg & Doering 2008*]. It may also be considered that, the network of prosthodontists may fulfill this task, but in this case, post-graduate education of prosthodontists should be completed with proper psychological and psychotherapeutical knowledge in a suitable manner.

In *acute cases*, the most important goal of initial psychosomatic therapy (IPT) is the avoidance of further useless invasive dental treatment [*Brodine & Hartshorn 2004, Sarlani et al. 2005/b, Reewes & Merrill 2007, Baad-Hansen 2008*], especially because aggravation or spread of symptoms following invasive dental interventions may occur frequently [*Lesse 1956, Köling 1988, Sarlani et al. 2005/b, Toyofuku & Kikuta 2006*]. The prevention of symptom chronification is also crucial, because chronification (especially with prolonged unsuccessful somatic/operative dental therapy in the history) frequently render pain and other symptoms intractable [*Harris et al. 1993, Wöstmann 1996, Fábián 1999/a,b, Fábián et al. 2004/a, Toyofuku & Kikuta 2006*]. Prevention of symptom chronification can be carried out efficiently with the simple avoidance of repeating unsuccessful dental treatments in many cases, in other cases symptom-centered psychosomatic treatment should also be used.

Symptom-centered psychosomatic treatment may also lead to recovery in many cases, and solve the problem finally (definitively) [*Pomp 1974, Harris et al. 1993, Staats & Krause 1995, Wöstmann 1996, Schmierer 1997, Bongartz & Bongartz 2000, Bálint et al. 2003, Fábián et al. 2004/a*]. In other acute cases, there is some significant improvement, but there is no recovery of the symptoms during IPT [*Fábián & Fábián 1998; Fábián et al. 2002, Toyofuku & Kikuta 2006*]. In such cases another important aim of initial psychosomatic therapy (IPT) is to keep these patients in a psychosomatic therapeutic relationship and motivate them to participate in a definitive psychosomatic therapy (see below in *paragraph 6.2.2.*) [*Pomp 1974, Fábián & Fábián 1998; Fábián et al. 2002*].

In *chronic cases* the prognosis of IPT is rather poor [*Harris et al. 1993, Dahlström et al. 1997, Fábián et al. 2004/a*]. There is no significant improvement during IPT in roughly half of chronic oral symptoms [*Dahlström et al. 1997; Fábián et al. 2004/a, Schwichtenberg & Doering 2008*]. Therefore, majority of chronic patients would need proper definitive psychosomatic therapy. Consequently, besides reaching some improvement of the symptoms (if any), major goal of IPT in chronic case is avoidance of repetition of unsuccessful futile somatic/operative dental treatment [*Brodine & Hartshorn 2004*] and obtaining motivation of patients to participate in a definitive psychosomatic therapy [*Brodine & Hartshorn 2004, Demmel 2007*].

Gradual escalation of therapy and avoidance of irreversible forms of treatment [*Laskin & Block 1986*] are "cornerstones" of the initial psychosomatic therapy. The *first goal* of IPT in the management of patients is to provide them with some understanding of their problem [*Laskin & Block 1986*], even if patients often have difficulty accepting a psychophysiologic explanation for their disease [*Laskin & Block 1986*]. During this phase of IPT use of placebo and/or palliative methods (physiotherapies, medication, medicinal herb therapy, diet therapy, CAM therapy etc.) combined with supportive communication techniques may be an appropriate way [*Green & Laskin 1974, Laskin & Block 1986*] to decrease the symptoms, and to develop a good patient-dentist relationship. At this phase of IPT some of the cases may be solved, others may be improved and at least an increase of patients' understanding related to their symptoms may be reached.

Based on patients' improved understanding, *second goal* of IPT is to administer any mind-body therapies, which are the "basic therapeutics" for psychosomatic disorders [*Iversen 1989, Binder & Bider 1989, Krause 1994*]. Mind-body therapies advantageously improves psychogenic symptoms in most of the cases [*Bálint et al. 2003, Kaán et al. 2003, Fábián et al. 2002, 2005/a, 2006/a, 2009/c*] leading *either* to a recovery [*Bálint et al. 2003, Kaán et al. 2003, Fábián et al. 2002, 2005/a, 2006/a, 2009/c*] *or* to an improvement, coupled with increased motivation of patients to take part in a definitive therapeutic processes [*Fábián & Fábián 1998; Fábián et al. 2002, 2005/a, 2009/c*].

The *third goal* of IPT is to refer the patient to definitive therapy and to make sure that patient enters and participate in definitive therapy [*Fábián et al. 2002, 2005/a, 2009/c, Demmel 2007*]. Although the efficiency of initial psychosomatic therapy (IPT) strongly depends on the improvement of symptoms; using efficient symptom-centered treatments it should be always considered that, any psychogenic symptom may represent a defense against psychiatric decompensation [*Lesse 1956, Delaney 1976, Marbach 1978, Violon 1980, Kaban & Belfer 1981, Fábián 1999/b*]. Therefore, symptom-centered interventions should be administered carefully, resulting in slow-going, gradual decrease of the symptoms to prevent decompensation of the patient during IPT [*Kaban & Belfer 1981, Fábián 1999/b*].

6.2.2. Definitive Psychosomatic Therapy

Definitive psychosomatic therapy (DPT) is a highest level care of PDI patients utilizing any available dental, medical and psychotherapeutical treatment possibilities in an evidence based manner. Definitive psychosomatic therapy should be offered for patients being refractory to IPT [*Laskin & Block 1986*], and for patients responding to IPT but without a stable treatment outcome in a long run (i.e. patients with frequent relapses). Definitive psychosomatic therapy (DPT) is clearly *not* a scope of *every* dentist's duties. Definitive psychosomatic therapy should be carried out by *specialized dental professionals* [*Dahlström et al. 1997, Hertrich & Joraschky 1996, Dworkin et al. 2002, Fejérdy 2007*] as members of a specialized *psychosomatic team* including *experienced* dentists and other medical and psychotherapeutical professionals [*Hertrich & Joraschky 1996, Dworkin et al. 1994, 2002, Turner et al. 2006, Fejérdy 2007*].

Although clinical experiences clearly indicate that there is a major role of specialized dental professionals also in DPT in most cases [*Pomp 1974, Fábián 1999/a,b, Bálint et al. 2003, Fábián et al. 2004/a, 2005/a, Kaán et al. 2004*]; close collaboration with medical professionals (especially with psychiatrists and neurologists) and with psychotherapists is clearly needed for DPT [*Dahlström et al. 1997, Hertrich & Joraschky 1996, Von Korff 2005, Turner et al. 2006, Fejérdy 2007, Schwichtenberg & Doering 2008*]. Dentists having full-qualification in *psychotherapy* and/or *psychosomatic dentistry* seem to be the most adequate professionals to organize definitive psychosomatic therapy for PDI patients, especially because continuation of a psychosomatic supportive dental care is needed in most of the cases [*Laskin & Block 1986*].

It should be also considered that, PDI patients usually display a lower level of psychopathology comparing to psychiatric patients [*Meldolesi et al. 2000*] (see also *paragraph 2.5.1.*); but in some cases severe psychopathologies including psychoses may also appear as a background of PDI symptoms [*Lesse 1956, Delaney 1976, Marbach 1978, Violon 1980, Kaban & Belfer 1981, Fábián 1999/b*] (see also *paragraph 2.5.1.*). In such cases referral to psychiatrist and definitive *psychiatric* therapy (instead of *psychosomatic* therapy) is crucial; although a supportive type psychosomatic dental care is usually also needed for proper definitive treatment and for stabilizing oral functions and oral health.

6.2.3. After-Care

All patients including PDI patients who wear any fixed or removable dentures should have an annual examination [*Woelfel 1983*]. This examination should include an evaluation of the health of the orofacial tissues. Health of the supporting teeth and other supporting tissues as well as the condition, retention, stability and other relevant properties and quality of dentures should also be controlled carefully [*Woelfel 1983*]. PDI related psychogenic symptoms of patients should also be examined.

Although there are rather few studies about the efficiency of treatment of oral psychosomatic patients, it is likely that at least 50-60% of such patients significantly improve in their complaints [*Schwichtenberg & Doering 2008*]. Sometimes, especially in not yet chronic cases the success rate may be even higher [*Bálint et al. 2003, Kaán et al. 2003, Fábián et al. 2002, 2005/a, 2006/a, 2009/c*]. However, there is still a relatively large amount of patients without any success or with suffering from several residual symptoms.

Therefore, patients should be made aware that it may not be possible to provide a permanent cure for the problem, but that they can learn to manage in a satisfactory manner [*Laskin & Block 1986*]. Home practice of most mind-body therapies (see *paragraph 6.4.*), diet- and medicinal herb therapy (see *chapter 7.*) as well as CAM therapies (see *chapter 8.*) regularly supervised by the dentist (and/or other professionals) are good tools to manage such residual symptoms as well as to maintain clinical results and to prevent relapse [*Laskin & Block 1986, Fábián in press*]. In the case of relapse (or exacerbation) of the PDI symptoms, patients should be treated as described in respect of initial therapy (see *paragraph 6.2.1*).

6.2.4. Individual and Group Therapies

Because of limitations in therapists' capacity, group therapy seems to be a promising possibility [*Dworkin et al. 1994, Moore et al. 1996, Dahlström et al. 1997, Fábián et al. 2006/a, 2009/c Meyer-Lückel & Schiffner 2009*], even if individual therapy is most frequently used in the field of psychosomatic dentistry at the present time [*Fábián & Fábián 1998, Dworkin et al. 2002, Fábián et al. 2004/a, 2006/a, Kaán et al. 2004*]. Initial psychosomatic therapy is usually carried out as an individual therapy, because of the patients' usual need to be treated as a "dental patient with somatic/technical dental problems". In many cases, definitive psychosomatic therapies are also carried out as individual therapy because of the patient's need, or because of the features of the problem.

However, because of limitations in insurance coverage of psychosomatic therapies and the fact that many patients attend fewer than six sessions of psychotherapy (i.e. initial therapy) [*Shapiro et al. 2003*], there is a need of highly efficient therapies achieving significant improvement of both behavior and symptoms of patients [*Dworkin et al. 1994, 2002, Fábián & Fábián 1998, Fábián et al. 2002, 2005/a, Von Korff et al. 2005, Turner et al. 2005, 2006*]. Although such efficiency may also be achieved via individual therapies [*Fábián & Fábián 1998, Dworkin et al. 2002, Fábián et al. 2004/a, 2006/a*], utilization of the "group effect" (group dynamics) appearing under group therapies [*Wentz 1972, Moore & Brødsgaard 1994, Moore et al. 1996*] can be rather advantageous for keeping psychosomatic patients inside the therapy [*Fábián et al. 2006/a, 2009/c*].

In general, efficiency of mind-body therapies may be significantly increased when used as a group therapy [*Krause 1994, 2000, Fábián et al. 2005/a, 2006/a*]. Even the efficiency of biofeedback-based therapies may be improved in groups using portable biofeedback devices [*Hörnlein-Rummel 2001, Reiner 2008*]. Patients' clubs and online support groups are other promising possibilities of group therapy, which may be utilized for patient education, for after care purposes and for prevention of relapse.

6.3. PSYCHOTHERAPEUTIC APPROACHES

6.3.1. Client-Centered Therapy

The *client-centered therapy* emphasizes the *autonomy* of clients (and thus avoids the use of term "patient") and the healing effect of the *encounter* during psychotherapy [*Rogers 1965*]. It also emphasizes the *attitudinal qualities of the therapist* such as *warmth*, *empathy* and *genuineness* (congruence) [*Rogers 1965, Smith 2000*] as well as the ability of therapist to emphatically recognize and reflect ("mirror") the real sense behind the client's communication [*Rogers 1965*]. Autonomy of client together with the encounter and the attitudinal qualities of the therapist help patient (client) to remove inside obstacles of personality development, and to become their best possible self [*Rogers 1965, Smith 2000*]. Client-centered therapy is a basic approach, which can be used as an individual therapy as well as a group therapy (*encounter groups*). It also serves as an important base for many other more specific approaches, and for any professional interpersonal relationship including patient-dentist relationship [*Bensing 2000*]. Client-centered approach can be used in psychosomatic dentistry as well especially for PDI patients [*Fábián et al. 2004/a, 2006/a, in press*].

6.3.2. Behavioral Therapy

Behavioral therapy is an operationalized approach, which has its roots in classical learning theory and other findings of experimental psychology [Watson & Rayner 1920, Millner & Dollard 1941, Skinner 1953, Wolpe 1958, Bandura & Walters 1963]. It focuses on current determinants of behavior and draws on the principles of learning to develop individual treatment strategies [de Silva 2000, Smith 2000]. The focus in behavior therapy is the presenting problem itself; and it is not assumed that the presenting problem is a manifestation of an underlying primary problem [de Silva 2000, Smith 2000]. The aim of behavior therapy is to modify the problem behavior at a behavioral level [de Silva 2000, Smith 2000].

The key cornerstones of this approach are the principles of Pavlov's classical conditioning and those of operant or instrumental conditioning [Skinner 1953] as well as reciprocal inhibition (desensitization) [Wolpe 1958] and social learning [Millner & Dollard 1941, Bandura & Walters 1963]. Although in this approach more emphasis is placed on "what patients do than what they say"; however it does not avoid completely the issue of the meaning of the behavior targeted or the meaning of the relationship between the therapist and the patient [Smith 2000]. The incorporation of cognitive therapy principles also occurred in the sixties and seventies of last century, which eventually led to what is today referred to as cognitive-behavioral therapy [de Silva 2000] (see also paragraph 6.3.3.).

Behavioral approach was used efficiently in dentistry, for the treatment of myofascial pain [Komiyama et al. 1999], to decrease clenching and clenching induced pain symptoms [Gale & Carlsson 1977] to treat gagging [Eli & Kleinhauz 1997] and to treat TMD patients [Dahlström 1989] as well as to reduce dental fear and odontophobia [Berggren & Linde 1984, Hammarstrand et al. 1995, Moore et al. 1996, Mehrstedt 1997, Jöhren et al. 2009]. Behavioral therapy may also be utilized efficiently for oral health education programs [Meyer-Lückel & Schiffner 2009]. This approach may also be used highly efficiently for pain management, in combination with other therapies such as relaxation (see paragraph 6.4.1.), biofeedback (see paragraph 6.4.6.) breathing exercises (see paragraph 8.4.) and posture correction exercises [Komiyama et al. 1999]. Behavior therapy may also be used efficiently in combination with hypnotherapy [Fábián 1996/a, Eli & Kleinhauz 1997, Mehrstedt 1997] (see also paragraph 6.4.2.).

6.3.3. Cognitive Therapy and Cognitive-Behavioral Therapy

Cognitive therapy is based on the assumption that, the person's feelings and behavior are determined by the way in which their experiences are processed cognitively [*Ellis 1962, Beck 1976*]. In this approach, *irrational determinants* of thoughts (i.e. *spontaneously appearing negative thoughts, errors of logical thoughts*, and *depressive cognitive schemes* [*Beck 1976*]) are assumed as a major cause of several pathopsychological conditions [*Ellis 1962, Beck 1976*]. Therefore, cognitive therapy aims to decrease premised maladaptive irrational cognitions and to increase adaptive cognitions of patients [*Fava 2000, de Silva 2000, Smith 2000*]. Cognitive therapy can be advantageously combined with behavioral therapy (see *paragraph 6.3.2.*) and these two approaches are often so interwoven with each other that the term *cognitive-behavioral therapy* (CBT) is used [*Fava 2000, de Silva 2000, Smith 2000*].

Cognitive-behavioral therapy includes a number of diverse therapeutic procedures such as cognitive therapy [*Ellis 1962, Beck 1976*] including rational emotive psychotherapy [*Ellis 1977*] as well as problem solving interventions, persuasion, exposure (desensitization) based techniques, and well-being therapy [*Fava 2000*]. Similarly, to behavioral therapy, cognitive-behavioral therapy may also be combined advantageously with several other therapies [*Lazarus 1971*] including relaxation (see *paragraph 6.4.1.*), hypnosis (see *paragraph 6.4.2.*)

meditation (see *paragraph 6.4.4.*) biofeedback (see *paragraph 6.4.6.*) and breathing exercises (see *paragraph 8.4.*).

Cognitive-behavioral therapy (CBT) was efficient to reduce pain [*Dworkin et al. 1994, 2002, Von Korff et al. 2005*], activity limitations due to pain (pain-activity inference) [*Dworkin et al. 1994, 2002, Von Korff et al. 2005*] and pain related fear (fear avoidance) [*Von Korff et al. 2005*] of chronic pain patients in randomized controlled trials. Accordingly, CBT with progressive muscle relaxation (PMR) and abdominal/diaphragmatic breathing [*Turner et al. 2005, 2006*] was highly efficient to reduce pain-activity interference, pain intensity, depression, maladaptive pain beliefs, catastrophizing and to improve masticatory jaw function of TMD related orofacial pain patients in a randomized controlled trial (RCT) [*Turner et al. 2006*]. Cognitive-behavioral approach may also be used to treat idiopathic environmental intolerance [*Giardino & Lehrer 2000, Staudenmayer 2000*] including "amalgam illness" and other psychogenic symptoms attributed to dental materials. Depressive symptoms and relapse to major depression can be prevented efficiently using meditation treatment combined with cognitive therapy (MBCT) as well [*Teasdale et al. 2000, Barnhofer et al. 2007*]. CBT may also be used efficiently to reduce dental fear and to treat dental phobia [*Hammarstrand et al. 1995, Moore et al. 1996*].

6.3.4. Psychoanalysis and Psychoanalytic Psychotherapy

Psychoanalysis is a dept-psychological theory, focusing on unconscious psychological processes and their interrelationships with conscious psychological function, as well as on their role in pathopsychological phenomena. There are various theoretical streams of psychoanalysis, all of which have been integrated as psychoanalytic theory. Besides the fundamental *libido-theory* [*Freud 1923/a*] and *ego-psychology* [*Freud 1923/b, Freud 1936, Hartmann 1964, Mahler et al. 1975, Kernberg 1980*], *object-relationships theory* [*Klein 1932, Winnicott 1953, Guntrip 1969, Kernberg 1976*] and *self-theory* [*Kohut 1971*] are the most important such theories. Major therapeutical interventions of psychoanalysis are analysis of free associations [*Freud 1900*], analysis of resistance [*Freud 1920*], analysis of transference [*Freud 1912*], analysis of counter-transference [*Freud 1910*] and the related interpretations [*Freud 1900*]; whereas interventions that contain suggestions or directions are usually avoided [*Roazen 2000, Smith 2000*].

Psychoanalytic psychotherapy (also referred to as *dynamic psychotherapy* or *psychodynamic psychotherapy* [*Smith 2000*]) is a collective noon of those psychotherapeutic methods; which are strongly linked derivatives of psychoanalysis but with some significant modifications related to technique and goal [*Alexander & French 1946, Bálint 1949, 1956, Bálint et al. 1972, Ferenczi 1980, Smith 2000*]. This kind of therapies are usually less intense in frequency and length comparing to psychoanalysis, they can be explicitly supportive, and utilize modified analytic techniques which may be mixed also with some non-analytic techniques [*Alexander & French 1946, Bálint 1949,1956, Bálint et al. 1972, Ferenczi 1980, Smith 2000*]. There are also several short-term forms of psychoanalytic therapy (referred to as *brief dynamic psychotherapy*) which are explicitly problem focused and focal [*Alexander &*

French 1946, Malan 1963, Sifneos 1972, Bálint et al. 1972, Mann 1973, Davanloo 1978, Smith 2000].

There are some other psychotherapies, which are clearly rooted in (interrelated with) the psychoanalytic theory, but also have an own independent theoretical development; therefore are not referred to as "psychoanalytic" anymore [*Roazen 2000, Smith 2000, Fábián et al. 2005/b, Fábián et al. 2006/c*]. The most important such therapeutical approaches are *individual psychotherapy* [*Adler 1920*], *Jung's analytic psychology* [*Jung 1926, 1968*], *logotherapy* [*Frankl 1994*] and *existential psychotherapy* [*Yalom 1980, 1995*]. The psychoanalytic approach was also combined with hypnotherapy referred to as *hypnoanalysis* [*Kinzel 1993*]. It was also applied to religious thinking and used for treatment of religious patients within the frame of *pastoral-psychotherapy* [*Baumgartner 1990, Fábián et al. 2005/b, Fábián 2007*]. The psychoanalytic approach was also used efficiently in dentistry for the treatment of several psychosomatic symptoms [*Somer 1991, 1997, Eli & Kleinhaus 1997, Gáspár et al. 2002, Bálint et al. 2003, Kaán et al. 2003, 2004, Fábián et al. in press*].

6.3.5. Contraindication of Psychotherapy

Although in general there is no contraindication of psychotherapy, however level of qualification of the dentist (or other professionals) should determine the depth of psychotherapeutic intervention used for psychosomatic therapy. Deeper psychotherapeutic interventions targeting psychological structural changes of the personality should be avoided in the absence of full psychotherapeutic qualification. Deeper psychotherapeutic interventions should also be avoided in the case of severe pathologies in the absence of psychiatric support and professional background. Refusal of psychotherapy by the patient may also be considered as a contraindication. Some specific methods such as mind-body therapy based psychotherapeutic approaches may also have some specific contraindications (see more detailed in *paragraph 6.4.7.*)

6.4. MIND-BODY THERAPIES

6.4.1. Relaxation

Relaxation belongs to the natural behavior repertoire of human, but can also be induced by several methods following a learning process [*Tóth & Fábián 2006, Fábián in press*]. The most frequently used basic methods are simple eye-closure, standard exercises of Autogenic Training (sAT) [*Schultz 1932*], progressive muscle relaxation (PMR) [*Jacobson 1938*], and biofeedback assisted relaxation (BAR) [*Ray et al 1979*]. Relaxation induces a relaxing feeling, reduced arousal level, and reduced stress [*Benson 1975, Orne & Whitehouse 2000*]. Relaxation usually increases the alpha level of EEG comparing to stress conditions [*Benson et al. 1974*] and other non-stressful eye opened alert states [*Wallace 1970, Edmonston & Grotevant 1975, Morse et al. 1977*]. There are also some rare theta waveforms displayed in relaxation [*Warrenburg et al. 1980*]. Relaxation training seems to be coupled with activation of a discrete set of brain regions such as left anterior cingulate, globus pallidus, and inferior parietal lobule [Critchley et al. 2001]. Further, an area of the right anterior medial temporal lobe may also be activated correlating with the decrease of sympathetic tone [*Critchley et al. 2001*].

Besides brain correlates, relaxation decreases breath- and heart rate and also blood pressure [*Mathews & Gelder 1969, Morse et al. 1977, Nava et al. 2004*]. There is also a significant increase of respiratory sinus arrhythmia (HRV) in the high frequency band indicating increased parasympathetic cardiac control [*Cowan et al. 1990, Sakakibara et al. 1994, Nava et al. 2004*]. Relaxation also significantly increases skin resistance as a consequence of decreased sympathetic activity [*Wallace 1970, Morse et al. 1977, O'Halloran et al. 1985*]; and significantly decreases level of stress related hormones including cortisol [*Pawlow & Jones 2002; 2005*] and catecholamines [*Davidson et al. 1979*].

In relation with oral psychosomatic symptoms, relaxation may be used efficiently for the therapy of bruxism, myofascial pain and TMD symptoms of muscular dysfunction origin [*Biondi & Picardi 1993, Sarlani et al. 2005/a*]. Somatoform chronic pain may also be treated efficiently using progressive muscle relaxation (PMR) [*Kröner-Herwig et al. 1998, Derra 2003, Rehfisch & Basler 2004*]. Dental fear and dental phobia can also be treated with relaxation based methods [*Hammarstrand 1995, Moore et al. 1996*]. Relaxation may also be combined advantageously with numerous psychotherapeutic approaches. Accordingly, combination of progressive muscle relaxation with cognitive behavioral therapy (see in *paragraph 6.3.3.*) and abdominal/diaphragmatic breathing (see in *paragraphs 8.4.*) was highly efficient to reduce pain-activity interference, pain intensity, depression, maladaptive pain beliefs, catastrophizing and to improve masticatory jaw function of TMD related orofacial pain patients in a randomized controlled trial (RCT) [*Turner et al. 2006*].

6.4.2. Hypnosis

Hypnosis may be defined as an altered state of consciousness (ASC) achieved by suggestions. Numerous important theories were developed to explain hypnosis [*Orne 1959; Shor 1962, Bányai & Hilgard 1976, Hilgard 1991, Bányai 1991, Crawford & Gruzelier 1992*]. However, there is currently consensus only on that the real essence of hypnosis lies in the experienced subjective alteration of consciousness (ASC) [*Orne 1959; Varga et al. 2001*]. In this relation, altered state of consciousness (ASC) can be defined as sudden and transient subjective experience significantly different from those of common everyday experiences [*Ludvig 1966, Tart 1970, Kihlstrom 1984, Farthing 1992*].

ASC may induce significant changes of most *psychological functions* including attention, perceptions, sense of time, body image, self image, imagination, fantasy, cognition, emotions, arousal, memory, self-control, suggestibility, identity etc. [*Ludvig 1966, Tart 1970, Bányai 1980, Kihlstrom 1984, Pekala & Kumar 1989, Farthing 1992, Varga et al. 2001, Halsband et al. in press*]. Importantly, significant *pain relieving effect* also occur following induction of hypnotic state [*Zeltner & LeBaron 1982; Gokli et al. 1994; Faymonville et al. 1995, 1997; Fábián & Fábián 1998*]; which can be influenced (i.e. increased or decreased) significantly using specific suggestions [*Meier et al. 1993; Rainville et al. 1997, 1999; Fábián & Fábián 1998; Castel et al. 2007, Gáspár et al. 2003*].

Functional neuroanatomical studies of pain modulation indicated that, alteration of nociception under hetero-hypnotic state are primarily mediated by the midcingulate area of anterior cingulate cortex (ACC) [*Rainville et al. 1997, 1999; Faymonville et al. 2000, 2006*]; in functional connectivity with left and right insula, perigenual cortex of ACC, pre-supplementary motor cortex, superior frontal gyrus, right thalamus, right caudate nucleus, midbrain and brainstem [*Faymonville et al. 2003, 2006*]. Anticipations and expectations related to both painfulness [*Larbig et al. 1982*] and painlessness [*Benedetti et al. 2003, 2006*] likely play pivotal role under hypnotic conditions as well. Similarly, learning- [*Colloca & Benedetti 2006*] and conditioning processes [*Benedetti et al. 2003*] and also released placebo/nocebo responses [*Benedetti et al. 2003, 2005, Benedetti 2006*] may also be crucial factors. Some environmental circumstances like restricted environmental stimulation may also play important role [*Barabasz 1982, Barabasz & Barabasz 1989*]. Distraction or engagement of attention also significantly influences pain perception [*Miltner et al. 1989, Larbig 2004, Kingston et al. 2007*].

Data indicate that, changes of attentional function during hypnosis may induce dissociation of several psychological functions [*Hilgard 1991, 1994*] including dissociation of sensory and affective components of pain [*Meier et al. 1993*] as well as other pain related functions including generation of pain at the periphery, sensitization of secondary sensory neurons, modulation of endocrine-, immune- or autonomic responses and modulation of psychological functions [*Miltner et al. 1992, Larbig 2004, Carli 2009, Vanhaudenhuyse et al. 2009*]. Besides pain perception, *other physiological functions* such as autonomic and hormonal responses, neuromuscular function, immune surveillance [*Gruzelier et al. 2001, Gruzelier 2002, Mawdsley et al. 2008*] and immune/inflammatory reactions [*Black et al. 1963, Fábián 1996/c, Gruzelier 2002, Mawdsley et al. 2008*] may also be advantageously influenced using hypnosis.

Hypnosis can also be used efficiently in dentistry. Dental hypnosis can be used as a noninvasive therapeutic option to increase treatment comfort and operative circumstances [*Ament & Ament 1970, Fábián 1996/b, Fábián & Fábián 1998, Fejérdy et al. 2003, Fábián et al. 2009/c, Rauch & Hermes 2008*]. It is also frequently used in prevention and treatment of needle phobia [*Gokli et al. 1994, Staats & Krause 1995, Schmierer 1997, Cyna et al. 2007*] and other dental phobias [*Staats & Krause 1995, Schmierer 1997, Fábián & Fábián 1998; Hermes et al. 2003*]. Hypnotherapy may also be used efficiently to avoid occurrence of panic attacks during dental treatment of panic disorder patients [*Fabian 1996/a, Fábián 1999/a*]. Gagging may also be improved efficiently using hypnosis [*Ament & Ament 1970, Staats & Krause 1995, Schmierer 1997, Gáspár et al. 2002*].

Hypnosis may also be used for the treatment of bruxism [*Clarke 1997, Eli & Kleinhaus 1997, Fábián & Fábián 1998*] and other neuromuscular symptoms [*Staats & Krause 1995, Chaves 1997, Eli & Kleinhaus 1997, Schmierer 1997*]. Myofascial pain, atypical facial pain oropyrosis and other psychogenic pain may also be treated efficiently [*Staats & Krause 1995, Chaves 1997, Eli & Kleinhaus 1997, Schmierer 1997, Fábián & Fábián 1998, 2000, Fábián et al. 2007/a*] Trigeminal neuralgia pain was also efficiently improved with hypnosis in a case [*Schmierer 2004*]. Hypnosis may be used highly efficiently also in the treatment of PDI [*Ament & Ament 1970, Staats & Krause 1995, Barsby 1997, Eli & Kleinhaus 1997, Schmierer 1997, Fábián & Fábián 2000, Fábián et al. 2007/a*]. Hypnoanalytic methods may also be used to uncover and resolve orofacial symptom-causing psychoemotional conflicts [*Ament & Ament 1970, Somer 1991, 1997, Eli & Kleinhaus 1997*].

6.4.3. Self-Hypnosis

Self-hypnosis may be defined as an altered state of consciousness (ASC) achieved by self-suggestions [*Anbar & Savedoff 2005*]. During practicing self-hypnosis, a deep hypnoid trance state (altered state of consciousness) develops [*Barolin 1990, Leuner 1990/b, Krause 1994*] similarly to those of hypnosis (see above). Autosuggestive techniques have been widely used from the earliest time of history [*Heinze 1993, Hoppál 1993/a,b*] but self-suggestions stood in the limelight of scientific interest in the last century only [*Baudouin 1920, Coué 1922, Schultz 1932, Salter 1941, Mészáros 1984*]. There are several methods may be classified as self-hypnosis including (self)imagination techniques [*Jung 1916, Amman 1978, Simonton et al. 1982, Achtenberg 1987*], active-graded-(self)hypnosis [*Kretschmer 1946, Langen 1969*], and biofeedback coupled techniques [*Leuner 1997, Barolin 2001, Egner et al. 2002*]. Photo-acoustic stimulation (see in *paragraph 6.4.5.*) may also be used to induce peculiar self-hypnotic states. The prototype of self-hypnotic methods is Autogenic Training (AT) [*Schultz 1932*], which is based on giving suggestions toward phenomena spontaneously occurring under relaxation to amplify and control them [*Schultz 1932, Krause 1994*].

Self-hypnosis practice can be resulted in prolonged increase of overall mental health [*Kröner & Beitel 1980*], including decrease of depression scores [*Hidderley & Holt 2004, Hudacek 2007*], (trait)anxiety level [*Benson et al. 1978, Whitehouse et al. 1996, Hidderley & Holt 2004*], perceived stress scores [*Whitehouse et al. 1996*] and increase of self-observed level of mental energy [*Gruzelier et al. 2001*] as well as improved sleep quality under stress conditions [*Whitehouse et al. 1996, Anbar & Slothower 2006*]. Sleeplessness (light sleep, disturbed sleep, insomnia) of patients can also be improved significantly using several self-hypnotic methods [*Krause 1994, Anbar & Slothower 2006*].

Self-hypnosis may be used for the treatment of anxiety disorder [*Benson et al. 1978; Leuner & Schroeter 1997*], several phobias [*Leuner & Schroeter 1997*], and to reduce dental treatment related acute fear reactions [*Taylor 1995/a, Shaw & Niven 1996*]. There is also a significant pain relieving effect of self-hypnosis [*Larbig 1994, Jenkins 1995, Burkle et al. 2005*], which may be used for reducing procedural pain effectively [*Jenkins & Pritchard 1994, Jenkins 1995*]. Post-operative pain can also be reduced efficiently with self-hypnotic methods [*Jenkins 1995*]. Wound healing may also be improved using self-hypnosis [*Rucklidge & Saunders 1999*].

Self-hypnosis may also be used efficiently for most forms of somatoform disorders; including somatoform chronic pain [*Leuner & Schroeter 1997, Fábián & Fábián 1998, Derra 2003, Pielsticker 2004*], pseudoneurological symptoms, autonomic dysfunction, pruritus (itching), several motor symptoms, fatigue (etc.) [*Leuner & Schroeter 1997, Bongartz & Bongartz 2000, Winkler & Krause 1989, Gerber 1990, Stetter 1985*]. Muscle activity may also be decreased promptly under self-hypnotic condition [*Morse et al. 1977*]. Myoclonic movements [*Sugimoto et al. 2007*] and tic-disorder [*Lang 2004*] can also be decreased efficiently using self-hypnotic methods. Self- hypnosis was also reported as an efficient method for the treatment of certain forms of tinnitus [*Leuner & Schroeter 1997*]. Allergic symptoms [*Wyler-Harper et al. 1994; Langewitz et al. 2005*] and allergic activity evaluated *via* skin test [*Teshima et al. 1982*] can also be improved using self-hypnosis.

Self-hypnosis training may also improve immune function including *prompt* increase of salivary immunoglobulin A (sIgA) [*Olness et al. 1989*], prompt increase of adherence of neutrophile granulocytes (PMN cells) [*Hall et al. 1993*], and *sustained* elevation (or prevention of the decline) of NK cell count [*Gruzelier et al. 2001, Naito et al. 2003, Hudacek 2007*] and $CD8^+$ cell count [*Gruzelier et al. 2001, Naito et al. 2003, Hidderley & Holt 2004*] under stress conditions. Self-hypnosis also increased the numbers of NK, $CD3^+$, and $CD8^+$ cells and increased herpes (HSV-2) virus specific functional NK cell activity with significant overall reduction in the number of reported episodes of recurrent mucosal (genital) herpes [*Fox et al. 1999, Gruzelier et al. 2006*].

6.4.4. Meditation

Although there are several forms of meditation, and no two meditation practices are alike in all features [*Ospina et al. 2007, Halsband et al. in press*] meditation can be defined as *volitional self-induced altered state of consciousness* (ASC), *established by mental faculties*, without *dominant* contribution of other persons, *highly intense* body exercises or use of *drugs* [*Fábián in press*]. Practices of meditation may be divided into two subgroups such as *concentrative type* and *nonconcentrative type* methods [*Orne & Whitehouse 2000, Fábián in press*]. Although concentrative and nonconcentrative approaches differ from each other, the subjective experience of *deeper* stages seems to be rather similar phenomenologically. Finally both group of meditation techniques, lead to a state of "Being", a state of "Knowing" or "Experiencing" without objectification and discursive thinking [*Maharishi 1963, Heinze 1993, Newberg & Iversen 2003, von Brück 2003; Kabat-Zinn 2005, Deskmuth 2006, Fábián in press*]. In religious form of meditation (see also *paragraph 8.2.*), premised deep meditative states and experiences have certain religious overtones [*Fábián in press*].

Deep meditative states usually induce highly increased theta activity roughly in all regions of the brain [*Banquet 1973, Coromaldi et al. 2004*]. Alpha activity also frequently shows significant increase under meditation [*Morse et al 1977, Coromaldi et al. 2004, Takahasi et al 2005, Halsband et al. in press*]; however transition of alpha waves to theta with consequent relative decrease of alpha power may also occur [*Banquet 1973, Jacobs & Lubar 1989, Jacobs & Friedmann 2004*]. Beta activity shows a global tendency toward decrease [*Tebécis 1975, Coromaldi et al. 2004*], whereas there is no general tendency related to gamma activity [*Lehmann et al. 2001, Coromaldi et al. 2004*] and lateralization [*Travis & Wallace 1999, Aftanas & Golocheikine 2001, Takahashi et al. 2005, Previc 2006*]. Local activations of certain brain areas as well as prompt autonomic and hormonal changes are strongly dependent on technique of meditation [*Fábián in press*].

There is also an overall improvement of *psychological abilities* of meditators [*Gaylord et al. 1989, Davis & O'Neill 2005, Shapiro et al. 2007*] leading to more efficient social functioning [*Esch et al. 2007, Smith et al. 2007*] and improved stress tolerance [*Benson 1996, 1997, Esch et al. 2002/a,b*] coupled with decreased level of neuroticism [*Gaylord et al. 1989*], depression [*Weber et al. 2002*], (trait)anxiety [*Benson et al. 1978, Gaylord et al. 1989,*

Walton et al. 1995, Galvin et al. 2006], trait negative affect [*Davidson et al. 2003*], stress induced emotional irritability [*Carlson et al. 2003*] and stress induced anger [*Weber et al. 2002*]. Long-run training of meditation also shortens habituation of stressful stimuli [*Orme-Johnson 1973, Gaylord et al. 1989*], and decreases the level of perceived stress [*Jain et al. 2007; Smith et al. 2007, Lucini et al. 2007*]. Meditation may also be used to treat anxiety disorder [*Benson et al. 1978, Raskin et al. 1980*]. Relapse to major depression [*Teasdale et al. 2000, Barnhofer et al. 2007*] can also be prevented using nonconcentrative type (MBCT) meditation treatment. There is also a possible anti-ageing neuroprotective effect of meditation [*Pagnoni & Cekic 2007*] including improved correlation of gray matter volume with age [*Pagnoni & Cekic 2007*] and increased cortical thickness [*Lazar et al. 2005*] which may offset cognitive decline associated with normal ageing [*Lazar et al. 2005, Pagnoni & Cekic 2007*].

Meditative states also possess highly efficient *anti-nociceptive effects* [*Larbig 1988, 1994, 2004, Jenkins 1995, Burkle et al. 2005, Kakigi et al. 2005, Peper et al. 2006*]. Sustained increase of pain tolerance [Kingston et al. 2007], reduction of pain induced distress [*Mills & Farrow 1981*] and reduced reactivity to pain in total brain [*Orme-Johnson et al. 2006*], thalamus [*Kakigi et al. 2005, Orme-Johnson et al. 2006*], prefrontal cortex [*Orme-Johnson et al. 2006*], anterior cingulate cortex (ACC) [*Kakigi et al. 2005, Orme-Johnson et al. 2006*] and insula [*Kakigi et al. 2005*] was also reported following meditation training. There is also a decrease of neuropeptide induced (neurogenic) inflammatory reactions under meditative state [*Lutgendorf et al. 2000*], which may be an important pathway of certain antinociceptive effects as well. Chronic pain can also be reduced significantly via meditation [*Castel et al. 2007*].

There are also significant sustained changes of *autonomic functions*. Frequency of rapid transient changes of skin resistance decreases following long-run practicing meditation [*Orme-Johnson 1973*]. Accordingly, decreased level of norepinephrine metabolites in urine [*Walton et al. 1995*] and decreased morning and evening serum levels and absence of diurnal rhythm of norepinephrine were found in long-run practitioners of meditation [*Infante et al. 2001*]. Decrease of morning (but not evening) serum level of epinephrine and consequent absence of diurnal rhythm also occurred [*Infante et al. 2001*], and daily rhythm of serum dopamine level was disappeared [*Infante et al. 2001*]. Premised changes of skin resistance and level of catecholamines are likely to indicate a more balanced and significantly decreased sympathetic activity as a result of meditation practice.

Level of *stress hormone cortisol* can also be decreased significantly using meditation practices. Baseline plasma [*MacLean et al. 1997*] and urine [*Walton et al. 1995*] level of cortisol can also be decreased following long-run practice of meditation [*Walton et al. 1995, MacLean et al. 1997*]. Salivary cortisol values under stress condition may also be decreased [*Cruess et al. 2000*]. Cortisol response to metabolic stressor (measured in both saliva and urine) was also decreased in long-term practitioners of meditation [*Walton et al. 2004*].

Prompt [*Travis et al. 1976, Morse et al. 1977, Delmonte 1984*] and also sustained [*Warrenburg et al. 1980, Shaw & Dettmar 1990*] decrease of *muscle tension* also occurs rather consistently in relation with meditation training, and most kinds of meditation also improve *complex motor functions* and neuromuscular coordination [*Shaw & Dettmar 1990, Egner & Gruzelier 2003, Raymond et al. 2005*], including also coordination of masticatory

[*Shaw & Dettmar 1990*] and craniomandibular [*Shaw & Dettmar 1990*] function. Importantly, improvement of motor functions are clearly not because of any specific movement exercises [*Shaw & Dettmar 1990*] indicating that, muscular function can be improved by mental faculties alone [*Egner & Gruzelier 2003, Raymond et al. 2005*].

Immune functions also shows rather consequent *immediate* and also *sustained* enhance of immune surveillance under most type of meditation [*Gruzelier 2002, Fábián in press*], including *prompt* increase of secretory immunoglobulin A (sIgA) [*Janoski & Kugler 1987, Pawlow & Jones 2005*] and HSP70/HSPA type chaperokines [*Fábián et al. 2004/b, in press*] in the saliva as well as *sustained* increase of NK cell function [*Zachariae et al. 1990*].

6.4.5. Photo-Acoustic Stimulation

Early studies demonstrated that turning the light or sound on and off induce alpha desynchronization on EEG [*Berger 1930, Walter et al. 1946*], leading to powerful stimulating effect on the central nervous system for a short time. In contrast, long lasting stimulation with flash light and tone signals (5-10 Hz frequency) leads to drowsiness and mixed alpha-theta activity [*Williams & West 1975*] coupled with body relaxation [*Brauchli 1993*] and appearance of significantly altered state of consciousness [*Fábián et al. 2002*]. These data indicate that, photo-acoustic stimulation whereas helps to keep the body relaxed, activates psychophysiological functions conducive to meditation (ASCs) coupled with somewhat increased arousal level [*Fábián et al. 2005/a, in press*]. Photo-acoustic stimulation also exerts anti-depressive properties [*Fábián et al. 2005/a, in press*].

Besides premised effects, flash light stimuli interact with the visual imagination leading to spontaneous appearance of various aspecific colored simple forms (i.e.: line, curve, web, lattice, spiral, cloud, tunnel etc.) [*Fábián et al. 2005/a, in press*] similar to those induced by several hallucinogens in the phase of non-complex images [*Siegel & Jarvik 1975, Siegel 1977*]. (Using lower light intensities real visual imaginations may also appear [*Fábián et al. 2005/a, in press*].) Since such visual imaginations appear spontaneously, a delightful experience of altered state of consciousness can be achieved even in case of patients with low motivation such as PDI patients [*Fábián et al. 2005/a, 2006/a, in press*].

Photo-acoustic stimulation also improves immune surveillance. Both secretory immunoglobulin A [*Brauchli 1993*] and salivary chaperokine HSP70/HSPA [*Fábián et al. 2004/b*] (a salivary defense protein, molecular chaperone and cytokine [*Fábián et al. 2003, 2007/b, 2008/a,b,c*]) were increased significantly under photo-acoustic stimulation induced meditative state. Similarly, other oral defense proteins such as salivary amylase [*Fábián et al. 2002, 2004/b*] and salivary lysozyme [*authors' unpublished data*] were also increased under premised meditative state. (Please note that: salivary amylase is proposed to inhibit microbial growth [*Shugars & Wahl 1998*]; whereas lysozyme is bacteriolytic for gram-positive bacteria and enhances phagocytic activity of PMN cells and macrophages [*Kokoshis et al. 1978; Dommett et al. 2005*].) All premised changes induced by photo-acoustic stimulation are advantageous and significantly improve general health and defense of the oral cavity [*Fábián et al. 2007/b, 2008/a,b,c,d*]; leading to clinical improvement of several oral mucosal symptoms especially of psychosomatic origin [*Fábián & Fábián 2000, Fábián et al. 2005/a; 2007/a, in press*].

Somatoform orofacial chronic pain can also be treated efficiently using photo-acoustic stimulation [*Fábián et al. 2002, 2005/a, 2006/a, in press, Bálint et al. 2003*]. Improvement of salivary gland function including significant increase of both flow rate and protein concentration following photo-acoustic stimulation treatment was also reported [*Kaán et al. 2003, Fábián et al. in press*]. Premised improvement of salivary gland function is likely because of a prolonged decrease of sympathetic activity following treatment [*Kaán et al. 2003*]; notwithstanding that, there is a prompt, but short-term sympathetic activation under photo-acoustic stimulation. Tinnitus was also improved using photo-acoustic stimulation [*Tönnies 2006*]. Photo-acoustic stimulation was also used efficiently in the treatment of PDI cases [*Fábián et al. 2004/a, 2006/a, in press*]. Photo-acoustic stimulation may be used highly efficiently also as a group-therapy [*Fábián et al. 2006/a, in press*].

6.4.6. Biofeedback Methods

Biofeedback methods alter patient's physiological processes using devices that amplify signs of physiological processes that are ordinarily difficult to perceive without some type of amplification [*Forgione & Mehler 2006*]. Patients use the provided feedback signals as a guide. Measurable parameters of body functions coupled with relaxation such as muscle tension (EMG), skin conductance level (GSR or SCL), heart rate, heart rate variability (HRV) and skin temperature may be used efficiently for biofeedback treatment of orofacial psychosomatic patients [*Forgione & Mehler 2006*]. Feedback of breathing with light and sound signals called *respiratory feedback* (RFB) [*Leuner 1984, 1997, Barolin 2001*] may also be used efficiently, because advantageous psychophysiological effects of breathing exercises (see *paragraph 8.4.*) and photo-acoustic stimuli (see *paragraph 6.4.5.*) also succeed in this case. Spontaneous appearance of altered state of consciousness was reported in significant proportion of subjects learning relaxation with the assistance of biofeedback equipment [*McKee 1980, Leuner 2001*] indicating that, therapeutic suggestions given under biofeedback may also be used highly efficiently [*Leuner 2001*].

Biofeedback methods, (especially EMG-biofeedback)   decrease muscle tension [*Zaichkowsky & Kamen 1978, McGrady et al. 1981, Dahlström et al. 1982, Forgione & Mehler 2006*], and may be used efficiently for the therapy of bruxism and TMD symptoms of muscular dysfunction origin [*Carlson et al. 1975, Carlsson & Gale 1977, Biondi & Picardi 1993, Korn 2005, Forgione & Mehler 2006*], as well as for the treatment of myofascial pain [*Forgione & Mehler 2006, Kreiner et al. 2001, Glaros 2006*]. Myoclonic movements may also be decreased efficiently with EMG-biofeedback methods [*Sugimoto et al. 2007*]. Feedback of evoked occlusal sonographic signals [*Watt 1966/a,b*] may also be used to improve patients' motor abilities for closure movements [*Fábián et al. 2005, Fábián 2007*]; which may lead to the decrease of perceived occlusal interferences and improvement of occlusal dysesthesia.

Importantly, EMG feedback signals of normal (chewing, speaking, swallowing, laughing) and abnormal (grinding, clenching) masseter activity can be recognized and clearly distinguish from each other *via* pattern recognition programs on computer [*Gallo et al. 1998*]. This provides the opportunity to monitor parafunction (and to warn patient when parafunction occur) all day long and during sleep also in natural environment (home, workplace) using portable long-term EMG biofeedback devices [*Gallo et al 1998, 1999, Glaros 2006, Mizumori et al. 2009*]. Accordingly, EMG biofeedback (monitoring) may also be used in the daily practice to identify artificial premature occlusal contact induced disturbance of muscle function after insertion of a new denture [*Learreta et al. 2007*].

Somatoform chronic pain may also be treated efficiently using several biofeedback methods [*Collett et al. 1986, Blanchard 1992, Flor & Birbaumer 1993, Leuner 2001, Loesch 2001, Derra 2003; Kröner-Herwig 2004*]. Other somatoform symptoms including pseudoneurological symptoms, autonomic dysfunction, pruritus (itching), several motor symptoms, fatigue (etc.) may also be treated efficiently with several biofeedback methods [*Winkler & Krause 1989, Basotti & Whitehead 1997, Martin & Rief 2006, Leuner 2001, Horinek 2001*]. Tinnitus may also be improved with several biofeedback methods [*Grossan 1976, House et al. 1977, Ganz 1983, White et al. 1986, Leuner 2001*]. Sleeplessness (light sleep, disturbed sleep, insomnia) of patients can also be improved with biofeedback [*Krause 1983, Niepoth & Korn 2006*]. Biofeedback methods may also be used for the treatment of anxiety disorder [*Raskin et al. 1980, Rice et al. 1993, Kroymann 2006, Reiner 2008*], panic disorder [*Bergdorf 2001, Kroymann 2006*], as well as for the treatment of high dental fear and dental phobia [*Hammarstrand et al 1995*]. Biofeedback can also be used efficiently to reduce treatment related acute fear reactions [*Litt et al. 1993, Hammarstrand et al 1995*]. Biofeedback (RFB) was also reported as an efficient method to reduce depressive symptoms [*Leuner 2001*]. Biofeedback methods may also improve immune function [*Taylor 1995/b*].

6.4.7. Contraindication of Mind-Body Therapies

Contraindications of mind-body therapies include several prepsychotic- and psychotic conditions [*Walsh & Roche 1979; Leuner 1990/a; Leuner & Schroeter 1997; Sethi & Bhargava 2003; Peter 2006; Kuijpers et al. 2007*], dementia and other deficiency of intelligence [*Leuner 1990/a; Leuner & Schroeter 1997*] and also narcolepsy [*Mészáros 1984; Leuner & Schroeter 1997*]. Mind-body therapies may also be contraindicated under acute psychic trauma (crisis) because of increased liability toward regression of the patient [*Fábián in press*]. Treatment of borderline and narcissistic patients [*Leuner 1990/a; Leuner & Schroeter 1997; Peter 2006*], strongly depressive or hysteric patients [*Leuner 1990/a*], introverted patients [*Leuner & Schroeter 1997*] and also hypochondria patients [*Leuner & Schroeter 1997*] may also be contraindicated.

Great care should be taken with somatic diseases of unknown origin [*Leuner & Schroeter 1997*], because palliation of symptoms via mind-body techniques may impede definitive diagnosis of dangerous diseases (if any) [*Leuner & Schroeter 1997*]. A possible disadvantageous parasympathetic "rebound" effect (parasympathetic "overshoot") induced by generalized relaxation of asthmatic patients was also expected in a study [*Lehrer et al. 1997*]. For the sake of completeness it can be noted that, increased epilepsy risk of meditation was also expected [*Jaseja 2005, 2006/a,b, Nicholson, 2006*]; but these expectations are likely exaggerated [*Barnes 2005, Orme-Johnson 2005, Fábián in press*].

Photo-acoustic stimulation induced ASCs should be avoided in case of epileptic patients (danger of visually induced seizure) [*Lindemuth et al. 2000; Fábián et al. 2005/a, in press*], in several eye disorders (especially glaucoma) [*Kreyer 1996; Fábián et al. 2005/a, in press*] and also in case of blepharospasm [*Kaji et al. 1999, Fábián et al. 2005/a, in press*]. Photo-acoustic stimulation should also be used carefully in case of pregnancy, cardiac problems, pacemaker patients and other strongly compromised health conditions because of its strong influence on the central and autonomic nervous system [*Kreyer 1996, Fábián et al. 2005/a, in press, Fábián in press*].

6.5. PHYSICOTHERAPIES

6.5.1. Massage

Massage is a therapeutic friction, stroking, kneading or shaking of a part of the body [*Laney 1983, Lund et al. 2006*]. Massage aid the return of venous blood, lymph, and catabolites into the main circulation and therefore may reduce muscle pain [*Laskin & Block 1986*] or other symptoms. *Facial massage* therapy may reduce chronic orofacial pain [*Gellrich et al. 2002, Lund et al. 2006*]. Massage of painful masticatory muscles of myofascial pain patients may also be helpful to reduce muscle pain and spasm [*Laskin & Block 1986, Sarlani et al. 2005/a, Lund et al. 2006*]. Function of the salivary glands (including secretion of total protein, amylase and salivary chaperone HSPA/HSP70) may also be improved due to massage treatment [*Fejérdy et al. 2004*]. Besides amelioration of chronic pain, level of anxiety and depression of patients may also be decreased due to massage treatment [*Lund et al. 2006*].

Massage may also be used intraorally for mucosal conditioning of edentulous patients [*Laney 1983*], which may be especially advantageous before fabrication of the first complete denture. The simplest method involves digital stimulation and can be done by the patient at regular intervals over the ridge tissues and border areas to be contacted by the denture base [*Laney 1983*]. Massage of the ridge mucosa with an automatic tooth brush with soft bristles used daily for 15 seconds may also used for mucosal conditioning [*Kapur & Shklar 1962, Laney 1983*]. Massage of intraoral soft tissues may also be carried out due to chewing bubble gum (chewing gum, an amount of 4 to 6 pieces) for 15 minutes twice a day with the denture out of the mouth [*Laney 1983*]. (Importantly, this latter method is likely to improve oral mucosal defense as well, since chewing significantly increases the level of salivary sIgA [*Proctor & Carpenter 2001*], salivary chaperone HSPA/HSP70 [*Fábián et al. 2003*] as well as salivary amylase [*Fábián et al. 2003*] levels.)

A unique way of intraoral massage treatment is the intra oral "mouth douche" (*hydro-massage*) using high-pressure water administration. Use of warm saline solution for such intraoral hydro-massage usually soothes the intraoral tissues, and may be used efficiently for mucosal conditioning of complete denture wearers [*Laney 1983*]. Administration of a *hot* water "douche" intraorally may lead to a combined effect of intra oral hydro-massage and intraoral heat treatment (see also *paragraph 6.5.5.*).

6.5.2. Muscle Exercises (Masticatory and Facial Muscles)

Muscle exercises of masticatory muscles may be used efficiently for the initial therapy of muscular dysfunctions of both psychogenic and occlusal origin [*Boos 1959, Mikami 1977, Laney 1983, Schulte 1988, Dahlström 1992*], including PDI coupled muscular dysfunctions. Their goal is to re-train the incoordinated masticatory musculature [*Boos 1959, Laney 1983, Schulte 1988*] and to improve the metabolic processes of the muscles. Maximum biting force and chewing performance may also be increased with certain chewing exercises [*Kawamura & Horio 1989*]. Physicokinetic therapy may also reduce chronic orofacial pain [*Gellrich et al. 2002*]. Careful daily stretching of painful masticatory muscles of myofascial pain and/or myospasm patients may also be useful [*Boos 1959, Clark 1981, Laney 1983, Sarlani et al. 2005/a*]. Careful jaw exercises may also be used for the treatment of TMJ osteoarthritis patients [*Boos 1959, Laney 1983, Sarlani et al. 2005/a*]. Muscle exercises may also be used for conditioning muscles before the fabrication of new dentures [*Boos 1959, Laney 1983*].

For most purposes above, three patterns of sequential movements of the mandible may be used 4 times daily for periods of 2 to 3 minutes as follows [*Boos 1959, Laney 1983*]: (1) maximal opening position held for 30 seconds and followed by relaxation (without tooth contact); (2) jaw movements to the right (and subsequently to the left) in a slow continuous stretch held for 30 seconds and followed by returning to the rest position; (3) the mandible is protruded held for 30 seconds and then retruded to the resting posture [*Boos 1959, Laney 1983*]. Further, a practice of forced bite (bite as hard as "possible" for a minute and then relax for a minute) repeated five times during each of six sessions scattered throughout a day may *extinguish* bruxist behavior, and may lead to significant improvement of bruxism patients after few weeks [*Mikami 1977*].

Training the patients to try to keep their teeth in light contact with their tongue resting against their palate may be helpful to improve occlusal discomfort or dysesthesia or to prevent several related tongue-parafunctions like storing a thick wedge of tongue in between their teeth [*Mew 2004*]. Similarly, constant repetition of coordinated muscle exercises can help patients to learn muscular activity patterns that aid in the retention of a "loose" mandibular denture [*Bohnenkamp & Garcia 2007*]. Importantly, such muscle training tasks were shown to induce significant increase of the representation of involved muscles in the motor cortex [*Svensson et al. 2003*]; which is likely to be an indication of *activity dependent neuronal plasticity* based adaptive changes in the brain.

Although exercises of masticatory and facial muscles are the most important forms of muscular exercises in dentistry, other body exercises to improve cervical range of motion [*Bell 1969/b, Lotzmann 2002*] as well as to improve gait or to correct posture [*Komiyama et al. 1999, Lotzmann 2002*] may also be reasonable [*Silverman 1961, Komiyama et al. 1999*] also in relation with PDI problems (see also in *paragraph 8.5. and 8.6*).

6.5.3. Ultrasound Treatment

Ultrasound produces vibrations within the tissue that cause particle collision and the release of energy resulting in the production of heat [*Laskin & Block 1986*]. Therefore, ultrasonic treatment induces a combined *deep* effect of vibration ("micromassage") and *deep* heat effect (to a dept of 4 - 5 cm) [*Bell 1969/b, Laskin & Block 1986*]. Ultrasound therapy may be used to reduce muscle tension [*Bell 1969/b, Laskin & Block 1986*] and to improve myofascial pain symptoms [*Bell 1969/b, Clark 1981, Esposito et al. 1984, Laskin & Block 1986*]. Ultrasound treatment also increases tissue elasticity [*Laskin & Block 1986*] and improve circulation [*Laskin & Block 1986*].

The sound head is used over the involved muscles (i.e. masseter or temporal muscles) and should be moved slowly to avoid excessive heat build up [*Laskin & Block 1986*]. Treatments last 10 to 15 minutes, and can be applied twice a day for 1 to 2 weeks [*Laskin & Block 1986*]. Ultrasound should not be applied over the eye, over the ear, over an area of *acute* inflammation [*Bell 1969/b, Laskin & Block 1986*] and over metallic implants [*Laskin & Block 1986*]. Ultrasound therapy is also contraindicated in patients with cardiac pacemaker, vascular insufficiency and malignancy [*Laskin & Block 1986*]. Use of ultrasound should also be avoided in the condylar area during the growth period [*Bell 1969/b*].

6.5.4. Cold Therapy

Cold effects can be applied as ice pack, cold water bag, cold gel bag, moist cold (wet hand-towel) or due to vapor-coolant sprays (i.e. ethyl chloride or fluorimethane) [*Clark 1981, Gibilisco 1983, Laskin & Block 1986, Sarlani et al. 2005/a*]. In general, cold application causes local analgesia, has anti-inflammatory effects, and can diminish muscle spasm [*Clark 1981, Laskin & Block 1986*]. The analgesic effect is likely to be due to a decrease in end organ activity and pain fiber conduction [*Laskin & Block 1986*]. The muscle spasm reducing effect is likely to occur due to a cold-induced reduction of the myoneural transmission [*Laskin & Block 1986*]. Although the cooling effect creates vasoconstriction *during* the treatment [*Laskin & Block 1986*], a reactive hyperemia also appear *following* cold application (especially when ice-cold is applied) [*Laskin & Block 1986*].

Application of ice cold (vapor-coolant spray, ice pack) is used for the *acute phases* of orofacial disorders including muscle spasm symptoms [*Clark 1981, Laskin & Block 1986*], myositis [*Sarlani et al. 2005/a, Gibilisco 1983*] as well as synovitis or capsulitis of the TMJ. They may be applied either 4 to 6 times daily for the first 24-36 hours, followed by moist heat application [*Sarlani et al. 2005/a*]; or 2 times daily for 2 to 3 days [*Laskin & Block 1986*]. Ice packs are usually applied for 10 to 15 minutes, and the packs should be placed onto the skin over the involved area [*Laskin & Block 1986*].

Vapor-coolant sprays are usually applied from roughly 30 cm away from the target area in a circular motion for 10 seconds repeated three times with a 10 second interval [*Laskin & Block 1986*]. The application should be done under careful protection of eyes and ears because of the volatile nature of the sprays [*Laskin & Block 1986*], and should be stopped when slight frosting appears on the skin [*Laskin & Block 1986*]. In case of muscle spasm, *moderate* stretch exercises should also be instituted after the treatment [*Laskin & Block 1986, Sarlani et al. 2005/a*]. In such cases ice-cold application may be used for the inactivation of muscle trigger points [*Bell 1969/b, Sarlani et al. 2005/a*].

Moderate cold application (i.e. cold water bag, cold gel bag, moist cold) may be used for acute posttraumatic or postsurgical injuries. Advantage of the use of moderate cold application may be that, there is only a moderate reactive hyperemia (if any) following treatment, which may be advantageous for control of such inflammations.

6.5.5. Heat Therapy

Heat effects can be applied as hot water bag, hot gel bag, moist heat (hot wet hand-towel) or due to infrared lamps. A unique way of warm application is the intra oral "mouth douche" due to administration of a hot water "douche" intraorally (see also *paragraph 6.5.1.*). Hyperemia frequently appears *during* treatment, which may help to return catabolites into the main circulation [*Laskin & Block 1986*]. Heat effect strongly induce the expression and consequent release [*Wang et al. 2004*] of HSP70/HSPA type stress proteins as well [*Ito et al. 2005, Ruell & Thompson 2008*]. (The use of *alkaline* water in the case of "mouth douche" may even further increase the up-regulation of HSP70/HSPA expression of oral mucosal cells [*Merne et al. 2001*].) Importantly, upregulation of HSP70/HSPA type stress proteins may lead to somewhat "Janus-faced" character of thermal treatment when used for inflammatory processes [*Fábián et al. 2009/a,b*] (see also *paragraphs 3.4.7.* and *3.4.8.*). On the other hand, increased expression HPS70/HSPA type stress proteins may improve cytoprotection of the oral tissues [*Ito et al. 2005, Fábián et al. 2009/a,b*].

Moist heat or hot water/gel bag can be applied over the involved muscle for half an hour (3 times 10 minutes followed by 5 minutes pause each, utilized for mild muscle stretching) at least twice daily to treat myofascial pain [*Laskin & Block 1986*] and other muscular pain symptoms. Heat effects may also be applied for 10-15 minutes 3 to 4 times a day (following an ice cold application see *paragraph 6.5.4.*) for the treatment of several TMJ symptoms [*Sarlani et al. 2005/a*].

Heat application may be used for the treatment of synovitis, capsulitis and osteoarthritis of the TMJ [*Sarlani et al. 2005/a*]. Heat effects also decreases pain and spasm of muscles [*Bell 1969/b, Clark 1981, Laskin & Block 1986*] including certain myalgic and myofascial forms of muscular pain as well [*Gibilisco 1983, Sarlani et al. 2005/a*]. Accordingly, heat effects may also be used advantageously as a prepreparation for muscle massage and muscle stretching exercises [*Gibilisco 1983, Laskin & Block 1986*]. Function of the salivary glands (including secretion of total protein, amylase and salivary chaperone HSPA/HSP70) may also be improved due to local heat application [*Fejérdy et al. 2004*].

6.5.6. Transcutaneous Electrical Nerve Stimulation (TENS)

Transcutaneous electrical nerve stimulation (*TENS*) refers to commercially available devices that apply electric impulses to the peripheral nerves via electrodes placed on the skin [*Bishop 1986, Curcio et al. 1987*]. Although electrodes of TENS devices were originally placed on the skin, in dentistry "*intraoral TENS*" (intraoral electrostimulation therapy) utilizing *electrodes placed intraorally* may also be used [*Bishop 1986, Curcio et al. 1987, Wilder-Smith & Zimmermann 1989, Wilder-Smith 1990*].

Based on the gate-control theory [*Melzack & Wall 1965*] it is hypothesized that stimulation of the branches of the trigeminal nerve due to TENS creates an inhibitory effect on the trigeminal nucleus and thereby reduces awareness of pain and helps (indirectly) to induce muscle relaxation [*Black 1986, Laskin & Block 1986, Hochman 1988*]. It is also hypothesized that, TENS induces release of endorphins, norepinephrine and serotonin in the central nervous system, which may also be responsible for the clinical effects [*Black 1986, Hochman 1988*]. Further, TENS increases circulation in the areas where electrodes are placed [*Hochman 1988*]. It is also very likely that, TENS increases the circulation of those muscles, which belong to the stimulated nerve [*Laskin & Block 1986*] and therefore reduces muscle pain and increases muscles' resistance to fatigue [*Laskin & Block 1986*]. There is also a rather significant placebo effect (see also *paragraph 6.6.8.*) coupled with TENS therapy [*Gold et al. 1983, Dahlström 1992, Green & Laskin 2000*].

TENS may be used for the treatment of myofascial pain problems [*Black 1986, Laskin & Block 1986, Dahlström 1992*]. Myofascial pain patient are usually treated by placing the electrode directly over the area of most discomfort for 30 minutes daily [*Laskin & Block 1986*]. Similarly, stimulation of the trigeminal branches may also improve certain form of trigeminal neuralgias [*Black 1986*]. Intraoral stimulation of the trigeminal branches results in significant intraoral analgesic effects that may be utilized for control of *minor* dental operative pain [*Bishop 1986, Black 1986, Curcio et al. 1987, Hochman 1988, Malamed & Quinn 1988*], as well as for the treatment of certain intraoral pain symptoms. Further, stimulation of the facial nerve may improve certain forms of facial paresis.

Importantly, TENS treatment is contraindicated for certain patients including pregnant patients and pacemaker patients as well as for patients with cerebral convulsive disorders (possibility of initiating seizure), with pathologic hypotension (TENS lowers blood pressure) and with cerebral vascular disorders (blood flow increases in the areas where electrodes are applied) [*Hochman 1988*].

6.5.7. Occlusal Splint Therapy

Occlusal splints are frequently used for the therapy of bruxism [Mikami 1977, Dahlström 1989, 1992, Biondi & Picardi 1993, Glaros 2006] and temporomandibular symptoms [Gibilisco 1983, Laskin & Block 1986, Dahlström 1989, 1992, Harris et al. 1993, Biondi & Picardi 1993] as well as for the treatment of orofacial pain of muscular dysfunction origin [Laskin & Block 1986, Dahlström 1989, Harris et al. 1993, Biondi & Picardi 1993] including myofascial pain [Laskin & Block 1986, Kreiner et al. 2001, Glaros 2006].

Reflex splints (occlusal disengagement) trigger mouth opening reflex (see paragraph 3.3.6.) due to functioning as an "artificial early contact" and as such may be used for reducing stress induced muscle spasm and parafunction activity [Mikami 1977, Laskin & Block 1986]. In such splints, a flat and nonguiding plateau of acrylic resin built up behind the maxillary anterior teeth serves as a stop for the lower incisor teeth; which prevent the occlusion of posterior teeth resulted in a separation (et maximum up to 2 mm) of posterior occlusal surfaces [Bell 1969/b, Green & Laskin 1972/a, Laskin & Block 1986].

Reflex splints should be used for short run (at maximum for 2 weeks [Freesmeyer 1995]), because if such a splint were worn too long, a "new series" of muscle spasm and parafunction could be triggered [Freesmeyer 1995]. Further, there is a danger of elongation (supereruption) of teeth [Bell 1969/b, Laskin & Block 1986, Griffin 1975], remodeling of the temporomandibular joint [Griffin 1975], as well as other severe and irreversible complications [Widmalm 1999] when wearing reflex splints too long. Premised risks can be reduced when reflex splints are not worn continuously, but only at night and for 5 to 6 hours during the day [Laskin & Block 1986]. Patients should also be instructed not to clench against the splint [Laskin & Block 1986]. Following these instructions, reflex splints may be used somewhat longer (at maximum for 4 to 6 weeks) under regular control [Bell 1969/b, Laskin & Block 1986].

Reflex splints may be equilibrated and transformed into equilibrated splints due to filling up the existing space between the molars [Green & Laskin 1972/a]. Following this adjustment, high spots should be detected with articulating paper and removed until simultaneous tooth contacts are achieved on both sides and frontal area (on complete occlusal coverage) of the arch [Bell 1969/b, Green & Laskin 1972/a, Griffin 1975, Laskin & Block 1986]. Such equilibrated splints may be used for harmonizing muscle function including improvement of certain altered EMG patterns [McNamara 1976, Mikami 1977, Dahlström et al. 1982, 1985, Dahlström 1989].

Equilibrated splints may also be used to determine (and/or try out) optimal and comfortable position of maximal intercuspidation of dentures under preparation for patients with neuromuscular symptoms [Griffin 1975, Griffin et al. 1975, Gibilisco 1983, Laney 1983, Freesmeyer 1995]. Equilibrated splints may also be used for similar purposes also in the case of patients undergoing bite opening procedures [Griffin 1975, Griffin et al. 1975, Laney 1983].

Equilibrated splints may also be used to prevent or limit the attrition of teeth of patients with bruxism [Mikami 1977, Laskin & Block 1986, Glaros 2006]. For such purposes equilibrated splints may be used for longer run (from several months to years) when regularly controlled [Laskin & Block 1986, Freesmeyer 1995, Widmalm 1999, Glaros 2006], and the equilibration procedure is regularly repeated [Laskin & Block 1986, Freesmeyer 1995].

Importantly, splint therapy may also be utilized for edentulous patients with neuromuscular dysfunction using sliding plates [Zuccolotto et al. 2007] for harmonizing muscle function. Although the efficiency of splint therapy is expected to be based (at least partially) on placebo effects [Green & Laskin 1972/a, 2000, Laskin & Block 1986, Molin 1999] (see also paragraph 6.6.8.), it clearly exerts certain specific therapeutic effects as well [Green & Laskin 1972/a, Dahlström 1992, Karppinen et al. 1999]. Especially when used as a repositioning appliance (due to positioning of condyles) in conservative therapy of disc displacements [Freesmeyer 1995, Sarlani et al. 2005/a].

6.5.8. Pulsed Electromagnetic Field Therapy (PEMF)

Pulsed electromagnetic field (*PEMF*) therapy seems to be a highly promising method for psychosomatic dentistry, even if the mechanisms behind its efficiency are mostly not yet clear. PEMF induces local vasodilatation [*Smith et al. 2004*]. PEMF increases angiogenesis likely due to stimulation of endothelial release of fibroblast growth factor beta-2 (FGF-2) inducing paracrine and autocrine changes in the surrounding tissues [*Tepper et al. 2004*]. PEMF alters the expression and functionality of adenosine receptors in human neutrophile granulocytes [*Varani et al. 2002, 2003*]. PEMF reverses the proliferative defects of lymphocytes from aged subjects [*Cossarizza et al. 1989/a,b*]; likely due to acting on the expression of IL-2 receptor on the plasma membrane and consequent increase of interleukin-2 (IL-2) utilization [*Cossarizza et al. 1989/b*]. It is also likely that, PEMF induces the expression and release of HSP70/HSPA type stress proteins [*authors unpublished data*].

PEMF enhances healing of bone fractures [*Gossling et al. 1992, Pienkowski et al. 1992, Inoue et al. 2002*], and decreases the rate of residual ridge resorption following tooth extraction [*Ortman et al. 1992*]. PEMF also increases the rate of orthodontic tooth movement and coupled bone deposition [*Stark & Sinclair 1987, Darendeliler et al. 1995*]. Bone formation around dental implants (osteointegration of implants) can also be promoted due to PEMF treatment [*Matsumoto et al. 2000, Fini et al. 2002*]. PEMF can also accelerate bone formation in bone defects filled with hydroxyapatite (HA) [*Shimizu et al. 1988, Ottani et al. 2002*] or with demineralized bone-matrix [*Takano-Yamamoto et al. 1992*]. Similarly, PEMF can also accelerate bone graft incorporation [*Kold et al. 1987*]. Osteoporitic symptoms may aslo be improved using PEMF [*Mishima 1988, Chang & Chang 2003, Tabrah et al. 1990*]. PEMF also improves the symptoms of osteoarthritis patients [*Trock et al. 1993, 1994, Pipitone & Scott 2001, Kumar et al. 2005*].

Besides the important bone-related effects, PEMF also improves tendon inflammation and returns to histological normality as well [*Binder et al. 1984, Lee et al. 1997*]. PEMF also improves wound healing of the gastrointestinal mucosa [*Mentes et al. 1996*] and the skin [*Patino et al. 1996, Scardino et al. 1998*]. Similarly, ulcerations may also be improved due to PEMF therapy [*Stiller et al. 1992*]. PEMF also improves regeneration of injured nerve [*Raji & Bowden 1983, Raji 1984, Zienowicz et al. 1991, Kanje et al. 1993*]. PEMF also improves clinical symptoms (i.e. pain, decrease of conductive function, decrease of reflex excitability) of several neuropathic conditions [*Musaev et al. 2003, Weintraub & Cole 2004*]. PEMF may also be used for acupuncture therapy (see *paragraph 8.3.*). Authors' preliminary data indicate that, PEMF can be utilized highly efficiently for the treatment of various PDI cases [*Fábián et al. 2006/b, Fábián & Sőti 2007*].

6.5.9. Low Level Laser (Soft-Laser) Therapy

Low level laser therapy (LLLT; also referred to as soft laser therapy) is a treatment with athermic low power lasers. There are many different types of low level laser (LLL) may be used for LLLT including either pulsed or continuous LLL, and with wavelength in both visible and invisible range [*Khullar et al. 1995, Kimura et al. 2000*]. The most commonly used laser types are HeNe laser (wavelength: 632 nm), Ar laser (wavelength: 514 nm),

GaAlAs laser (wavelengths: 780 or 830 or 900 nm), ruby laser (wavelength: 694 nm) Nd:YAG laser (wavelength: 1060 nm) and CO_2 laser (wavelength 10600 nm) [*Khullar et al. 1995, Kimura et al. 2000*]. Although the usual output power of CO_2 lasers [*Kimura et al. 2000*], Nd:YAG lasers [*Kimura et al. 2000*] and Ar lasers are mostly at middle level or higher (therefore these lasers are typically *not* referred to as low level lasers), they may be used at lower level output powder suitable for LLLT as well.

In general, increase of cell metabolism, collagen synthesis and activity of immune cells are the most important pathways behind the efficiency of low level laser therapy [*Qadri et al. 2005*]. LLLT also inducing long-lasting expression of HSP70/HSPA type stress proteins [*Souil et al. 2001*]. There is also a prominent placebo effect coupled with low level laser therapy [*Kimura et al. 2000, Payer et al. 2005*]. Importantly, it is very likely that, both wavelength (of a laser) and the cell type (of the irradiated tissue) significantly influence the biological effect [*Moore et al. 2005*]. Therefore, no wonder that, there is still controversy regarding which wavelength would be the most appropriate for various orofacial symptoms [*Khullar et al. 1995*].

LLLT may be used advantageously to control periodontal inflammation [*Qadri et al. 2005, de Almeida et al. 2008, Schwarz et al. 2008*] and more severe inflammatory and/or necrotizing bone pathologies [*Vescovi et al. 2008*]. LLLT may also be used to improve implant-tissue interaction in the bone [*Khadra 2005, Kim et al. 2007, Lopes et al. 2007*] and at the implant-soft tissue interface [*Khadra et al. 2005/a,b, Schwarz et al. 2005*]. LLLT may also be used to facilitate orthodontic tooth movement and related alveolar bone remodeling as well [*Kawasaki & Shimizu 2000, Fujita et al. 2008, Kim et al in press/b*]. LLLT may also facilitate bone metabolism during bone healing at the sites of deproteinized bone grafts [*Kim et al. in press/a*] and bone defects filled with hydroxyapatite (HA) [*Pinheiro et al. 2009*] or enamel matrix protein derivatives [*Ozcelik et al. 2008/a*].

Besides its advantageous effect in the bone, LLLT improves myofascial pain [*de Medeiros et al. 2005, Shirani et al. in press*], temporomandibular joint pain [*Dahlström 1992, Mazzetto et al. 2007*] and other TMD symptoms [*Carrasco et al. 2008*] as well as post surgical trismus and facial swelling [*Aras & Hüngörmüş in press*]. LLLT may also be used to improve functional recovery of injured peripheral nerves [*Khullar et al. 1995, Ozen et al. 2006*]. LLLT also accelerates oral wound healing [*Neiburger 1999, Amorim et al. 2006, Ozcelik et al. 2008/b*] as well as healing of oral ulcerations [*Sharon-Buller & Sela 2004, Navarro et al. 2007*]. Dentinal hypersensitivity of exposed dentin (i.e. because of gingival recession and following scaling or root planing) may also be treated efficiently [*Gerschman et al. 1994, Kimura et al. 2000, Pesevska et al. in press*]. Low level lasers may also be used for acupuncture therapy (see *paragraph 8.3.*).

6.5.10. Contraindication of Physiotherapies

Besides certain specific contraindications and precautions of physiotherapies (mentioned above), there can be numerous other contraindications of physiotherapies. In general, physiotherapy is contraindicated in the case of patients with any severe systemic diseases and with strongly compromised health. In the case of such patients, use of physiotherapy should be avoided in the absence of a clear agreement of the medical professional(s) responsible for the treatment of the systemic disease(s) at issue (and/or responsible for the medical care of strongly compromised health). Similarly, physiotherapy is usually contraindicated in the cases of patients with any hemorrhagic diathesis, precancerosis, and malignancy as well as in the case of patients having any oncological treatment in the anamnesis (at least in the absence of a clear agreement of the oncologist or other responsible medical professional).

Importantly, use of *any* physiotherapy should be *strictly* avoided near to a naevus. In the absence of clear evidences about the innocuity, several forms of physiotherapy may be contraindicated for patients with pacemaker (or with another implanted electric instruments) as well as in the case of patients with any implants including also dental implants. Similarly, physiotherapeutic treatment should be avoided near to the ear, eye, brain or spinal cord (i.e. temporal or paravertebral use) in the absence of clear evidence about the innocuity of the chosen treatment modality. (Especially those modalities utilizing electric impulses or irradiative energy with significant heat generating effect like laser or ultrasound should be considered for such contraindication.)

6.6. MEDICAMENTOUS THERAPIES

6.6.1. Pain Killers and Anti-Inflammatory Drugs

There is frequently no significant improvement of chronic orofacial psychosomatic symptoms after treatment with pain killers and non-steroidal anti-inflammatory drugs (NSAIDs) [*Gellrich et al. 2002*]. In other cases, drug tolerance and dependence may appear [*Israel & Scrivani 2000*]. Therefore, pain killers and NSAIDs are used primarily for the initial therapy of not yet chronic cases in psychosomatic dentistry. Since most of the orofacial pain symptoms are also (at least partially) of inflammatory origin, in most cases NSAIDs (instead of exclusive pain killers) are used for such purposes.

Trigger point sensitivity of myofascial pain patients may be reduced with NSAIDs [*Sarlani et al. 2005/a*], and administration of NSAIDs may also be a part of myositis [*Sarlani et al. 2005/a*] and myofascial pain therapy [*Green & Laskin 1972/b, Biondi and Picardi 1993*]. NSAIDs may also be used efficiently for orofacial pain of vascular origin [*Benoliel et al. 1997*]. Painful TMD cases including painful disc displacement, synovitis, capsulitis or osteoarthritis can also be improved using NSAIDs [*Gibilisco 1983, Biondi and Picardi 1993, Sarlani et al. 2005/a*]. Importantly, NSAIDs can also be applied locally [*King 1988*]. There are numerous NSAID *gels* and plasters available for *local application*, which may be used advantageously when applied onto the skin surface over the painful area. A certain NSAID (namely indomethacine) can also be used for diagnostic purposes as a drug trial to exclude/verify the diagnosis of chronic paroxysmal hemicrania (CPH) based on the robust response (improvement) of CPH to this specific drug [*Sarlani et al. 2005/b*].

6.6.2. Muscle Relaxants

Spasm produces pain that in turn produces more spasm in many cases [*Laskin & Block 1986*]. Thus, muscle relaxants may be used to interrupt this *vicious cycle*, especially when used in conjunction with a pain-relieving medication [*Laskin & Block 1986*]. Accordingly, muscle relaxants may be used for the treatment of myofascial pain patients [*Green & Laskin 1969, Laskin & Block 1986, Ryan et al. 1985, Dahlström 1992; Sarlani et al. 2005/a*]. Muscle relaxants may also be used for the therapy of bruxism and TMD symptoms of muscular dysfunction origin [*Gibilisco 1983, Dahlström 1992, Biondi & Picardi 1993*].

Importantly, certain anxiolytics (especially benzodiazepines, see *paragraph 6.6.3.* below) also exert significant myorelaxant properties [*Chaco, 1973, Laskin & Block 1986, Dahlström 1989, 1992*]. Since tranquilizing (anxiolytic) properties can be beneficial in relieving muscle tension too [*Laskin & Block 1986*], premised anxiolytics (benzodiazepines) are the drugs most often prescribed as muscle relaxants [*Laskin & Block 1986, Dahlström 1992*]. Again, benzodiazepines should also be taken in conjunction with an analgesic for the best effect [*Laskin & Block 1986*]. Interestingly, drugs with only muscle relaxant properties (i.e. without any anxiolytic effects) seem to be not as successful as premised anxiolytics (benzodiazepines) for the treatment of myofascial pain [*Laskin & Block 1986*].

6.6.3. Anxiolytics

Anxiolytics (especially benzodiazepines) may be used for prevention of dental fear [*Lu 1994, Fábián & Fábián 2000, Fábián et al. 2007/a*]; and may also be used for decreasing treatment induced pain (i.e. conscious sedation) [*Fábián & Fábián 2000, Fábián et al. 2007/a*]. Benzodiazepines may also be used as an adjunct for the initial treatment of PDI patients with high background anxiety level [*Bell 1969/b*]. Because of their significant antidepressive properties [*Köhler 2005*] benzodiazepines may also be used advantageously for PDI patients with depression [*Bell 1969/a*], although cases with *severe* depression can not be managed with the use of benzodiazepines by itself [*Köhler 2005*]. Based on their myorelaxant effect, benzodiazepines may also be used advantageously as an adjunct to the initial therapy of patients with myofascial pain [*Bell 1969/b, Green & Laskin 1972/b, Ryan et al. 1985, Laskin & Block 1986*] and functional (neuromuscular dysfunction related) TMD problems [*Bell 1969/b, Chaco 1973, Dahlström 1989*] (see also *paragraph 6.6.2.* above). Benzodiazepines may also be used for the treatment of burning mouth syndrome [*Sarlani et al. 2005/b*].

6.6.4. Antidepressants

Tricyclic antidepressants (inhibit reuptake of *both* serotonin *and* norepinephrine) [*Sarlani et al. 2005*] and *selective* serotonin reuptake inhibitors (SSRIs) [*Maina et al. 2003*] may be used for the treatment of various PDI symptoms. There are also some antidepressive effects of benzodiazepines [*Laskin & Block 1986, Köhler 2005*] (see also *paragraph 6.6.3.*) and Ltriptophan (see also *paragraph 7.3.2.*) which may also be utilized for such purposes [*Köhler 2005*]. Although a definitive medicamentous treatment of affective disorders (including depression) is clearly a scope of psychiatrist; *short run* (1 to 2 weeks, or maximum 3 to 4 weeks) administration of *low doses* antidepressants (see also below) can be carried out also by the dentist in the frame of initial psychosomatic therapy [*Miyamoto & Ziccardi 1998, Laskin & Block 1986, Toyofuku & Kikuta 2006*]. Especially pain symptoms including myofascial pain [*Laskin & Block 1986, Derra & Egle 2003, Sarlani et al. 2005/a*] atypical facial pain [*Köling 1998, Sarlani et al. 2005/b*], atypical odontalgia [*Sarlani et al. 2005/b*], phantom tooth pain [*Sarlani et al. 2005/b*] burning mouth syndrome [*Maina et al. 2003*], fibromyalgia [*Derra & Egle 2003*], neuropathic pain [*Derra & Egle 2003*] and vascular pain [*Benoliel et al. 1997*] may be improved in this way. Similarly, certain somatosensory symptoms may also be improved due to low dose antidepressant administration (see also below).

Importantly, *antidepressants can be used for pain reduction even if there are no current symptoms of depression* [*Maina et al. 2003, Derra & Egle 2003*]; because they also exert a significant *direct analgesic effect* which is likely to be independent from the antidepressive effect [*Derra & Egle 2003*]. In contrast to antidepressive effect (appearing earliest after 2-4 weeks *at best* [*Köhler 2005*]) premised analgesic effect appears after 3-7 days [*Miyamoto & Ziccardi 1998, Derra & Egle 2003*]; and importantly, *low doses* are also sufficient to reach the premised analgesic effect [*Miyamoto & Ziccardi 1998, Derra & Egle 2003, Sarlani et al. 2005*]. For such low dosage administration, especially serotonin-norepinephrine reuptake inhibitors may be useful [*Miyamoto & Ziccardi 1998, Derra & Egle 2003*], because their direct analgesic effect seems to be stronger comparing to other groups of antidepressants [*Miyamoto & Ziccardi 1998, Derra & Egle 2003*].

Similarly, serotonin-norepinephrine reuptake inhibitors exert a *direct effect on the somatosensory system* as well; which is also likely to be independent from the antidepressive effect [*Toyofuku & Kikuta 2006*] and can be utilized efficiently for treating occlusal dysesthesia [*Toyofuku & Kikuta 2006*]. Similarly to pain treatment, *low doses* are likely to be sufficient to reach this kind of somatosensory effect too [*Toyofuku & Kikuta 2006*], however, this effect likely appears somewhat later (after 2-4 weeks) [*Toyofuku & Kikuta 2006*].

6.6.5. Local Anesthetics

Local anesthetics may be used for reducing spasm (and consequent pain) of trigger points [*Clark 1981, Dunteman & Swarm 1995, Sarlani et al. 2005/a*] and/or of the whole muscle (myospasm) [*Clark 1981, Sarlani et al. 2005/a*] before stretching exercises of the muscles [*Dunteman & Swarm 1995, Sarlani et al. 2005/a*]. Local anesthetics, when injected to a muscle, exert their effect on hypertonus by preferential paralysis of both alpha- and gamma motoneurons (fusimotor fibers) as well as endings and afferent fibers leaving the muscle spindles [*Mathews & Rushworth 1957, Harris & Griffin 1975*].

Therefore, there is no need to infiltrate muscle tissues directly, when the innervating nerve is available for block anaesthesia (conduction anaesthesia) [*Mathews & Rushworth 1957*]. If block anaesthesia is unaccomplishable, 0.5 ml anesthetics should be injected into the painful muscle area [*Laskin & Block 1986*]. Importantly, local anesthetics *without any vasoconstrictor* should be used [*Bell 1969/b, Clark 1981, Laskin & Block 1986, Dunteman & Swarm 1995*] to promote the infiltration of the tissues, to decrease of the time span of treatment, and especially to prevent the decrease of *blood flow* in the muscle.

Following application of local anesthetics, relieve of pain and decrease of muscle spasm occur, which may be utilized for gentle muscle stretch exercises [*Laskin & Block 1986*]. The *muscular exercises should be carried out very carefully during the period of anaesthesia*, because the protective reflexes of muscles are inhibited (see *paragraph 3.3.3.*). Since too frequent injection can be injurious to the muscle, local application of local anesthetics can be repeated several times within a week if effective; but thereafter other treatment modalities should be used [*Laskin & Block 1986*].

Besides treatment of muscle spasm, lidocain patch may also be used for the treatment of postherpetic neuralgia [*Sarlani et al. 2005/a*]. Further, local anesthetics may also be used for diagnostic purposes to differentiate between peripheral- and central origin as well as between somatic- and psychogenic origin of pain (or other sensory symptoms) [*Laskin & Block 1986, Sarlani et al. 2005/a*]. Primary and secondary (referred) pain may also be differentiated using local anesthetics [*Bell 1969/a*] based on the *frequently* occurring phenomenon that applied local anesthetic that interrupts the primary pain stops both primary and referred pain; whereas local anesthetic applied to the nerve trunk giving sensory innervation to the site of referred pain may not stop the pain because it does not arise there but only seems to [*Bell 1969/a*].

6.6.6. Anticonvulsant Drugs

The use of anticonvulsant drugs is especially reasonable under neuropathic pain such as neuralgia of several origin [*Derra & Egle 2003, Grond & Lehman 2003, Sarlani et al. 2005/a*], although they may also be used for the treatment of severe atypical facial pain and atypical odontalgia [*Benoliel et al. 1997, Derra & Egle 2003, Grond & Lehman 2003, Sarlani et al. 2005/b*]. They may be used also for the treatment of severe PDI related pain symptoms occasionally. In general carbamazepine, clonazepam or gabapentin may be used [*Derra & Egle 2003, Grond & Lehman 2003, Sarlani et al. 2005/a*]. In the orofacial region, carbamazepine seems to be significantly more efficient than other anticonvulsant drugs [*Derra & Egle 2003, Grond & Lehman 2003*], although in the case of herpetic and postherpetic neuralgia gabapentin can also be offered [*Sarlani et al. 2005/a*].

6.6.7. Vitamins

In general, the lack of *water-soluble vitamins* (i.e. vitamins of vitamin B group and vitamin C) affects tissues that are growing or metabolizing rapidly [*Nestle 1985*] such as skin, gastrointestinal mucosa (including oral mucosa), blood and the nervous system [*Nestle 1985, Bourre 2006*]. Further, vitamin C is also involved in the synthesis of collagen and intercellular matrix [*Martin 1985/b*]. Therefore, administration of vitamin C and members of vitamin B group such as Thiamin (B$_1$), riboflavin (B$_2$), pantothenic acid (B$_5$), niacin, pyridoxine (B$_6$), biotin, cobalamin (B$_{12}$) and folic acid (folate) could be advantageous in case of most idiopathic and/or psychosomatic symptoms appearing in the orofacial region. Folate, thiamine and pyridoxine also advantageously influence cognitive and emotional functions [*Riggs et al. 1996, Young 1993, Benton & Donohoe 1999*]. Similarly, vitamin C is likely to improve coping ability with stress [*Peeters et al. 2005*].

Although all water-soluble vitamins serve as specific coenzymes or cofactors in several enzymatic reactions, their effects are strongly interrelated [*Martin 1985/b*]. Therefore, the use of their *mixture* (rather than use of a certain one) seems to be more advantageous for psychosomatic therapies. Moreover, it should be also considered that, *serious* water-soluble vitamin deficiencies are rare in orofacial *psychosomatic* cases, whereas *moderate* deficiencies occur rather frequently especially in the case of folate [*Martin 1985/b*]. Taking together all above aspects it can be concluded that, administration of *slightly elevated doses* (up to five times of recommended daily dietary intake) of a *mixture* of water-soluble vitamins *for few weeks* is recommended for the *initial therapy* of *most* oral psychosomatic cases (except patients with vitamin abuse).

In contrast to water-soluble vitamins, deficiencies of *fat-soluble vitamins* (i.e. vitamins A, D, E and K) are rare in adults [*Nestle 1985*]. However, they require normal fat absorption, therefore biliary system disorders, pancreatic dysfunctions and any other steatorrhea may result in vitamin deficiency [*Martin 1985/a*]. Since they are not excreted in the urine and the body is able to store excess fat-soluble vitamins, the risk of overdosage is higher [*Martin 1985/a, Nestle 1985*]. Therefore fat-soluble vitamins should not be used in a mixture for *therapeutical* purposes (i.e. in higher doses than recommended for daily dietary intake); but they should be used aimed.

Vitamin A (retinol, and its provitamin β-carotene) is necessary for vision, reproduction mucus secretion, and the maintenance of differentiated epithelia [*Martin 1985/a*]. Therefore vitamin A may be used advantageously for the treatment of mucosal symptoms (could also be administered locally) and may be for salivation problems.

Vitamins D are a group of sterol compounds that occur in animals in humans and also in plants. Vitamin D of human and animal origin is called *cholecalciferol* (vitamin D_3), which is generated from 7-dehydrocholesterol via photolysis in the skin, and stored as 25-hydroxy cholecalciferol (25-hydroxy-D_3) in the liver [*Martin 1985/a*]. Therefore, exposure to sunlight, and ingestion of animal liver (especially fish liver) in the diet are main sources of vitamin D_3. Vitamin D of plant origin is called *ergocalciferol* (vitamin D_2) which may also be ingested in vegetarian diet. Importantly, ergocalciferol and cholecalciferol are of *equal biologic potency* as D vitamins [*Martin 1985/a*].

Inadequate intake of vitamin D (and/or inadequate sun exposure) may contribute to low bone mineral density, increases risk of osteoporosis and related (pain)symptoms [*Dawson-Huges et al. 1991*], and also increases risk of insufficient healing of most bone-related pathologies. Therefore, in such cases, administration of vitamin D and/or adequate sun exposure should be considered. A possible role of vitamin D supplementation in the prevention of various aspects of neurodegenerative and neuroimmune diseases may also be expected based on preliminary findings [*Garcion et al. 2002, Zittermann 2003, Bourre 2006*].

Vitamin E (α-tocopherol) is an oil present in plants (particularly wheat germ, rice and cotton seeds), which is required (likely also in human) for fertility and for proper muscular function. Vitamin E is also required for the prevention of peroxidative damage of cellular and subcellular elements under coping with disease, physical and chemical insults or other cellular stresses [*Martin 1985/a*]. Vitamin E is also likely to improve cognitive functions

[*Bourre 2006*] including coping ability with stress [*Peeters et al. 2005*] and may improve impaired immune function too [*Tucker 1995*]. Premised cellular stress related defense functions and possible psychological and immunological function of vitamin E could be rather advantageous in the treatment of orofacial symptoms. Therefore, slightly increased intake of vitamin E for few weeks should be considered for the therapy of such cases.

Vitamin K is a group of polyisoprenoid substituted naphthoqinones with similar biological functions. Menadione (vitamin K_3), menaquinone-n (vitamin K_2) and phylloquinone (vitamin K_1) belong to this group [*Martin 1985/a*]. Vitamin K is known to be required for the maintenance of normal levels of several blood clotting factors. It is also used as an antidote to certain anticoagulant drugs [*Martin 1985/a*]. Because of its rather specific effects, vitamin K is not used for therapeutical purposes in relation with oral psychosomatic disorders.

It should be also considered that, vitamins are primarily administered for therapy via capsules, tablets, or injections. However, they could be ingested in high amounts also in the diet. Therefore, patients' diet should also be considered before therapeutic administration of vitamins. For related *diet-therapeutic aspects* of vitamins, see also *paragraph 7.3.7.*

6.6.8. Placebos and Placebo Effect

The placebo effect is the effect that follows the administration of an inert treatment (the placebo) [*Benedetti 2006*]. It is a psychobiological phenomenon that can be due to different mechanisms [*Benedetti et al. 2005*]. Placebo effect is primarily induced due to expectation and conditioning [*Benedetti 2006*], which strongly indicates the important role of the psychosocial context of a therapy [*Laskin & Green 1972, Benedetti 2006*]. The placebo effect is additive to *any* specific treatment [*Benedetti 2006, Benedetti et al. 2006*], therefore it is a highly important phenomenon that brings to fullness *any* treatment modalities [*Laskin & Green 1972, Benedetti 2006*].

Although there is a great difference of success between "responders" and "nonresponders" [*Benedetti et al. 2004, 2005*] and prior experiences may also influence the efficiency of therapeutic suggestions and patients' expectations strongly [*Colloca & Benedetti 2006*]; majority of patients would benefit from placebos [*Green & Laskin 1969, 1972/a,b, 2000, Laskin & Block 1986, Benson 1996, 1997*]. It should be emphasized that, not only medicamentous therapies but *any other therapies are coupled with placebo effect* [*Green & Laskin 1972/a, 2000, Laskin & Green 1972, Goodman et al. 1976, Gold et al. 1983, Laskin & Block 1986, Benson 1997, Molin 1999*]; and dentists should purposefully improve this effects (*via* proper communication and suggestions) when using any psychosomatic therapies [*Laskin & Green 1972, Green & Laskin 2000*].

However, it should be also emphasized that, the effects of suggestions and expectations on *conscious* and *unconscious* physiological functions can be rather different [*Benedetti et al. 2003*]. Further, patients' beliefs and expectancies may also lead to negative aspects and worsening of symptoms, which is referred to as *nocebo effect* [*Benson 1997*]. Similarly to placebo effect, nocebo effect may also be coupled with any form of therapies, and should be carefully avoided primarily due to the avoidance of negative suggestions and utilization of positive suggestions [*Benson 1997*].

6.6.9. Contraindication of Medicamentous Therapy

There are various specific medical contraindications and possible side effects of medicamentous therapies, which should be considered very carefully [*Bell 1969/b, Laskin & Block 1986, Friedlander et al. 2004*]. Utilizing pharmacological databases and an *up-to-date* pharmacological knowledge, dentists should be familiar with the potential hazards before prescribing a medication [*Bell 1969/b, Laskin & Block 1986, Friedlander et al. 2004*]. Considering premised precautions, *short run* (1 to 2 weeks, or maximum 3 to 4 weeks) administration of several medicaments can be carried out by the dentist in the frame of initial psychosomatic therapy [*Bell 1969/b, Miyamoto & Ziccardi 1998, Laskin & Block 1986, Toyofuku & Kikuta 2006*].

Long-run medicamentous treatment of long-standing PDI symptoms and/or any systemic disorders (if any) behind them, is clearly a scope of medical professionals such as psychiatrists, neurologists, rheumatologists, internists, family doctors (etc.). Therefore, *if long-run medication is needed because of any reasons, it is necessary to place the patient under physicians' care* [*Laskin & Block 1986*]. In the case of pregnancy, lactation, any serious systemic disease or strongly compromised health, referral to medical professional(s) responsible for the treatment of the systemic disease(s) at issue (and/or responsible for the medical care of strongly compromised health) is highly recommended before starting any medicamentous therapy (even if short run therapy). It should be also considered that, not only administration but also removal of a medication may be contraindicated. In the case of medication abuse, the removal of a medication should be carried out by that professional being regularly responsible for the administration of the medication at issue.

6.7. Conclusion

Besides reaching improvement or recovery of symptoms using symptom-centered treatment; psychosomatic dental therapy also induce changes towards an over-all improvement of psychological abilities, social functioning, and stress resistance, which may support the healing process and stabilize treatment outcome. Mind-body therapies may also induce stress related autonomic and hormonal changes, including decrease of sympathetic activity, blood pressure, HPA axis hormones and catecholamine levels and advantageous changes of heart rate variability (HRV) [*Fábián in press*]; all of which can be highly important for the treatment of stress related orofacial symptoms. General improvement of musculoskeletal functions [*Shaw & Dettmar 1990, Egner & Gruzelier 2003, Raymond et al 2005*] as well as improvement of pain tolerance may also occur as highly important results of the psychosomatic treatment. Further, psychosomatic therapies may upregulate immune system and increase immune surveillance [*Gruzelier 2002*] leading to improved defense against several local or systemic infections, oral microbes and tumor formation. Immunomodulator effects may also occur [*Hall et al. 1996*], indicating that, exaggerated immunological reactions such as allergy [*Teshima et al. 1982, Wyler-Harper et al. 1994, Langewitz et al. 2005*] or autoimmune conditions [*Collins & Dunn 2005*] may also be balanced with such methods. Salivation problems, and pseudoneurological symptoms may also be treated efficiently in many cases.

REFERENCES

[1] Achtenberg, J. *Die heilende Kraft der Imagination*. Bern: Scherz; 1987.
[2] Adler, A. Theroie und Praxis der Individualpsychologie. Frankfurt am Main: Fischer; 1920.
[3] Aftanas, LI. & Golocheikine, SA. Human anterior and frontal midline theta and lower alpha reflect emotionally positive state and internalized attention: high-resolution EEG investigation of meditation. *Neurosci Letters*, 2001 310, 57-60.
[4] Alexander, F. & French, TM. *Psychoanalytic therapy*. New York: Rolan Press; 1946
[5] Ament, P. & Ament, A. Body image in dentistry. *J Prosthet Dent*, 1970 24, 362-366.
[6] Amman, AN. *Aktive Imagination*. Freiburg: Walter; 1978.
[7] Amorim, JC; de Sousa, GR; de Barros Silveira, L; Prates, RA, Pinotti, M; Ribeiro, MS. Clinical study of the gingiva healing after gingivectomy and low-level laser therapy. *Photomed Laser Surg*, 2006 24, 588-594.
[8] Anbar, RD. & Savedoff, AD. Hypnosis-associated blue-tinted vision: a case report. *BMC Ophthalmology*, 2005 5, 28.
[9] Anbar, RD. & Slothower, MP. Hypnosis for treatment of insomnia in school-age children: a retrospective chart review. *BMC Pediatrics*, 2006 6, 23.
[10] Aras, MH. & Güngörmüş, M. Placebo-controlled randomized clinical trial of the effect of two different low-level laser therapies (LLLT) - intraoral and extraoral - on trismus and facial swelling following surgical extraction of the lower third molar. *Lasers Med Sci*, in press. DOI: 10.1007/s10103-009-0684-1
[11] Baad-Hansen, L. Atypical odontalgia - pathophysiology and clinical management. *J Oral Rehabil*, 2008 35, 1-11.
[12] Bálint, M. *Changing therapeutical aims and techniques in psychoanalysis*. (1949). In: Balint M. *Primary love and psychoanalytic technique*. London: Imago; 1952.
[13] Bálint, M. *The doctor, his patient and the illness*. London: Pitman Med Publisher; 1956.
[14] Bálint, M; Ornstein, PH; Bálint E. *Focal therapy*. London: Tavistock; 1972
[15] Bálint, M; Krause, M; Krause W-R; Kaán, B; Fejérdy, L; Gáspár, J; Fábián. TK. Modification of the photo-acoustic stimulation in the psychotherapy of oral psychosomatic patients. Preliminary experiences. *Fogorv Szle*, 2003 96, 171-174.
[16] Bandura, A. & Walters, RH. *Social learning and personality development*. New York: Holt-Rinehart-Winston; 1963.
[17] Banquet JP. Spectral analysis of the EEG in meditation. *Electroencephal Clin Neurophysiol*, 1973 35, 143-151.
[18] Bányai, ÉI. A new way to induce a hypnotic-like altered state of consciousness: Active alert induction. In: Kardos L, Pléh Cs editors. *Problems of the regulation of activity*. Budapest: Akadémiai Kiadó; 1980. 261-273.
[19] Bányai, ÉI. Toward a social-psychobiological model of hypnosis. In: Lynn SJ, Rhue JW editors. *Theories of hypnosis: Current models and perspectives*. New York - London: Quildford Press; 1991. 564-598
[20] Bányai, ÉI. & Hilgard ER. A comparison of active-alert hypnotic induction with traditional relaxation induction. *J Abnorm Psychol*, 1976 85, 218-224.

[21] Barabasz, AF. Restricted environmental stimulation and the enhancement of hypnotizability: pain, EEG alpha, skin conductance and temperature responses. *Int J Clin Exp Hypn*, 1982 30, 147-166.

[22] Barabasz, AF. & Barabasz, M. Effects of restricted environmental stimulation: enhancement of hypnotizability for experimental and chronic pain control. *Int J Clin Exp Hypn*, 1989 37, 217-231.

[23] Barnes, VA. EEG, hypometabolism, and ketosis during transcendental meditation indicate it does not increase epilepsy risk. *Med Hypothesis*, 2005 65, 202-203.

[24] Barnhofer, T; Duggan, D; Crane, C; Hepburn, S; Fennell, MJV; Williams, JMG. Effects of meditation on frontal α-asymmetry in previously suicidal individuals. *NeuroReport*, 2007 18, 709-712.

[25] Barolin, GS. Das Hypnoid in der Behandlung organischer Leiden und Krankheiten, insbesondere in der Neuro-Rehabilitation. In: Gerber G, Sedlak F editors. *Autogenes Training mehr als Entspannung*. München: Ernst-Reinhardt Verlag; 1990. 36-58.

[26] Barolin, GS. Das Respiratorische Feedback (RBF) - Basis und Praxis. In: Barolin GS, editor. *Das Respiratorische Feedback nach Leuner*. Berlin: VWB Verlag für Wissenschaft und Bildung; 2001. 9-32.

[27] Barsby, M. Hypnosis in the management of denture intolerance. *Hypn Int Monographs*, 1997 3, 71-78.

[28] Bassotti, G. & Whitehead, WE. Biofeedback, relaxation training, and cognitive behavior modification as treatments for lower functional gastrointestinal disorders. *Q J Med*, 1997 90, 545-550.

[29] Baudouin, C. *Suggestion and autosuggestion*. London: Allen; 1920.

[30] Baumgartner, I. *Pastoralpsychologie*, Düsseldor: Patmos Verlag; 1990.

[31] Beck, AT. *Cognitive theory and emotional disorders*. New York: International University Press; 1976.

[32] Bell, WE. Clinical diagnosis of the pain-dysfunction syndrome. *JADA*, 1969/a 79, 154-160.

[33] Bell, WH. Nonsurgical management of the pain-dysfunction syndrome. *JADA*, 1969/b 79, 161-170.

[34] Benedetti, F. Placebo analgesia. *Neurol Sci*, 2006 27, S100-S102.

[35] Benedetti, F; Pollo, A; Lopiano, L; Lanotte, M; Vighetti, S; Rainero, I. Conscious expectation and unconscious conditioning in analgesic, and hormonal placebo/nocebo responses. *J Neurosci*, 2003 23, 4315-4323.

[36] Benedetti, F; Colloca, L; Torre, E; Lanotte, M; Melcarne, A; Pesare, M; Bergamasco, B; Lopiano, L. Placebo-responsive Parkinson patients show decreased activity in single neurons of subthalamic nucleus. *Nat Neurosci*, 2004 7, 587-588.

[37] Benedetti, F; Mayberg, HS; Wager, TD; Stohler, CS; Zubieta, J-K. Neurobiological mechanisms of the placebo effect. *J Neurosci*, 2005 25, 10390-10402.

[38] Benedetti, F; Arduino, C; Costa, S; Vighetti, S; Tarenzi, L; Rainero, I; Asteggiano, G. Loss of expectation-related mechanisms in Alzheimer's disease makes analgesic therapies less effective. *Pain*, 2006 121, 133-144.

[39] Benoliel, R; Elishoov, H; Sharav, Y. Orofacial pain with vascular-type features. *Oral Surg Oral Med Oral Pathol Oral Radiol Endod*. 1997 84, 506-512.

[40] Bensing, J. Bridging the gap. The separate worlds of evidence-based medicine and patient-centered medicine. *Patient Education Counseling*, 2000 39, 17-25.

[41] Benson, H. *The relaxation response*. New York: Morrow; 1975.

[42] Benson, H. *Timeless healing: the power and biology of belief*. New York: Scribner; 1996.

[43] Benson, H. The nocebo effect: History and physiology. *Preventive Med*, 1997 26, 612-615.

[44] Benson, H; Beary, JF; Carol, MP. The relaxation response. *Psychiatry*, 1974 37, 37-46.

[45] Benson, H; Frankel, FH; Apfel, R; Daniels, MD; Schniewind, HE; Nemiah, JC; Sifneos, PE; Crassweller, KD; Greenwood, MM; Kotch, JB; Arns, PA; Rosner, B. Treatment of anxiety: a comparison of the usefulness of self-hypnosis and a meditational relaxation technique. An overview. *Psychother Psychosom*, 1978 30, 229-242.

[46] Benton, D. & Donohoe, RT. The effects of nutrients on mood. *Public Health Nutr*, 1999 2, 403-409.

[47] Bergdorf, A. Psycho-Onkologie und Schmerzbehandlung mit dem Respiratorischen Feedback. In: Barolin GS, editor. *Das Respiratorische Feedback nach Leuner*. Berlin: VWB Verlag für Wissenschaft und Bildung; 2001. 125-135.

[48] Berger, H. Über das Elektro-Enkephalogram des Menschen. II. *J Psychol Neurol* (Lpz), 1930 40; 160-169.

[49] Berggren, U. & Linde, A. Dental fear and avoidance: A comparison of two modes of treatment. *J Dent Res*, 1984 63, 1223-1227.

[50] Binder, H. & Binder, K. *Autogenes Training, Basispsychotherapeutikum*. Köln: Deutscher Ärzteverlag; 1989.

[51] Binder, A; Parr, G; Hazleman, B; Fitton-Jackson, S. Pulsed electromagnetic field therapy of persistent rotator cuff tendinitis. A doble-blind controlled assessment. *Lancet*, 1984 1(8379), 695-698.

[52] Biondi, M. & Picardi, A. Temporomandibular joint pain-dysfunction syndrome and bruxism: etiopathogenesis and treatment from a psychosomatic integrative viewpoint. *Psychother Psychosom*, 1993 59, 84-98.

[53] Bishop, TS. High frequency neural modulation in dentistry. *JADA*, 1986 112, 176-177.

[54] Black, RR. Use of transcutaneous electrical nerve stimulation in dentistry. *JADA*, 1986 113, 649-652.

[55] Black, S; Humphrey, JH; Niven, JSF. Inhibition of mantoux reaction by direct sugestion under hypnosis. *Brit Med J*, 1963 22, 1649-1652.

[56] Blanchard, EB. Psychological treatment of benign headache disorders. *J Consult Clin Psychol*, 1992 60, 537-551.

[57] Bohnenkamp, DM. & Garcia, LT. Phonetics and tongue position to improve mandibular denture retention: A clinical report. *J Prosthet Dent*, 2007 98, 344-347.

[58] Bongartz, W. & Bongartz, B. *Hypnosetherapie* 2-nd edition. Göttingen - Bern -Toronto - Seattle: Hogrefe; 2000; 252-254, 312.

[59] Boos, RH. Preparation and conditioning of patients for prosthetic treatment. *J Prosthet Dent*, 1959 9, 4-10.

[60] Bourre, JM. Effects of nutrients (in food) on the structure and function of the nervous system: update on dietary requirements for brain. Part 1: Micronutrients. *J Nutr Health Aging*, 2006 10, 377-385.

[61] Brauchli, P. Comparative study of the psychophysiologic relaxation effects of an optic-acoustic mind machine with relaxation music. *Z Exp Angew Psychol*, 1993 40, 179-193.

[62] Brodine, AL. & Hartshorn, MA. Recognition and management of somatoform disorders. *J Prosthet Dent*, 2004 91, 268-273.

[63] Burkle, CM; Jankowski, CJ; Torsher, LC; Rho, EH; Degnim, AC. BIS monitor findings during self-hypnosis. *J Clin Monit Comput*, 2005 19, 391-393.

[64] Carli, G. An update on pain physiology: the relevance of Craig's and Jäning's hypotheses for hypnotic analgesia. *Contemp Hypnosis*, 2009 26, 4-14.

[65] Carlsson, SG; Gale, EN; Öhman, A. Treatment of temporomandibular joint syndrome with biofeedback training. *JADA*, 1975 91, 602-605.

[66] Carlsson, SG. & Gale, EN. Biofeedback in the treatment of long-term temporomandibular joint pain: An outcome study. *Biofeedback Self-Regul*, 1977 2, 161-171.

[67] Carlson, LE; Speca, M; Patel, KD; Goodey, E. Mindfulness-based stress reduction in relation to quality of life, mood, symptoms of stress, and immune parameters in breast and prostate cancer outpatients. *Psychosom Med*, 2003 65, 571-581.

[68] Carrasco, TG; Mazzeto, MO; Mazzetto, RG; Mestriner Jr., W. Low intensity laser therapy in temporomandibular disorder: a phase II double-blind study. *Cranio*, 2008 26, 274-281.

[69] Castel, A; Pérez, M; Sala, J; Padrol, A; Rull, M. Effect of hypnotic suggestion on fibromyalgic pain: Comparison between hypnosis and relaxation. *Eur J Pain*, 2007 11, 463-468.

[70] Chaco, J. Electromyography of the masseter muscles in Costen's syndrome. *J Oral Med*, 1973 28, 45-46.

[71] Chang, K. & Chang, WH. Pulsed electromagnetic fields prevent osteoporosis in an ovarectomized female rat model: a prostaglandin E2-associated process. *Bioelectromagnetics*, 2003 24, 189-198.

[72] Chaves, JF. Hypnosis in dentistry: Historical overview and current appraisal. *Hypn Int Monographs*, 1997 3, 5-24

[73] Clark, GT. Management of muscular hyperactivity. *Int Dent J*, 1981 31, 216-225.

[74] Clarke, JH. The role of hypnosis in treating bruxism. *Hypn Int Monographs*, 1997 3, 79-86.

[75] Collet, L; Cottraux, J; Juenet, C. GSR feedback and Schultz relaxation in tension headaches: a comparative study. *Pain*, 1986 25, 205-213.

[76] Collins, MP. & Dunn, LF. The effects of meditation and visual imagery on an immune system disorder: dermatomyositis. *J Altern Complement Med*, 2005 11, 275-284.

[77] Colloca, L. & Benedetti, F. How prior experiences shape placebo analgesia. *Pain*, 2006 124, 126-133.

[78] Coromaldi, E; Basar-Eroglu, C; Stadler, MA. EEG-Rythmen während tiefer Meditation: Eine Einzelfallstudie mit einem Zen-Meister. *HyKog*, 2004 21, 61-76.

[79] Cossarizza, A; Monti, D; Bersani, F; Cantini, M; Cadossi, R; Sacchi, A; Franceschi, C. Extremely low frequency pulsed electromagnetic fields increase cell proliferation in lymphocytes from young and aged subjects. *Biochem Biophys Res Commun*, 1989/a 160, 692-698.

[80] Cossarizza, A; Monti, D; Bersani, F; Paganelli, R; Montagnani, G; Cadossi, R; Cantini, M; Franceschi, C. Extremely low frequency pulsed electromagnetic fields increase interleukin-2 (IL-2) utilization and IL-2 receptor expression in mitogen-stimulated human lymphocytes from old subjects. *FEBS Lett*, 1989/b 248, 141-144.

[81]   Coué, E. *Self-mastery through conscious autosuggestion.* London: Allen; 1922.

[82]   Cowan, MJ; Kogan, H; Burr, R; Hendershot, S; Buchanan, L. Power spectral analysis of heart rate variability after biofeedback training. *J Electrocardiol*, 1990 23, Suppl: 85-94.

[83]   Crawford, HE. & Gruzelier, JH. A midstream view of the neuropsychology of hypnosis: Recent research and future directions. In: Fromm E, Nash MR editors. *Contemporary hypnosis research.* New York - London: Guilford Press, 1992, 227-266.

[84]   Critchley, HD; Melmed, RN; Featherstone, E; Mathias, CJ; Dolan, RJ. Brain activity during biofeedback relaxation. A functional neuroimaging investigation. *Brain*, 2001 124, 1003-1012.

[85]   Cruess, DG; Antoni, MH; Kumar, M; Schneiderman, N. Reduction in salivary cortisol is associated with mood improvement during relaxation training among HIV-seropositive men. *J Behavioral Med*, 2000 23, 107-122.

[86]   Curcio, FB; Tackney, VM; Berweger, R. Transcutaneous electrical nerve stimulation in dentistry: A report of a double-blind study. *J Prosthet Dent*, 1987 58, 379-383.

[87]   Cyna, AM; Tomkins, D; Maddock, T; Barker, D. Brief hypnosis for severe needle phobia using switch-wire imagery in a 5-year old. *Pediatr Anesth*, 2007 17, 800-804.

[88]   Dahlsröm, L. Electromyographic studies of craniomandibular disorders: a review of the literature. *J Oral Rehabil*, 1989 16, 1-20.

[89]   Dahlström, L. Conservative treatment methods in craniomandibular disorder. *Swed Dent J*, 1992 16, 217-230.

[90]   Dahlström, L; Carlsson, GE; Carlsson, SG. Comparison of effects of electromyographic biofeedback and occlusal splint therapy on mandibular dysfunction. *Scand J Dent Res*, 1982 90, 151-156.

[91]   Dahlström, L; Haraldson, T; Janson, ST. Comparative electromyographic study of bite plates and stabilization splints. *Scand J Dent Res*, 1985 93, 262-268.

[92]   Dahlström, L; Lindvall, AM; Milthon, R; Widmark, G. Management of chronic orofacial pain: attitudes among patients and dentists in a Swedish county. *Acta Odontol Scand*, 1997 55, 181-185.

[93]   Darendeliler, MA; Sinclair, PM; Kusy, RP. The effects of samarium-cobalt magnets and pulsed electromagnetic fields on tooth movement. *Am J Orthod Dentofacial Orthop*, 1995 107, 578-588.

[94]   Davanloo, H. *Basic principles and techniques in short-term dynamic psychotherapy.* New York: Spectrum Publ.; 1978

[95]   Davidson, DM; Winchester, MA; Taylor, CB; Alderman, EA; Ingels, NB. Effects of relaxation therapy on cardiac performance and sympathetic activity in patients with organic heart disease. *Psychosom Med*, 1979 41, 303-309.

[96]   Davidson, RJ; Kabat-Zinn, J; Schumacher, J; Rosenkranz, M; Muller, D; Santorelli, SF; Urbanowski, F; Harrington, A; Bonus, K; Sheridan, JF. Alterations in brain and immune function produced by mindfulness meditation. Psychosom Med, 2003 65, 564-570.

[97]   Davis, KE. & O'Neill, SJ. A focus group analysis of relapse, prevention strategies for persons with substance use and mental disorders. *Psychiat Services*, 2005 56, 1288-1291.

[98] Dawson-Huges, B; Dallal, GE; Krall, EA; Harris, S; Sokoll, LJ; Falconer, G. Effect of vitamin D supplementation on wintertime and overall bone loss in healthy postmenopausal women. *Ann Intern Med*, 1991 115, 505-512.

[99] de Almeida, JM; Theodoro, LH; Bosco, AF; Nagata, MJH; Oshiiwa, M; Garcia, VG. In vivo effect of photodynamic therapy on periodontal bone loss in dental furcations. *J Periodontol*, 2008 79, 1081-1088.

[100] Delaney, JF. Atypical facial pain as a defense against psychosis. *Am J Psychiat*, 1976 133, 1151-1154.

[101] Delmonte, MM; Physiological responses during meditation and rest. *Biofeedback Self Regul*, 1984 9, 181-200.

[102] de Medeiros, JS; Vieira, GF; Nishimura, PY. Laser application effects on the bite strength of the masseter muscle, as an orofacial pain treatment. *Photomed Laser Surg*, 2005 23, 373-376.

[103] Demmel, HJ. Die Überweisung psychosomatisch kranker Patienten. *Zahnärztl Mitteilungen*, 2007 97, 40-44.

[104] Derra, C. Entspannungsverfahren und Hypnose. In: Egle UT, Hoffmann SO, Lehmann KA, Nix WA editors. *Handbuch chronischer Schmerz. Grundlagen, Pathogenese, Klinik und Therapie aus bio-psycho-socialer Sicht.* Stuttgart-New York: Schattauer GmbH; 2003. 392-403.

[105] Derra C. & Egle, UT. Psychopharmaka in der Schmerztherapie. In: Egle UT, Hoffmann SO, Lehmann KA, Nix WA editors. *Handbuch Chronischer Schmerz. Grundlagen, Pathogenese, Klinik und Therapie aus bio-psycho-sozialer Sicht.* Stuttgart - New York: Schattauer GmbH; 2003; 352-359.

[106] de Silva, P. *Behavior therapy.* In: Fink G, editor in chief. *Encyclopedia of stress. (vol. 1.).* San Diego: Academic Press; 2000. 300-304.

[107] Deskmuth, VD. Neuroscience of meditation. *TSW Journal*, 2006 6, 2239-2253.

[108] Dommett, R; Zilbauer, M; George, JT; Bajaj-Elliott, M. Innate immune defense in the human gastrointestinal tract. *Molecular Immunol*, 2005 42, 903-912.

[109] Dunteman, E. & Swarm, R. Atypical facial "neuralgia". (Case reports). *Anesth Analg*, 1995 80, 188-190.

[110] Dworkin, SF; Turner, JA; Mancl, L; Wilson, L; Massoth, D; Huggins, KH; LeResche, L; Truelove, E. A randomized clinical trial of a tailored comprehensive care treatment program for temporomandibular disorders. *J Orofac Pain*, 2002 16, 259-276.

[111] Dworkin, SF; Turner, JA; Wilson, L; Massoth, D; Whitney, C Huggins, Burgess, J; Sommers, E; Truelove, E. Brief group cognitive-behavioral intervention for temporomandibular disorders. *Pain*, 1994 59, 175-187.

[112] Edmonston Jr, WE. & Grotevant WR. Hypnosis and alpha density. *Am J Clin Hypn*, 1975 17, 221-232.

[113] Egner, T. & Gruzelier, JH. Ecological validity of neurofeedback: Modulation of slow-wave EEG enhances musical performance. *Neuroreport*, 2003 14, 1221-1224.

[114] Egner, T; Strawson, E; Gruzelier, JH. EEG signature and phenomenology of alpha/theta neurofeedback training versus mock feedback. *Appl Psychophysiol Biofeedback*, 2002 27, 261-270.

[115] Eli, I. & Kleinhauz, M. Hypnosis and dentistry. *Hypn Int Monographs*, 1997 3, 59-70.

[116] Ellis, AT. *Reason and emotion in psychotherapy.* New York: Lyle Stuart; 1962.

[117] Ellis, A. *Die Rational-Emotiven Therapie.* München: Pfeiffer; 1977.

[118] Esch, T; Stefano, GB; Fricchione, GL; Benson, H. Stress-related diseases -- a potential role of nitric oxide. *Med Sci Monitor*, 2002/a 8, RA103-RA118.

[119] Esch, T; Stefano, GB; Fricchione, GL; Benson, H. Stress in cardiovascular diseases. *Med Sci Monitor*, 2002/b 8, RA93-RA101.

[120] Esch, T; Duckstein, J; Welke, J; Stefano, GB; Braun, V. Mind/body techniques for physiological and psychological stress reduction: Stress management via Tai Chi training - a pilot study. *Med Sci Monitor*, 2007 13, CR488-CR497.

[121] Esposito, CJ; Veal, SJ; Farman, AG. Alleviation of myofascial pain with ultrasonic therapy. *J Prosthet Dent*, 1984 51, 106-108.

[122] Fábián G. Psychosomatic aspects of orthodontics. [Az orthodontia pszichoszomatikus vonatkozásai]. In: Fábián TK, Vértes G editors. *Psychosomatic dentistry [Fogorvosi pszichoszomatika]*. Budapest: Medicina; 2007; 137-146.

[123] Fábián, G; Bálint, M; Fábián, TK. Psychology and psychosomatics of the orthodontic treatment. *Fogorv Szle*, 2005 98, 113-119.

[124] Fábián, TK. Hypnotic desensitization as a supplemental method in dental care of patients with panic disorder. Report of a case. *Fogorv Szle*, 1996/a 89, 57-62.

[125] Fábián TK. Anxiety as a dynamic factor of dental hypnosis. *Fogorv Szle*, 1996/b 89, 153-157.

[126] Fábián, TK. The use of hypnosis in the dental practice. A symbolic method. *Fogorv Szle*, 1996/c 89, 295-299.

[127] Fábián, TK. *Possibilities of medical hypnosis in operative and psychosomatic dentistry [Az orvosi hipnózis alkalmazásának lehetőségei a klinikai fogászatban, fogászati pszichoszomatikában]*. Ph.D. thesis. Budapest: Hungarian Academy of Sciences; 1999/a.

[128] Fábián, TK. Treatment possibilities of denture intolerance. Use of photo-acoustic stimulation and hypnotherapy in a difficult clinical case. [Adalékok a protézis intolerancia gyógyításához. Fény-hang kezeléssel kombinált hipnoterápia alkalmazásának szokatlan módja egy eset kapcsán.] *Hipno Info*,1999/b 38, 81-88.

[129] Fábián, TK. Mental health and pastoral counsealing [Mentálhigiéné és lelkigondozás]. In: Fábián TK, Vértes G editors. *Psychosomatic dentistry [Fogorvosi pszichoszomatika]*. Budapest: Medicina; 2007; 158-168.

[130] Fábián, TK. *Mind-body connections. Pathways of psychosomatic coupling under meditation and other altered states of consciousness*. New York: Nova Science Publishers; in press.

[131] Fábián, TK. & Fábián, G. Stress of life, stress of death: Anxiety in dentistry from the viewpoint of hypnotherapy. *Ann NY Acad Sci*, 1998 851, 495-500.

[132] Fábián, TK. & Fábián, G. Dental stress. In: Fink G, editor in chief. *Encyclopedia of stress. (vol. 1.)*. San Diego: Academic Press; 2000; 567-659.

[133] Fábián, TK. & Sőti, Cs. Low induction value pulsed electromagnetic field stimulation. [Alacsony indukció értékű mágneses impulzus tér stimuláció] In: Vértes G, Fábián TK editors. *Psychosomatic dentistry [Fogorvosi Pszichoszomatika]* Budapest: Medicina; 2007; 201-210.

[134] Fábián, TK; Vértes, G; Szabó, A; Varga, K. Photo-acoustic stimulation and hypnotherapy. An effective combination for treatment of oral psychosomatic disorders. *Hypn Int Monographs*, 2002 6, 199-207.

[135] Fábián, TK; Gáspár, J; Fejérdy, L; Kaán, B; Bálint, M; Csermely, P; Fejérdy, P. Hsp70 is present in human saliva. *Med Sci Monit*, 2003 9, BR62-65.

[136] Fábián, TK; Kaán, B; Fejérdy, L; Tóth, Zs; Fejérdy, P. Effectiveness of psychotherapy in the treatment of denture intolerance. Evaluation of 25 cases. *Fogorv Szle*, 2004/a 97, 163-168.

[137] Fábián, TK; Tóth, Zs; Fejérdy, L; Kaán, B; Csermely, P; Fejérdy, P. Photo-acoustic stimulation increases the amount of 70 kDa heat shock protein (Hsp70) in human whole saliva. A pilot study. *Int J Psychophysiol*, 2004/b 52, 211-216.

[138] Fábián, TK; Krause, WR; Krause, M; Fejérdy, P. Photo-acoustic stimulation and hypnotherapy in the treatment of oral psychosomatic disorders. *Hypnos*, 2005/a 32, 198-202.

[139] Fábián, TK; Vértes, G; Fejérdy, P. Pastoralpsychology in dentistry. *Fogorv Szle*, 2005/b 98. 37-42.

[140] Fábián, TK; Mierzwińska-Nastalska, E; Fejérdy P. Photo-acoustic stimulation. A suitable method in the treatment of psychogenic denture intolerance. *Protet Stomatol*, 2006/a 56, 335-340.

[141] Fábián, TK; Sőti, Cs; Fejérdy, P. Low induction value pulsed electromagnetic field stimulation. A minimal-invasive possibility in the treatment of several idiopathic symptoms of denture intolerance. *Fogorv Szle*, 2006/b 99, 66.

[142] Fábián, TK; Kovács, Sz; Müller, O; Fábián, G; Marten, A; Fejérdy, P. Some aspects of existential psychotherapy in dentistry. *Fogorv Szle*, 2006/c 99, 246.

[143] Fábián, TK; Fábián, G; Fejérdy, P. Dental stress. In: Fink G, editor in chief. *Encyclopedia of stress. Second edition. (vol. 1.)* .Oxford: Academic Press; 2007/a; 733-736.

[144] Fábián, TK; Fejérdy, P; Nguyen, MT; Sőti, Cs; Csermely, P. Potential immunological functions of salivary Hsp70 in mucosal and periodontal defense mechanisms. *Arch Immunol Ther Exp*, 2007/b 55, 91-98.

[145] Fábián, TK; Sőti, Cs; Nguyen, MT; Csermely, P; Fejérdy, P. Expected functions of salivary HSP70 in the oral cavity. In: Morell E, Vincent C editors. *Heat shock proteins: New research*. New York: Nova Science Publishers; 2008/a; 321-340.

[146] Fábián, TK; Sőti, Cs; Nguyen, MT; Csermely, P; Fejérdy, P. Expected functions of salivary HSP70 in the oral cavity. *Int J Med Biol Frontiers*, 2008/b 14, 289-308.

[147] Fábián, TK; Fejérdy, P; Csermely, P. Salivary genomics, transcriptomics and proteomics: The emerging concept of the oral ecosystem and their use in the early diagnosis of cancer and other diseases. *Current Genomics*, 2008/c 9, 11-21.

[148] Fábián, TK; Fejérdy, P; Csermely, P. Chemical biology of saliva in health and disease. In: Begley T, editor in chief. Wiley encyclopedia of chemical biology. Hoboken: John Wiley & sons; 2008/d; DOI: 10.1002/9780470048672.wecb643

[149] Fábián, TK; Gótai, L; Beck, A; Fábián, G; Fejérdy, P. The role of molecular chaperones (HSPAs/HSP70s) in oral health and oral inflammatory diseases: A review. *Eur J Inflammation*, 2009/a 7, 53-61.

[150] Fábián, TK; Csermely, P; Fábián, G; Fejérdy, P. Spondyloarthropathies and bone resorption: A possible role of heat shock protein (Hsp70). (Review). *Acta Physiol Hungarica*, 2009/b 96, 149-155.

[151] Fábián, TK; Gótai, L; Krause, WR; Fejérdy, P. Zahnärztliche Hypnoseforschung an der Semmelweis Universität Budapest. *Deutsche Z Zahnärztl Hypn*, 2009/c 8, 9-14.

[152] Fábián, TK; Kovács, JK; Gótai, L; Beck, A; Krause, WR; Fejérdy, P. Photo-acoustic stimulation: Theoretical background and ten years of clinical experience. *Contemporary Hypnosis*, in press, DOI: 10.1002/ch.389

[153] Farthing, GW. *The psychology of consciousness*. Prentice Hall New Jersey: Englewood Cliffs; 1992; 202-219, 478-497.

[154] Fava, GA. Cognitive behavioral therapy. In: Fink G, editor in chief. *Encyclopedia of stress. (vol. 1.)*. San Diego: Academic Press; 2000; 484-487.

[155] Faymonville, ME; Fissette, J; Mambourg, PH; Roediger, L; Joris, J; Lamy, M. Hypnosis as adjunct therapy in conscious sedation for plastic surgery. *Reg Anest*, 1995 20, 145-151.

[156] Faymonville, ME; Mambourg, PH; Joris, J; Vrijens, B; Fissette, J; Albert, A; Lamy, M. Psychological approaches during conscious sedation. Hypnosis versus stress reducing strategies: A prospective randomized study. *Pain*, 1997 73, 361-367.

[157] Faymonville, ME; Laureys, S; Degueldre, C; DelFiore, G; Luxen, A; Franck, G; Lamy, M; Maquet, P. Neural mechanisms of antinociceptive effects of hypnosis. *Anesthesiology*, 2000 92, 1257-1267.

[158] Faymonville, ME; Roediger, L; Del Fiore, G; Degueldre, C; Phillips, C; Lamy, M; Luxen, A; Maquet, P; Laureys, S. Increased cerebral functional connectivity underlying the antinociceptive effects of hypnosis. *Cogn Brain Res*, 2003 17, 255-262.

[159] Faymonville, ME; Boly, M; Laureys, S. Functional neuroanatomy of the hypnotic state. *J Physiology Paris*, 2006 99, 463-469.

[160] Fejérdy, L; Gáspár, J; Kaán, B; Bálint, M; Fábián, TK. Time parameters of dental hypnosis. *Fogorv Szle*, 2003 96, 161-164.

[161] Fejérdy, L; Tóth, Zs; Kaán, B; Fábián, TK; Csermely, P; Fejérdy, P. The effect of heat stimulation and mechanical stress (massage) of salivary glands on the secretoric parameters of salivary Hsp70. A pilot study. *Fogorv Szle*, 2004 97, 204-210.

[162] Fejérdy, P. Compass of dental psychosomatic treatment and postgraduate education. [A fogorvosi pszichoszomatikus beavatkozások keretei, a továbbképzés formái]. In: Fábián TK, Vértes G editors. *Psychosomatic dentistry* [*Fogorvosi pszichoszomatika*]. Budapest: Medicina; 2007; 17-21.

[163] Ferenczi, S. *Final contributions to the problems and methods of psycho-analysis*. New York: Brunnel and Mazel; 1980.

[164] Fini, M; Cadossi, R; Cane, V; Cavani, F; Giavaresi, G; Krajewski, A; Martini, L; Aldini, NN; Ravaglioli, A; Rimondini, L; Torricelli, P; Giardino, R. The effect of pulsed electromagnetic fields on the osteointegration of hydroxyapatite implants in cancellous bone: a morphologic and microstructural in vivo study. *J Orthop Res*, 2002 20, 756-763.

[165] Flor, H. & Birbaumer, N. Comparison of the efficacy of electromyographic biofeedback, cognitive-behavioral therapy, and conservative medical interventions in the treatment of chronic musculoskeletal pain. *J Consult Clin Psychol*, 1993 61, 653-658.

[166] Forgione, AG. & Mehler, BL. Biofeedback in the treatment of myofascial pain disorder and temporomandibular joint pain. In: Mostofsky DI, Forgione AG, Giddon DB editors. *Behavioral dentistry*. Ames (Iowa): Blackwell Munksgaard; 2006; 51-64.

[167] Fox, PA; Henderson, DC; Barton, SE; Champion, AJ; Rollin, MS; Catalan, J; McCormack, SM; Gruzelier, J. Immunological markers of frequently recurrent genital herpes simplex virus and their response to hypnotherapy: a pilot study. *Int J STD AIDS*, 1999 10, 730-740.

[168] Frankl, VE. *Logotherapy and Existenzanalyse.* Berlin-München: Quintessenz; 1994.

[169] Freesmeyer, WB. Okklusionsschienen. In: Koeck B, editor. *Funktionsstörungen des Kauorgans.* München - Wien - Baltimore: Urban & Schwarzenberg; 1995; 215-241.

[170] Freud, S. *Die Traumdeutung* (1900) In: Strachey J, editor. *The standard edition of the complete psychological works of Sigmund Freud. Vol. IV-V.* London: Imago; 1953-1966.

[171] Freud, S. *Diezukünftigen Chancen der psychoanalytischen Therapie.* (1910) In: Strachey J, editor. *The standard edition of the complete psychological works of Sigmund Freud. Vol. XI.* London: Imago; 1953-1966.

[172] Freud, S. *Zur Dynamik der Übertragung* (1912) In: Strachey J, editor. *The standard edition of the complete psychological works of Sigmund Freud. Vol. XII.* London: Imago; 1953-1966.

[173] Freud, S. *Jenseits des Lustprinzips.* (1920) In: Strachey J, editor. *The standard edition of the complete psychological works of Sigmund Freud. Vol. XVIII.* London: Imago; 1953-1966.

[174] Freud, S. *"Psychoanalyse" und "Libidotheory".* (1923/a) In: Strachey J, editor. *The standard edition of the complete psychological works of Sigmund Freud. Vol. XVIII.* London: Imago; 1953-1966.

[175] Freud, S. *Das Ich und das Es.* (1923/b) In: Strachey J, editor. *The standard edition of the complete psychological works of Sigmund Freud. Vol. XIX.* London: Imago; 1953-1966

[176] Freud, A. Das Ich und die Abwehrmechanismen. London: Imago, 1936.

[177] Friedlander, AH; Marder, SR; Sung, EC. Panic disorder. Psychopathology, medical management and dental implications. *JADA*, 2004 135, 771-778.

[178] Fujita, S; Yamaguchi, M; Utsunomiya, T; Yamamoto, H; Kasai, K. Low-energy laser stimulates tooth movement velocity via expression of RANK and RANKL. *Orthod Craniofac Res*, 2008 11, 143-155.

[179] Gale, EN. & Carlsson, SG. Lemon juice: Whose reinforcer is what? *Behav Therapy*, 1977 8, 507-509.

[180] Gallo, LM; Guerra, PO; Palla, S. Automatic on-line one-channel recognition of masseter activity. *J Dent Res*, 1998 77, 1539-1546.

[181] Gallo, LM; Salis Gross, SS; Palla, S. Nocturnal masseter EMG activity of healthy subjects in a natural environment. *J Dent Res*, 1999 78, 1436-1444.

[182] Galvin, JA; Benson, H; Deckro, GR; Fricchione, GL; Dusek, JA. The relaxation response: Reducing stress and improving cognition in healthy aging adults. *Compl Ther Clin Pract*, 2006 12, 186-191.

[183] Ganz, FJ. *Ohrgeräusche. Ärztlicher Rat.* Stuttgart: Thieme; 1983. 95.

[184] Garcion, E; Wion-Barbot, N; Montero-Menei, CN; Berger, F; Wion, D. New clues about vitamin D functions in the nervous system. *Trends Endocrinol Metab*, 2002 13, 100-105.

[185] Gáspár, J; Fejérdy, L; Fábián, TK. The psychical aspects of overactive gag reflex (gagging): a case report. *Fogorv Szle*, 2002 95, 199-203.

[186] Gáspár, J; Linninger, M; Kaán, M; Bálint, M; Fejérdy, L; Fábián, TK. The effectivity of standardized direct suggestions under dental hypnotic conditions. *Fogorv Szle*, 2003 96, 205-210.

[187] Gaylord, C; Orme-Johnson, D; Travis, F. The effects of the transcendental meditation technique and progressive muscle relaxation on EEG coherence, stress reactivity, and mental health in black adults. *Int J Neurosci*, 1989 46, 77-86.

[188] Gellrich, NC; Schramm, A; Böckmann, R; Kugler, J. Follow-up in patients with oral cancer. *J Oral Maxillofac Surg*, 2002 60, 380-386.

[189] Gerber, G. Therapeutisches Setting und KB-Therapie bei psychosomatisch erkrankten Jugendlichen. In: Wilke E, Leuner H editors. *Das Katathyme Bilderleben in der Psychosomatischen Medizin*. Bern-Stuttgart-Toronto: Hans Huber Verlag; 1990; 302-307.

[190] Gerschman, JA; Ruben, J; Gebart-Eaglemont, J. Low level laser therapy for dentinal tooth hypersensitivity. *Aust Dent J*, 1994 39, 353-357.

[191] Giardino, ND. & Lehrer, PM. Behavioral conditioning and idiopathic environmental intolerance. *Occup Med*, 2000 15, 519-528.

[192] Gibilisco, JA. Manifestations of systemic disease of the temporomandibular joint. In: Laney WR, Gibilisco JA editors. *Diagnosis and treatment of prosthodontics*. Philadelphia: Lea & Febiger; 1983; 112-128.

[193] Glaros, AG. Bruxism. In: Mostofsky DI, Forgione AG, Giddon DB editors. *Behavioral dentistry*. Ames (Iowa): Blackwell Munksgaard; 2006; 127-137.

[194] Gokli, MA; Wood, AJ; Mourino, AP; Farrington, FH; Best, AM. Hypnosis as an adjunct to the administration of local anesthetic in pediatric patients. *J Dent Child*, 1994 61, 272-275.

[195] Gold, N; Greene, CS; Laskin, DM. TENS therapy for treatment of MPD (abstract). *IADR Progr & Abstracts*. 1983, 244.

[196] Goodman, P; Greene, CS; Laskin, DM. Response of patients with myofascial pain-dysfunction syndrome to mock equilibration. *JADA*, 1976 92, 755-758.

[197] Gossling, HR; Bernstein, RA; Abbott, J. Treatment of ununited tibial fractures: a comparison of surgery and pulsed electromagnetic fields (PEMF). *Orthopedics*, 1992 15, 711-719.

[198] Green, CS. & Laskin, DM. Meprobamate therapy for the myofascial pain-dysfunction (MPD) syndrome: a double-blind evaluation. *JADA*, 1969 82, 587-590.

[199] Green, CS. & Laskin, DM. Splint therapy for the myofascial pain-dysfunction (MPD) syndrome: a comparative study. *JADA*, 1972/a 84, 624-628.

[200] Green, CS. & Laskin, DM. Therapeutic effects of diazepam (valium) and sodium salicilate in myofascial pain-dysfunction (MPD) patients (abstract). *IADR Progr & Abstr*, 1972/b, 96.

[201] Green, CS. & Laskin, DM. Long-term evaluation of conservative treatment for myofascial pain-dysfunction syndrome. *JADA*, 1974 89, 1365-1368.

[202] Green, CS. & Laskin, DM. Temporomandibular disorders: Moving from a dentally based to a medically based model. *J Dent Res*, 2000 79, 1736-1739.

[203] Griffin, CJ: The treatment of the temporomandibular joint syndrome. In: Griffin CJ, Harris R editors. *The temporomandibular joint syndrome. The masticatory apparatus of man in normal and abnormal function*. (Monographs in oral science, Vol. 4.) Basel - München - Paris - London - New York - Sydney: Karger; 1975; 170-187.

[204] Griffin, CJ, Watson, JE; Marshall, WG: Electromyographic analysis of the effects of treatment in patients with the temporomandibular joint syndrome. In: Griffin CJ, Harris R editors. *The temporomandibular joint syndrome. The masticatory apparatus of man in normal and abnormal function.* (Monographs in oral science, Vol. 4.) Basel - München - Paris - London - New York - Sydney: Karger; 1975; 188-200.

[205] Grond, S. & Lehmann, KA. Analgetika: Anwendung, Nutzen und Probleme. In: Egle UT, Hoffmann SO, Lehmann KA, Nix WA editors. *Handbuch Chronischer Schmerz. Grundlagen, Pathogenese, Klinik und Therapie aus bio-psycho-sozialer Sicht.* Stuttgart - New York: Schattauer GmbH; 2003; 334-345.

[206] Grossan, M. Treatment of subjective tinnitus with Biofeedback. *Ear Nose Throat J,* 1976 55, 22-30.

[207] Gruzelier, JH. A review of the impact of hypnosis, relaxation, guided imagery and individual differences on aspects of immunity and health. *Stress,* 2002 5, 147-163.

[208] Gruzelier, J; Smith, F; Nagy, A; Henderson, D. Cellular and humoral immunity, mood and exam stress: the influences of self-hypnosis and personality predictors. *Int J Psychophysiol,* 2001 42, 55-71.

[209] Gruzelier, J; Champion, A; Fox, P; Rollin, M; McCormack, S; Catalan, P; Barton, S; Henderson, D. Individual differences in personality, immunology and mood in patients undergoing self-hypnosis training for the successful treatment of a chronic viral illness, HSV-2. *Contemp Hypnosis,* 2006 19, 149-166.

[210] Guntrip, HJS. Schizoid phenomena, object-relations and the self. New York: Int Univ Press; 1969.

[211] Hall, H; Minnes, L; Olness, K. The psychophysiology of voluntary immunomodulation. *Int J Neurosci.* 1993 69, 221-234.

[212] Hall, H; Papas, A; Tosi, M; Olness, K. Directional changes in neutrophil adherence following passive resting versus active imagery. *Int J Neurosci,* 1996 85, 185-194.

[213] Halsband, U; Mueller, S; Hinterberger, T; Strickner, S. Plasticity changes in the brain in hypnosis and meditation. *Contemp Hypn,* in press. DOI: 10.1002/ch.386

[214] Hammarstrand, G; Berggren, U; Hakeberg, M. Psychophysiological therapy vs. hypnotherapy in the treatment of patients with dental phobia. *Eur J Oral Sci,* 1995 103, 399-404.

[215] Harris, R. & Griffin, CJ. Neuromuscular mechanisms and the masticatory apparatus. In: Griffin CJ, Harris R editors. *The temporomandibular joint syndrome. The masticatory apparatus of man in normal and abnormal function.* (Monographs in oral science, Vol. 4.) Basel - München - Paris - London - New York - Sydney: Karger; 1975; 45-64.

[216] Harris, M; Feinmann, C; Wise, M; Treasure, F. Temporomandibular joint and orofacial pain: clinical and medicolegal management problems. *Brit Dent J,* 1993 174, 129-136.

[217] Hartmann, H. *Ego psychology and the problem of adaptation.* New York: Int Univ Press; 1964.

[218] Heinze, R-I. Shamanistic states of consciousness: Access to different realities. In: Hoppál M, Howard KD editors. *Shamans and cultures* (ISTOR books 5). Budapest - Los Angeles: Akadémiai Kiadó & International Society of Trans-Oceanic Research; 1993. 169-178.

[219] Hermes, D; Hakim, SG; Trübger, D; Sieg, P. Tape Recorded Hypnosis. Eine effiziente Therapieoption zur Verbesserung des Behandlungskomforts in der Oral- und Mund-Kiefer-Gesichtschirurgie. *Quintessenz,* 2003 54, 911-919.

[220] Hertrich, K. & Joraschky, P. Psychotherapie in der zahnärztlichen Praxis: Möglichkeiten der Integration und Kooperation. In: Sergl HG, editor. *Psychologie und Psychosomatik in der Zahnheilkunde*. München - Wien - Baltimore: Urban & Schwarzenberg; 1996; 261-279.

[221] Hidderley, M. & Holt, M. A pilot randomized trial assessing the effects of autogenic training in early stage cancer patients in relation to psychological status and immune system responses. *Eur J Oncol Nurs*, 2004 8, 61-65.

[222] Hilgard, ER. A neodissociation interpretation of hypnosis. In: Lynn SJ, Rhue JW editors. *Theories of hypnosis. Current models and perspectives*. New York - London: Guilford Press; 1991. 83-104.

[223] Hilgard, ER. Neodissociation theory. In: Lynn SJ, Rhue JW editors. *Dissociation: Clinical and theoretical perspectives*. New York: Guilford Press; 1994. 32-51.

[224] Hochman, R. Neurotransmitter modulator (TENS) for control of dental operative pain. *JADA*, 1988 116, 208-212.

[225] Hoppál, M. Shamanism: Universal structures and regional symbols. In: Hoppál M, Howard KD editors. *Shamans and cultures*. (ISTOR books 5). Budapest - Los Angeles: Akadémiai Kiadó & International Society of Trans-Oceanic Research; 1993/a. 181-192.

[226] Hoppál, M. Studies on Eurasian shamanism. In: Hoppál M, Howard KD editors. *Shamans and cultures*. (ISTOR books 5). Budapest - Los Angeles: Akadémiai Kiadó & International Society of Trans-Oceanic Research; 1993/b. 258-288.

[227] Horinek, H. Allgemeinmedizin und Psychosomatik. In: Barolin GS, editor. *Das Respiratorische Feedback nach Leuner*. Berlin: VWB Verlag für Wissenschaft und Bildung; 2001; 137-144.

[228] House, JW; Miller, L; House, PR. Severe tinnitus: treatment with biofeedback training (results in 41 cases). *Trans Am Acad Ophtalmol Otol*, 1977 84, 697-703.

[229] Hörnlein-Rummel, H. RFB als Gruppentherapie. In: Barolin GS, editor. *Das Respiratorische Feedback nach Leuner*. Berlin: VWB Verlag für Wissenschaft und Bildung; 2001; 145-161.

[230] Hudacek, KD. A review of the effects of hypnosis on the immune system in breast cancer patients: a brief communication. *Int J Clin Exp Hypn*. 2007 55, 411-425.

[231] Infante, JR; Torres-Avisbal, M; Pinel, P; Vallejo, JA; Peran, F; Gonzalez, F; Contreras, P; Pacheco, C; Roldan, A; Latre, JM. Catecholamine levels in practitioners of the transcendental meditation technique. *Physiol Behav*, 2001 72, 141-146.

[232] Inoue, N; Ohnishi, I; Chen, D; Deitz, LW; Schwardt, JD; Chao, EY. Effect of pulsed electromagnetic fields (PEMF) on late-phase osteotomy gap healing in a canine tibial model. *J Orthop Res*, 2002 20, 1106-1114.

[233] Israel, HA. & Scrivani, SJ. The interdisciplinary approach to oral, facial and head pain. *JADA*, 2000 131, 919-926.

[234] Ito, YH; Ippongi, S; Nakano, M; Kurabe, T; Kazaoka, Y. Ishiguchi, T. Bioprotection by local and whole-body preheating - bioprotection of damage to mice tongue from burning by local preheating of oral cavity and of radiation damage of small intestine from whole-body preheating. *Nippon Igaku Hoshasen Gakkai Zassi*, 2005 65, 255-262.

[235] Iversen, G. & Geleitwort. In: Binder H, Binder K editors. *Autogenes Training, Basispsychotherapeutikum*. Köln: Deutscher Ärzteverlag; 1989.

[236] Jacobs, GD. & Friedman, R. EEG spectral analysis of relaxation techniques. *Applied Physiol Biofeedback*, 2004 29, 245-254.

[237] Jacobs, GD. & Lubar, JF. Spectral analysis of the central nervous system effects of the relaxation response elicited by autogenic training. *Behav Med*, 1989 15, 125-132.

[238] Jacobson, E. *Progressive relaxation*. Chicago: Univ. of Chicago Press; 1938.

[239] Jain, S; Shapiro, SL; Swanick, S; Roesch, SC; Mills, PJ; Bell, I; Schwartz, GE. A randomized controlled trial of mindfulness meditation versus relaxation training: effects on distress, positive states of mind, rumination, and distraction. *Ann Behav Med*, 2007 33, 11-21.

[240] Janoski, ML. & Kugler, J. Relaxation, imagery, and neuroimmunomodulation. *Ann NY Acad Sci*, 1987 496, 722-730.

[241] Jaseja, H. Meditation may predispose to epilepsy: an insight into the alteration in brain environment induced by meditation. *Med Hypothesis*, 2005 64, 464-467.

[242] Jaseja, H. A brief study of a possible relation of epilepsy association with meditation. *Med Hypotheses*, 2006/a 66, 1036-1049.

[243] Jaseja, H. Meditation potentially capable of increasing susceptibility to epilepsy - A follow up hypotheses. *Med Hypotheses*, 2006/b 66, 925-928.

[244] Jenkins, MW. Teaching patients to block post-operative pain by self-hypnosis. *Eur J Clin Hypn*, 1995 2(3), 54-55.

[245] Jenkins, MW. & Pritchard, M. Practical applications and theoretical considerations of hypnosis in normal labour. *Eur J Clin Hypn*, 1994 1(3), 23-28.

[246] Jöhren, HP; Enkling, N; Heinen, R; Sartory, G. Klinischer Erfolg einer verhaltenstherapeutischen Kurzintervention zur Behandlung von Zahnbehandlungsphobie. *Deutsch Zahnärztl Z*, 2009 64, 377.

[247] Jung, CG. *The structure and dynamics of the psyche.* (1926) In: *Collected works* (Vol. 8). Princeton NJ: Princeton University press; 1960.

[248] Jung, CG. *Analytical psychology: its theory and practice.* New York: Pantheon; 1968.

[249] Jung, CG. Die transcendente Funktion. Cit. Amman, AN. *Aktive Imagination.* Freiburg: Walter; 1978. page 9.

[250] Kaán, B; Krause, W-R; Krause, M; Fejérdy, L; Gáspár, J; Bálint, M; Fábián, TK. Effects of photo-acoustic stimulation combined with hypnotherapy on saliva secretion. A pilot study. *Fogorv Szle*, 2003 96, 217-221.

[251] Kaán, B; Tóth, Zs; Fábián, TK. The role of sexual trauma as a cause of oro-facial symptoms. Case report. *Fogorv Szle*, 2004 97, 37-40.

[252] Kaban, LB. & Belfer, ML. Temporomandibular joint dysfunction: an occasional manifestation of serious psychopathology. *J Oral Surg*, 1981 39, 742-746.

[253] Kabat-Zinn, J. Wherever you go, there you are. Mindfullness meditation in Everyday life. New York: Hyperion; 2005.

[254] Kaji, R; Katayama-Hirota, M; Kohara, N; Kojima, Y; Yang, Q; Kimura, J. Blepharospasm induced by a LED flashlight. *Mov Disord*, 1999 14, 1045-1047.

[255] Kakigi, R; Nakata, H; Inui, K; Hiroe, N; Nagata, O; Honda, M; Tanaka, S; Sadato, N; Kawakami, M. Intracerebral pain processing in a yoga master who claims not to feel pain during meditation. *Eur J Pain*, 2005 9, 581-589.

[256] Kanje, M; Rusovan, A; Sisken, B; Lundborg, G. Pretreatment of rats with pulsed electromagnetic fields enhances regeneration of the sciatic nerve. *Bioelectromagnetics*, 1993 14, 353-359.

[257] Kapur, K. & Shklar, G. Effects of a power device for oral physiotherapy on the mucosa of the edentulous ridge. *J Prosthet Dent*, 1962 12, 762-769.

[258] Karppinen, K; Eklund, S; Suoninen, E; Eskelin, M; Kirveskari, P. Adjustment of dental occlusion in treatment of chronic cervicobrachial pain and headache. *J Oral Rehabil*, 1999 26, 715-721.

[259] Kawamura, Y. & Horio, T. Effect of chewing exercise on the maximum biting force and chewing. *Shika Kiso Igakkai Zasshi*, 1989 31, 281-290.

[260] Kawasaki, K. & Shimizu, N. Effects of low-energy laser irradiation on bone remodeling during experimental tooth movement in rats. *Lasers Surg Med*, 2000 26, 282-291.

[261] Kernberg, OF. *Object relations theory and clinical psychoanalysis*. New York: Jason Aronson; 1976.

[262] Kernberg, OF. *Internal world and external reality*. New York: Basic Books; 1980.

[263] Khadra, M. The effect of low level laser irradiation on implant-tissue interaction. In vivo and in vitro studies. *Swed Dent J Suppl*, 2005 172, 1-63.

[264] Khadra, M; Kasem, N; Lyngstadaas, SP; Haanæs HR; Mustafa, K. Laser therapy accelerates initial attachment and subsequent behavior of human fibroblasts cultured on titanium implant material. *Clin Oral Impl Res*, 2005/a 16, 168-175.

[265] Khadra, M; Lyngstadaas, SP; Hans, R; Haanæs, Mustafa, K. Effect of laser therapy on attachment, proliferation and differentiation of human osteoblast-like cells cultures on titanium implant material. *Biomaterials*, 2005/b 26, 3503-3509.

[266] Khullar, SM; Brodin, P; Messelt, EB; Haanæs, HR. The effects of low level laser treatment on recovery of nerve conduction and motor function after compression injury in the rat sciatic nerve. *Eur J Oral Sci*, 1995 103, 299-305.

[267] Kihlstrom, JF. Conscious, subconscious, unconscious: A cognitive perspective. In: Bowers KS, Meichenbaum D editors. *The unconscious reconsidered*. New York: John Wiley and Sons; 1984; 149-211.

[268] Kim, YD; Kim, SS; Hwang, DS; Kim, SG; Kwon, YH; Shin, SH; Kim, UK; Kim, JR; Chung, IK. Effect of low-level laser treatment after installation of dental titanium implant - immunohystochemical study of RANKL, RANK, OPG: an experimental study in rats. *Lasers Surg Med*, 2007 39, 441-450.

[269] Kim, YD; Song, WW; Kim, SS; Kim, GC; Hwang, DS; Shin, SH; Kim, UK; Kim, JR; Chung, IK. Expression of receptor activator of nuclear factor -κB ligand, receptor activator of nuclear factor -κB, and osteoprotegerin, following low-level laser treatment on deproteinized bovine bone graft in rats. *Lasers Med Sci*, in press/a. DOI: 10.1007/s10103-008-0614-7

[270] Kim, YD; Kim, SS; Kim, SJ; Kwon, DW; Jeon, ES; Son, WS. Low-level laser irradiation facilitates fibronectin and collagen type I turnover during tooth movement in rats. *Lasers Med Sci*, in press/b. DOI: 10.1007/s10103-008-0585-8

[271] Kimura, Y; Wilder-Smith, P; Yonaga, K; Matsumoto, K. Treatment of dentine hypersensitivity by lasers: a review. *J Clin Periodontol*, 2000 27, 715-721.

[272] King, RB. Concerning the management of pain associated with herpes zoster and of postherpetic neuralgia. *Pain*, 1988 33, 73-78.

[273] Kingston, J; Chadwick, P; Meron, D; Skinner, TC. A pilot randomized control trial investigating the effect of mindfulness practice on pain tolerance, psychological well-being, and physiological activity. *J Psychosom Res*, 2007 62, 297-300.

[274] Kinzel, C. *Psychoanalyse und Hypnose*. München: Quintessenz; 1993.

[275] Klein, M. *The psycho-analysis of children*. London: Hogarth; 1932.

[276] Kohut, H. *The analysis of the self.* New york: International University Press; 1971.

[277] Kokoshis, PL; Williams, DL; Cook, JA; Di Luzio, NR. Increased resistance to Staphylococcus aureus infection and enhancement in serum lysozyme activity by glucan. *Science,* 1978 199, 1340-1342.

[278] Kold, SE; Hickman, J; Meisen, F. Preliminary study of quantitative aspects and the effect of pulsed electromagnetic field treatment on the incorporation of equine cancellous bone grafts. *Equine Vet J,* 1987 19, 120-124.

[279] Komiyama, O; Kawara, M; Arai, M; Asano, T; Kobayashi, K. Posture correction as part of behavioral therapy in treatment of myofascial pain with limited opening. *J Oral Rehabil,* 1999 26, 428-435.

[280] Korn, HJ. Biofeedback und zahnmedizinische Behandlungsansätze bei temporomandibulären Störungen und Bruxismus. *Verhaltenstherapie,* 2005 15, 94-102.

[281] Köhler, T. Fortbildung: Psychopharmakotherapie (2. Teil). *Verhaltenstherapie & Verhaltensmedizin,* 2005 26, 141-168.

[282] Köling, A. Neurologist, otolaryngologist...? Which specialist should treat facial pain? *Lakartidningen,* 1998 95, 2320-2325.

[283] Krause, WR. Grundlagen der Biofeedback-Therapie und ihre therapeutischen Anwendungsmöglichkeiten. *Z ärztl Fortbild,* 1983 77, 493-494.

[284] Krause, WR. Hypnose und Autogenes Training (Selbsthypnose) in der Rehabilitation. Ergänzung in: Schultz, JH. *Hypnose-Technik. Praktische Anleitung zum Hypnotisieren für Ärzte.* 9. Auflage - bearbeitet und ergänzt von G. Iversen und W.-R. Krause. Stuttgart - Jena - New York: Gustav Fischer Verlag; 1994. 71-79.

[285] Krause, WR. Hypnose und Autogenes Training. *Mitteldeutsch Hausarzt,* 2000 2, 20-22.

[286] Kreiner, M; Betancor, E; Clark, GT. Occlusal stabilization appliances: evidence of their efficacy. *JADA,* 2001 132, 770-777.

[287] Kretschmer, E. Über gestufte aktive Hypnoseübungen und den Umbau der Hypnosetechnik. *Dtsch Med Wschr,* 1946 71, 281-283.

[288] Kreyer, G. Psychopathologische Krankheitsbilder und ihre Bedeutung für den Zahnarzt. In: Sergl HG, editor. *Psychologie und Psychosomatik in der Zahnheilkunde.* München-Wien-Baltimore: Urban & Schwarzenberg; 1996; 259.

[289] Kreyer, G. Psychosomatics of the orofacial system. *Wien Med Wochenschr,* 2000 150, 213-216.

[290] Kroymann, R. Angststörungen. In: Rief W, Birbaumer N editors. *Biofeedback. Grundlagen, Indikationen, Kommunikation, praktisches Vorgehen in der Therapie.* Stuttgart-New York: Schattauer Verlag; 2006; 97-127.

[291] Kröner, B. & Beitel, E. Longitudinal study of the effect of Autogenic Training on various forms of subjective perception of relaxation and the sense of well-being. *Z Klin Psychol Psychother,* 1980 28, 127-133.

[292] Kröner-Herwig, B; Mohn, U; Pothmann, R. Comparison of biofeedback and relaxation in the treatment of pediatric headache and the influence of parent involvement on outcome. *Appl Psychophysiol Biofeedback,* 1998 23, 143-157.

[293] Kröner-Herwig, B. Biofeedback. In: Basler H-D, Franz K, Kröner-Herwig B, Rehfisch H-P editors. *Psychologische Schmerztherapie.* Berlin-Heidelberg-New York: Springer; 2004; 551-565.

[294] Kuijpers, HJH; van der Heijden, FMAA; Tuinier, S; Verhoeven, WMA. Meditation-induced psychosis. *Psychopathology,* 2007 40, 461-464.

[295] Kumar, VS; Kumar, DA; Kalaivani, K; Gangadharan, AC; Raju, KV; Thejomoorthy, P; Manohar, BM; Puvanakrishnan, R. Optimization of pulsed electromagnetic field therapy for management of arthritis in rats. *Bioelectromagnetics*, 2005 26, 431-439.

[296] Laney, WR. Medical preparations of the mouth for prostheses. In: Laney WR, Gibilisco JA editors. *Diagnosis and treatment of prosthodontics*. Philadelphia: Lea & Febiger; 1983; 182-193.

[297] Lang, AM. Der Tic als Entwicklungs-Kick. Hypnosebehandlung eines 16-jähriges Jungen mit einer Tic-Störung. In: Ebell H, Schukall H editors. *Warum theraeutische Hypnose? Fallgeschichten aus der Praxis von Ärzten und Psychotherapeuten*. München-Berlin-Düsseldorf-Heidelberg: Richard Pflaum Verlag; 2004; 421-436.

[298] Langewitz, W; Izakovic, J; Wyler, J; Schindler, C; Kiss, A; Bircher, AJ. Effect of self-hypnosis on hay fever symptoms - a randomized controlled intervention study. *Psychoter Psychosom*, 2005 74, 165-172.

[299] Langen, D. *Die gestufte Aktivhypnose*, 3. Aufl. Stuttgart: Huber; 1969.

[300] Larbig, W. Transkulturelle und laborexperimentelle Untersuchungen zur zentralnervösen Schmerzverarbeitung: Empirische Befunde und klinische Konsequenzen. In: Miltner W, Larbig W, Brengelmann JC editors. *Psychologische Schmerzbehandlung*. München: Röttger; 1988; 1-17.

[301] Larbig, W. EEG-Korrelate der Schmerzkontrolle. *EEG-EMG*, 1994 25, 151-160.

[302] Larbig W. Hirnphysiologische Korrelate der Hypnoanalgesie. *HyKog*, 2004 21, 39-59.

[303] Larbig, W; Elbert, T; Lutzenberger, W; Rockstroh, B; Schnerr, G; Birbaumer, N. EEG and slow brain potentials during anticipation and control of painful stimulation. *Electroencephal Clin Neurophysiol*, 1982 53, 298-309.

[304] Laskin, DM. & Block, S. Diagnosis and treatment of myofacial pain-dysfunction (MPD) syndrome. *J Prosthet Dent*, 1986 56, 75-84.

[305] Laskin, DM. & Green, CS. Influence of the doctor-patient relationship on placebo therapy for patients with myofascial pain-dysfunction (MPD) syndrome. *JADA*, 1972 85, 892-894.

[306] Lazar, SW; Kerr, CE, Wasserman, RH; Gray, JR; Greve, DN; Treadway, MT; McGarvey, M; Quinn, BT; Dusek, JA; Benson, H; Rauch, SL; Moore, CI; Fischl, B. Meditation experience is associated with increased cortical thickness. *Neuroreport*, 2005 16, 1893-1897.

[307] Lazarus, AA. *Verhaltenstherapie im Übergang*. München: Reinhardt; 1971.

[308] Learreta, JA; Beas J; Bono, AE; Durst A. Muscular activity disorders in relation to intentional occlusal interferences. *Cranio*, 2007 25, 193-199.

[309] Lee, EW; Maffulli, N; Li, CK; Chan, KM. Pulsed magnetic and electromagnetic fields in experimental achilles tendonitis in the rat: a prospective randomized study. *Arch Phys Med Rehabil*, 1997 78, 399-404.

[310] Lehmann, D; Faber, PL; Achermann, P; Jeanmonod, D; Gianotti, LR; Pizzagalli, D. Brain sources of EEG gamma frequency during volitionally meditation-induced altered states of consciousness, and experience of the self. *Psychiatry Res: Neuroimaging*, 2001 108, 111-121.

[311] Lehrer, PM; Hochron, SM; Mayne, TM; Isenberg, S; Lasoski, AM; Carlson, V; Gilchrist, J; Porges, S. Relationship between changes in EMG and respiratory sinus arrhythmia in a study of relaxation therapy for asthma. *Appl Psychophysiol Biofeedback*, 1997 22, 183-191.

[312] Lesse, S. Atypical facial pain syndromes of psychogenic origin. Complications of their misdiagnosis. *J Nerv Ment Dis*, 1956 124, 346-351.

[313] Leuner, H. Zur Indikation und wissenschaftlichen Fundierung des Respiratorisches Feedbacks. Allgemeinarzt, 1984 6, 334-354.

[314] Leuner, H. Die Methode des Katahymen Bilderlebens. In: Wilke E, Leuner H editors. *Das Katathyme Bilderleben in der Psychosomatischen Medizin*. Bern-Stuttgart-Toronto: Hans Huber Verlag; 1990/a; 15-29.

[315] Leuner, H. Die Stellung des Katahymen Bilderlebens (KB) in psychosomatischer Forschung und Therapie. In: Wilke E, Leuner H editors. *Das Katathyme Bilderleben in der Psychosomatischen Medizin*. Bern-Stuttgart-Toronto: Hans Huber Verlag; 1990/b; 57-77.

[316] Leuner, H. Respiratorische Feedback (RFB) als atembezogene Selbsthypnose. (Anhang). In: Leuner H, Schroeter E editors. *Indikationen und spezifische Anwendungen der Hypnosebehandlung. Ein Überblick*. (2. erweiterte Auflage). Bern-Göttingen-Toronto-Seattle: Hans Huber Verlag; 1997; 204-209.

[317] Leuner, H. Manuskriptfragmente. In: Barolin GS, editor. *Das Respiratorische Feedback nach Leuner*. Berlin: VWB Verlag für Wissenschaft und Bildung; 2001; 39-105.

[318] Leuner, H. & Schroeter, E. *Indikationen und spezifische Anwendungen der Hypnosebehandlung*. Bern-Göttingen-Toronto-Seattle: Hans Huber Verlag; 1997; 24, 52, 66, 152-155, 158-160, 173-175.

[319] Lindemuth, R; Mayr, T; Schimrigk, K. Visually induced seizure caused by "opto-acoustic relaxation system". *J Neurol*, 2000 247, 303.

[320] Litt, MD; NYE, C; Shafer, D. Coping with oral surgery by self-efficacy enhancement and perceptions of control. *J Dent Res*, 1993 72, 1237-1243.

[321] Loesch, W. Erfahrugen mit dem Respiratorischen Feedback nach *Leuner* in der Therapie chronischer Schmerzpatienten. In: Barolin GS, editor. *Das Respiratorische Feedback nach Leuner*. Berlin: VWB Verlag für Wissenschaft und Bildung; 2001; 163-172.

[322] Lopes, CB; Pinheiro, AL; Sathaiah, S; Da Silva, NS; Salgado, MA. Infrared laser photobiomodulation (lambda 830 nm) on bone tissue around dental implants: a Raman spectroscopy and scanning electronic microscopy study in rabbits. *Photomed Laser Surg*, 2007 25, 96-101.

[323] Lotzmann, U. Okklusion, Kiefergelenk und Wirbelsäule. *Zahnärztl Mitteilungen*, 2002 92, 34-41.

[324] Lu, DP. The use of hypnosis for smooth sedation induction and reduction of postoperative violent emergencies from anesthesia in pediatric dental patients. *J Dentistry Children*, 1994, 182-185

[325] Lucini, D; Riva, S; Pizzinelli, P; Pagani, M. Stress management at the worksite. Reversal of symptoms profile and cardiovascular dysregulation. *Hypertension*, 2007 49, 291-297.

[326] Ludwig, AM. Altered states of consciousness. Arch Gen Psychiatry 1966. Reprinted in Tart, CT. *Altered state of consciousness*. Garden City, New York: Anchor Books - Doubleday and Co., Inc.; 1979. 11-24.

[327] Lund, I; Lundeberg, T; Carleson, J; Sönnerfors, H, Uhrlin, B; Svensson, E. Corticotropin releasing factor in urine - A possible biochemical marker of fibromyalgia responses to massage and guided relaxation. *Neurosci Letters*, 2006 403, 166-171.

[328] Lutgendorf, S; Logan, H; Kirchner, HL; Rothrock, N; Svengalis, S; Iverson, K; Lubaroff, D. Effects of relaxation and stress on the capsaicin-induced local inflammatory response. *Psychosom Med*, 2000 62, 524-534.

[329] MacLean, CRK; Walton, KG; Wenneberg, SR; Levitsky, DK; Mandarino, JP; Waziri, R; Hillis, SL; Schneider, RH. Effects of the transcendental meditation program on adaptive mechanisms: changes in hormone levels and responses to stress after 4 months of practice. *Psychoneuroendocrinology*, 1997 22, 277-295.

[330] Maharishi, MY. *The science of being and art of living*. Livingston Manor (NY): Maharishi International University Press; 1963. 288.

[331] Mahler, MS; Pine, F; Bergman, A. *The psychological birth of the human infant*. New York: Basic Books; 1975.

[332] Maina, G; Vitalucci, A; Gandolfo, S; Bogetto, F. Comparative efficacy of SSRIs and amisulpride in burning mouth syndrome: a single-blind study. *J Clin Psychiatry*, 2003 64, 336-337.

[333] Malan, DH. *A study of brief psychotherapy*. New York: Plenum Press; 1963.

[334] Malamed, SF. & Quinn, CL. Electronic dental anesthesia in a patient with suspected allergy to local anesthetics: report of a case. *JADA*, 1988 116, 53-55.

[335] Mann, J. *Time-limited psychotherapy*. Cambridge: Harvard Univ Press; 1973.

[336] Marbach, JJ. Phantom bite syndrome. *Am J Psychiatry*, 1978 135, 476-479.

[337] Martin Jr., DW. Fat-soluble vitamins. In: Martin DW, Mayes PA, Rodwell VW, Granner DK editors. *Harper's review of biochemistry*. Twentieth edition. Los Altos, California: Lange Medical Publications; 1985/a; 118-127.

[338] Martin Jr., DW. Water-soluble vitamins. In: Martin DW, Mayes PA, Rodwell VW, Granner DK editors. *Harper's review of biochemistry*. Twentieth edition. Los Altos, California: Lange Medical Publications; 1985/b; 101-117.

[339] Martin, A; Rief, W. Somatoforme Störungen. In: Rief W, Birbaumer N editors. *Biofeedback. Grundlagen, Indikationen, Kommunikation, praktisches Vorgehen in der Therapie*. Stuttgart-New York: Schattauer Verlag; 2006; 73-96.

[340] Mathews, AM. & Gelder, MG. Psycho-physiological investigations of brief relaxation training. *J Psychosom Res*, 1969 13, 1-12.

[341] Mathews, PBC. & Rushworth G. The selective effect of procaine on the stretch reflex and tendon jerk of soleus muscle when applied to its nerve. *J Physiol Lond*, 1957 135, 245-262.

[342] Matsumoto, H; Ochi, M; Abiko, Y; Hirose, Y; Kaku, T; Sakaguchi, K. Pulsed electromagnetic fields promote bone formation around dental implants inserted into the femur of rabbits. *Clin Oral Implant Res*, 2000 11, 354-360.

[343] Mawdsley, JE; Jenkins, DG; Macey, MG; Langmead, L; Rampton, DS. The effect of hypnosis on systemic and rectal mucosal measures of inflammation in ulcerative colitis. *Am J Gastroenterol*, 2008 103, 1460-1469.

[344] Mazzetto, MO; Carrasco, TG; Bidinelo, EF; de Andrade Pizzo, RC; Mazzetto, RG. Low intensity laser application in temporomandibular disorders: a phase I double- blind study. *Cranio*, 2007 25, 186-192.

[345] McGrady, AV; Yonker, R; Tan, SY; Fine, TH; Woerner, M. The effect of biofeedback-assisted relaxation training on blood pressure and selected biochemical parameters in patients with essential hypertension. *Biofeedback Self Regul*, 1981 6, 343-353.

[346] McKee, MG. Spontaneous hypnotic states induced during biofeedback training. In: Pajntar M, Roškar E, Lavrič M editors. *Hypnosis in psychotherapy and psychosomatic medicine.* Kranj: Slovenian Society for Clinical and Experimental Hypnosis; 1980; 347-351.

[347] McNamara, DC. Electrodiagnosis at median occlusal position for human subjects with mandibular joint syndrome. *Arch Oral Biol*, 1976 21, 325-

[348] Mehrstedt, M. Hypnosis and behavior therapy of dental fear in children. *Hypn Int Monographs*, 1997 3, 49-58.

[349] Meier, W; Klucken, M; Soyka, D; Bromm, B. Hypnotic hypo- and hyperalgesia: divergent effects on pain ratings and pain-related cerebral potentials. *Pain*, 1993 53, 175-181.

[350] Meldolesi, GN; Picardi, A; Accivile, E; Toraldo di Francia, R; Biondi, M. Personality and psychopathology in patients with temporomandibular joint pain-dysfunction syndrome. *Psychother Psychosom*, 2000 69, 322-328.

[351] Melzack, R. & Wall, P. Pain mechanisms: a new theory. *Science*, 1965 150, 971-979.

[352] Mentes, BB; Tascilar, O; Tatlicioglu, E; Bor, MV; Isman, F; Turkozkan, N; Celebi, M. Influence of pulsed electromagnetic fields on healing of experimental colonic anastomosis. *Dis Colon Rectum*, 1996 39, 1031-1038.

[353] Merne, ME; Syrjänen, KJ; Syrjänen, SM. Systemic and local effects of long-term exposure to alkaline drinking water in rats. *Int J Exp Pathol*, 2001 82, 213-219.

[354] Mészáros, I. *Hypnosis [Hipnózis].* Budapest: Medicina; 1984. 74, 153-160.

[355] Mew, J. Phantom bite. *Brit Dent J*, 2004 197, 660.

[356] Meyer-Lückel, H. & Schiffner, U. Effektivität und Effizienz verhaltensmodifizierender gruppenprophylaktischer Massnahmen bei Kindern. *Deutsch Zahnärztl Z*, 2009 64, 152-167.

[357] Mikami, DB. A review of psychogenic aspects and treatment of bruxism. *J Prosthet Dent*, 1977 37, 411-419.

[358] Millner, NE. & Dollard, J. *Social learning and imitation.* New Haven: Yale Univers Press; 1941.

[359] Mills, WW. & Farrow, JT. The transcendental meditation technique and acute experimental pain. *Psychosom Med*, 1981 43, 157-164.

[360] Miltner, W; Johnson, R; Braun, C; Larbig, W. Somatosensory event-related potentials to painful and non-painful stimuli: effects of attention. *Pain*, 1989 38, 303-312.

[361] Miltner, W; Braun, C; Revenstorf, D. Nozizeption ist nicht gleich Schmerz. Eine Studie über schmerzreizkorrelierte hirnelektrische Potentiale unter Hypnose. *HyKog*, 1992 10, 22-34.

[362] Mishima, S. The effect of long-term pulsing electromagnetic field stimulation on experimental osteoporosis of rats. *J UOEH*, 1988 10, 31-45.

[363] Miyamoto, SA. & Ziccardi, VB. Burning mouth syndrome. *Mt Sinai J Med*, 1998 65, 343-347.

[364] Mizumori, T; Inano, S; Sumiya, M; Kobayashi, Y; Watamoto, T; Yatani, H. An ambulatory bruxism recording system with sleep-stage analyzing function. *J Prosthodontic Res*, 2009 53, 150-154.

[365] Molin, C. From bite to mind: TMD -- a personal and literature review. *Int J Prosthodont*, 1999 12, 279-288.

[366] Moore, R. & Brødsgaard, I. Group therapy compared with individual desensitization for dental anxiety. *Community Dent Oral Epidemiol*, 1994 22, 258-262.

[367] Moore, R; Abrahamsen, R; Brødsgaard, I. Hypnosis compared with group therapy and individual desensitization for dental anxiety. *Eur J Oral Sci*, 1996 104, 612-618.

[368] Moore, P; Ridgway, TD; Higbee, RG; Howard, EW; Lucroy, MD. Effect of wavelength on low-intensity laser irradiation-stimulated cell proliferation in vitro. *Lasers Surg Med*, 2005 36, 8-12.

[369] Morse, DR; Martin, JS; Furst, ML; Dubin, LL. A physiological and subjective evaluation of meditation, hypnosis and relaxation. *Psychosom Med*, 1977 39, 304-324.

[370] Moulton, R; Ewen, S; Thieman, W. Emotional factors in periodontal disease. *Oral Surg Oral Med Oral Pathol*, 1957 5, 833-860.

[371] Musaev, AV; Guseinova, SG; Imamverdieva, SS. The use of pulsed electromagnethic fields with complex modulation in the treatment of patients with diabetic polyneuropathy. *Neurosci Behav Physiol*, 2003 33, 745-752.

[372] Naito, A; Laidlaw, TM; Henderson, DC; Farahani, L; Dwivedi, P; Gruzelier, JH. The impact of self-hypnosis and Johrei on lymphocyte subpopulation at exam time: a controlled study. *Brain Res Bulletin*, 2003 62, 241-253.

[373] Nava, E; Landau, D; Brody, S; Linder, L; Schächinger, H. Mental relaxation improves long-term incidental visual memory. *Neurobiol Learning Memory*, 2004 81, 167-171.

[374] Navarro, R; Marquezan, M; Cerqueira, DF; Silveira, BL; Correa, MS. Low-level-laser therapy as an alternative treatment for primary herpes simplex infection: a case report. *J Clin Pediatr Dent*, 2007 31, 225-228.

[375] Neiburger, EJ. Rapid healing of gingival incisions by helium-neon diode laser. *J Mass Dent Soc*, 1999 48, 8-13, 40.

[376] Nestle, M. Nutrition. In: Martin DW, Mayes PA, Rodwell VW, Granner DK editors. *Harper's review of biochemistry*. Twentieth edition. Los Altos, California: Lange Medical Publications; 1985; 661-680.

[377] Newberg, AB & Iversen, J. The neutral basis of the complex mental task of meditation: neurotransmitter and neurochemical considerations. *Med Hypotheses*, 2003 61, 282-291.

[378] Nicholson, P. Does meditation predispose to epilepsy? EEG studies of expert meditators self-inducing simple partial seizures. *Med Hypotheses*, 2006 66, 674-676.

[379] Niepoth, L. & Korn, HJ. Schlafstörungen. In: Rief W, Birbaumer N editors. *Biofeedback. Grundlagen, Indikationen, Kommunikation, praktisches Vorgehen in der Therapie*. Stuttgart-New York: Schattauer Verlag; 2006; 250-269.

[380] O'Halloran, JP; Jevning, R; Wilson, AF; Skowsky, R; Walsh, RN; Alexander, C. Hormonal control in a state of decreased activation: potentiation of arginine vasopressin secretion. *Physiol Behav*, 1985 35, 591-595.

[381] Olness, K; Culbert, T; Uden, D. Self-regulation of salivary immunoglobulin A by children. *Pediatrics*, 1989 83, 66-71.

[382] Orme-Johnson, DW. Autonomic stability and transcendental meditation. *Psychosom Med*, 1973 35, 341-349.

[383] Orme-Johnson, D. Transcendental meditation does not predispose to epilepsy. *Med Hypotheses*, 2005 65, 201-202.

[384] Orme-Johnson, DW; Schneider, RH; Son, YD; Nidich, S; Cho, ZH. Neuroimaging of meditation's effect on brain reactivity to pain. *Neuroreport*, 2006 17, 1359-1363.

[385] Orne, MT. The nature of hypnosis: Artifact and essence. *J Abnorm Social Psychol*, 1959 58, 277-299.

[386] Orne, MT. & Whitehouse, WG. Relaxation techniques. In: Fink G, editor in chief. *Encyclopedia of Stress*. Vol. III. San Diego: Academic Press; 2000; 341-348.

[387] Ortman, LF; Casey, DM; Deers, M. Bioelectric stimulation and residual ridge resorption. *J Prosthet Dent*, 1992 67, 67-71.

[388] Ospina, MB; Bond, TK; Karkhaneh, M; Tjosvold, L; Vandermeer, B; Liang, Y; Bialy, L; Hooton, N; Buscemi, N; Dryden, DM; Klassen, TP. Meditation practices for health: State of research. Evidence Report/Technology Assessment No. 155. (AHRQ Publication No. 07-E010). Rockville MD: Agency for Healthcare Research and Quality; 2007. 193-197, B1-B4.

[389] Ottani, V; Raspanti, M; Martini, D; Tretola, G; Ruggeri Jr, A; Franchi, M; Giuliani Piccari, G; Ruggeri, A. Electromagnetic stimulation on the bone growth using backscattered electron imaging. *Micron*, 2002 33, 121-125.

[390] Ozcelik, O; Cenk Haytac, M; Seydaoglu, G. Enamel matrix derivative and low-level laser therapy in the treatment of intra-bony defects: a randomized placebo-controlled clinical trial. *J Clin Periodontol*, 2008/a 35, 147-156.

[391] Ozcelik, O; Haytac, MC; Kunin, A; Seydaoglu, G. Improved wound healing by low-level laser irradiation after gingivectomy operations: a controlled clinical pilot study. *J Clin Periodontol*, 2008/b 35, 250-254.

[392] Ozen, T; Orhan, K; Gorur, I; Ozturk, A. Efficacy of low level laser therapy on neurosensory recovery after injury to the inferior alveolar nerve. *BMC Head Face Med*, 2006 2, 3.

[393] Pagnoni, G. & Cekic, M. Age effects on gray matter volume and attentional performance in Zen meditation. *Neurobiol Aging*, 2007 28, 1623-1627.

[394] Patino, O; Grana, D; Bolgiani, A; Prezzavento, G; Mino, J; Merlo, A; Benaim, F. Pulsed electromagnetic fields in experimental cutaneous wound healing in rats. *J Burn Care Rehabil*, 1996 17, 528-531.

[395] Pawlow, LA. & Jones, GE. The impact of abbreviated progressive muscle relaxation on salivary cortisol. *Biol Psychol*, 2002 60, 1-16.

[396] Pawlow, LA. & Jones, GE. The impact of abbreviated progressive muscle relaxation on salivary cortisol. *Appl Psychophysiol Biofeedback*, 2005 30, 375-387.

[397] Payer, M; Jakse, N; Pertl, C; Truschnegg, A; Lechner, E; Eskici, A. The clinical effect of LLLT in endodontic surgery: A prospective study on 72 cases. *Oral Surg Oral Med Oral Pathol Oral Radiol Endod*, 2005 100, 375-379.

[398] Peeters, E; Neyt, A; Beckers, F; De Smet, S; Aubert, AE; Geers, R. Influence of supplemental magnesium, tryptophan, vitamin C, and vitamin E on stress responses of pigs to vibration. *J Anim Sci*, 2005 83, 1568-1580.

[399] Pekala, RJ. & Kumar, VK. Phenomenological patterns of consciousness during hypnosis: Relevance to cognition and individual differences. *Aust J Clin Exp Hypn*, 1989 17, 1-20.

[400] Peper, E; Wilson, VE; Gunkelman, J; Kawakami, M; Sata, M; Barton, W; Johnston, J. Tongue piercing by a yogi: QEEG observations. *Appl Physiol Biofeedback*, 2006 31, 331-338.

[401] Pesevska, S; Nakova, M; Ivanovski, K. Angelov, N; Kesic, L; Obradovic, R; Mindova, S; Nares, S. Dentinal hypersensitivity following scaling and root planing: comparison

of low level laser and topical fluoride treatment. *Lasers Med Sci*, in press. DOI: 10.1007/s10103-009-0685-0

[402] Peter, B. *Einführung in die Hypnotherapie*. Heidelberg: Carl-Auer Verlag; 2006. 103-104.

[403] Pielsticker, A. Das Würfelexperiment. Die Behandlung eines Patienten mit atypischem Gesichtsschmerz. In: Ebell H, Schukall H editors. *Warum theraeutische Hypnose? Fallgeschichten aus der Praxis von Ärzten und Psychotherapeuten*. München-Berlin-Düsseldorf-Heidelberg: Richard Pflaum Verlag; 2004; 328-340.

[404] Pienkowski, D; Pollack, SR; Brighton, CT; Griffith, NJ. Comparison of asymmetrical and symmetrical pulse waveforms in electromagnetic stimulation. *J Orthop Res*, 1992 10, 247-255.

[405] Pinheiro, ALB; Martinez Gerbi, ME; de Assis Limeira Jr, F; Carneiro Ponzi, EA; Marques, AMC; Carvalho, CM; de Carneiro Santos, R; Oliveira, PC; Nóia, M; Ramalho, LMP. Bone repair following bone grafting hydroxyapatite guided bone regeneration and infra-red laser photobiomodulation: a histological study in a rodent model. *Lasers Med Sci*, 2009 24, 234-240.

[406] Pipitone, N. & Scott, DL. Magnetic pulse treatment for knee osteoarthritis: a randomized, double-blind, placebo-controlled study. *Curr Med Res Opin*, 2001 17, 190-196.

[407] Pomp, AM. Psychotherapy for the myofascial pain-dysfunction syndrome: a study of factors coinciding with symptom remission. *JADA*, 1974 89, 629-632.

[408] Previc FH. The role of the extrapersonal brain systems in religious activity. *Consciousness Cogn*, 2006 15, 500-539.

[409] Proctor, GB. & Carpenter, GH. Chewing stimulates secretion of human salivary secretory immunoglobulin A. *J Dent Res*, 2001 80, 909-913.

[410] Qadri, T; Miranda, L; Tunér, J; Gustafsson, A. The sort-term effects of low-level lasers as adjunct therapy in the treatment of periodontal inflammation. *J Clin Periodontol*, 2005 32, 714-719.

[411] Rainville, P; Duncan, GH; Price, DD; Carrier, B; Bushnell, MC. Pain affect encoded in human anterior cingulate but not somatosensory cortex. *Science*, 1997 277, 968-971.

[412] Rainville, P; Hofbauer, RK; Paus, T; Duncan, GH; Bushnell, MC; Price, DD. Cerebral mechanisms of hypnotic induction and suggestion. *J Cogn Neurosci*, 1999 11, 110-125.

[413] Raji, AM. An experimental study of the effects of pulsed electromagnetic field (Diapulse) on nerve repair. *J Hand Surg Br*, 1984 9, 105-112.

[414] Raji, AR. & Bowden, RE. Effects of high-peak pulsed electromagnetic field on the degeneration and regeneration of the common peroneal nerve in rats. *J Bone Joint Surg Br*, 1983 65, 478-492.

[415] Raskin, M; Bali, LR; Peeke, HV. Muscle biofeedback and transcendental meditation. A controlled evaluation of efficacy in the treatment of chronic anxiety. *Arch Gen Psychiatry*. 1980 37, 93-97.

[416] Rauch, C. & Hermes, D. Akzeptanz klinischer Hypnose in der allgemeiner-zahnärztlichen Praxis - Ergebnisse einer Umfrage. *Deutsche Zahnärztl Z*, 2008 63, 697.

[417] Ray, WR; Raczynski, JN; Rogers, T; Kimball, WH. *Evaluation of clinical biofeedback*. New York: Plenum Press; 1979.

[418] Raymond, J; Sajid, I; Parkinson, LA; Gruzelier, J. Biofeedback and dance performance: A preliminary investigation. *Appl Psychophysiol Biofeedback*, 2005 30, 65-73.

[419] Rehfisch, HP. & Basler, HD. Entspannung und Imagination. In: Basler HD, Franz K, Kröner-Herwig B, Rehfisch HP editors. *Psychologische Schmerztherapie*. Berlin-Heidelberg-New York: Springer; 2004. 537-550.

[420] Reeves 2nd, JL. & Merrill, RL. Diagnostic and treatment challenges in occlusal dysesthesia. *J Calif Dent Assoc*, 2007 35, 198-207.

[421] Reiner, R. Integrating a portable biofeedback device into clinical practice for patients with anxiety disorders: Results of a pilot study. *Appl Psychophysiol Biofeedback*, 2008 33, 55-61.

[422] Rice, KM; Blanchard, EB; Purcell, M. Biofeedback treatments of generalized anxiety disorders: preliminary results. *Biofeedback Self Regul*, 1993 18, 93-105.

[423] Riggs, KM; Spiro, A; Tucker, K; Rush, D. Relations of vitamin B_{12}, vitamin B_6, folate and homocysteine to cognitive performance in the Normative Aging Study. *Am J Clin Nutr*, 1996 63, 306-314.

[424] Roazen, P. Psychoanalysis In: Fink G, editor in chief. *Encyclopedia of stress. (vol. 3.)*. San Diego: Academic Press; 2000; 283-287.

[425] Rogers, CR. The therapeutic relationship: Recent therapy and research. *Australian J Psychol*. 1965 13, 95-108

[426] Ross, GL; Bentley, HJ; Greene Jr., GW. The psychosomatic concept in dentistry. *Psychosom Med*, 1953 15, 168-173.

[427] Rucklidge, JJ, & Saunders, D. Hypnosis in a case of long-standing idiopathic itch. *Psychosom Med*, 1999 61, 355-358.

[428] Ruell, PA, & Thompson, MW. The effect of temperature on HSP72 induction in mammals. In: Morell E, Vincent C editors. *Heat shock proteins: New research*. New York: Nova Science Publishers; 2008; 361-373.

[429] Ryan, W; Green, CS; Laskin, DM. Comparison of diazepam, chlorazepate, carisoprodol and placebo in the treatment of MPD syndrome (abstract). *J Dent Res*, 1985 64 (spec issue), 232.

[430] Sakakibara, M; Takeuchi, S; Hayano, J. Effect of relaxation training on cardiac parasympathetic tone. *Psychophysiology*, 1994 31, 223-228.

[431] Salter: Three techniques of autohypnosis. *J Gen Psychol*, 1941 24, 423-438.

[432] Sarlani, E; Balciunas, BA; Grace, EG. Orofacial pain - Part I. Assessment and management of musculoskeletal and neuropathic causes. *AACN Clin Issues*, 2005/a 16, 333-346.

[433] Sarlani, E; Balciunas, BA; Grace, EG. Orofacial pain - Part II. Assessment and management of vascular, neurovascular, idiopathic, secondary, and psychogenic causes. *AACN Clin Issues*, 2005/b 16, 347-358.

[434] Scardino, MS; Swaim, SF; Sartin, EA; Steiss, JE; Spano, JS; Hoffman, CE; Coolman, SL; Peppin, BL. Evaluation of treatment with a pulsed electromagnetic field on wound healing, clinicopathologic variables, and central nervous system activity of dogs. *Am J Vet Res*, 1998 59, 1177-1181.

[435] Schmierer, H. *Einführung in die zahnärztliche Hypnose*. Berlin: Quintesenz; 1997; 236-244, 245-250, 253-275, 283-286

[436] Schmierer, H. Rückmeldung nach 12 Jahren. Zahnextraction bei einer Patientin mit Trigeminusneuralgie. In: Ebell H, Schukall H editors. *Warum theraeutische Hypnose? Fallgeschichten aus der Praxis von Ärzten und Psychotherapeuten*. München-Berlin-Düsseldorf-Heidelberg: Richard Pflaum Verlag; 2004; 165-168.

[437] Schulte, W. Conservative treatment of occlusal dysfunctions. *Int Dent J*, 1988 38, 28-39.

[438] Schultz, JH: *Das Autogene Training. (Konzentrierte Selbstentspannung).* Leipzig: Georg Thieme Verlag; 1932.

[439] Schwarz, F; Sculean, A; Rothamel, D; Schwenzer, K; Georg, T; Becker, J. Clinical evaluation of an Er:YAG laser for nonsurgical treatment of peri-implantitis: a pilot study. *Clin Oral Implant Res*, 2005 16, 44-52.

[440] Schwarz, F; Aoki, A; Becker, J; Sculean, A. Laser application in non-surgical periodontal therapy: a systematic review. *J Clin Periodontol*, 2008 35(8 Suppl), 29-44.

[441] Schwichtenberg, J. & Doering, S. Success of referral in a psychosomatic-psychotherapeutic outpatient unit of a dental school. *Z Psychosom Med Psychother*, 2008 54, 285-292.

[442] Sethi, S. & Bhargava, S. Relationship of meditation and psychosis: case studies. *Aust N Z J Psychiatry*. 2003 37, 382.

[443] Shapiro, DA; Barkham, M; Stiles, WB; Hardy GE; Rees A; Reynolds, S; Startup, M. Time is of the essence: a selective review of the fall and rise of brief therapy research. *Psychol Psychother Theory Res Practice*, 2003 76, 211-235.

[444] Shapiro, D; Cook, IA; Davydov, DM; Ottaviani, C; Leuchter, AF; Abrams, M. Yoga as a complementary treatment of depression: effects of traits and moods on treatment outcome. *eCAM*, 2007 4, 493-502.

[445] Sharon-Buller, A. & Sela, M. CO_2-laser treatment of ulcerative lesions. *Oral Surg Oral Med Oral Pathol Oral Radiol Endod*, 2004 97, 332-334.

[446] Shaw, RM. & Dettmar, DM. Monitoring behavioral stress control using a craniomandibular index. *Aust Dent J*, 1990 35, 147-151.

[447] Shaw, AJ. & Niven, N. Theoretical concepts and practical applications of hypnosis in the treatment of children and adolescents with dental fear and anxiety. *Brit Dent J*, 1996 180, 11-16.

[448] Shimizu, T; Zerwekh, JE; Videman, T; Gill, K; Mooney, V; Holmes, RE; Hagler, HK. Bone ingrowth into porous calcium phosphate ceramics: influence of pulsing electromagnetic field. *J Orthop Res*, 1988 6, 248-258.

[449] Shirani, AM; Gutknecht, N. Taghizadeh, M; Mir, M. Low-level laser therapy and myofacial pain dysfunction syndrome: a randomized controlled clinical trial. *Lasers Med Sci*, in press. DOI: 10.1007/s10103-008-0624-5

[450] Shor, RE. Three dimensions of hypnotic depth. *Int J Clin Exp Hypn*, 1962 10, 23-38.

[451] Shugars, DC. & Wahl, SM. The role of the oral environment in HIV-1 transmission. *J Am Dent Assoc.* 1998 129, 851 - 858.

[452] Siegel, RK. Hallucinations. *Scientific American*, 1977 237, 132-140

[453] Siegel, RK. & Jarvik, ME. Drug induced hallucinations in animals and man. In: Siegel RK, West LJ editors. *Hallucinations: Behavior, experience, and theory.* New York: Wiley; 1975; 81-161.

[454] Sifneos, PE. Short-term psychotherapy and emotional crisis. Cambridge: Harvard Univ Press; 1972.

[455] Silverman, SI. *Oral physiology.* St Louis: Mosby; 1961; 447

[456] Simonton, OC; Matthews-Simonton, S; Creighton, J. *Wieder gesund werden.* Hamburg: Rowohlt; 1982.

[457] Skinner, BF. *Science and human behavior.* New York: The Free Press; 1953.

[458] Smith, GC. Psychotherapy. In: Fink G, editor in chief. *Encyclopedia of stress. (vol. 3.)*. San Diego: Academic Press; 2000; 310-315.

[459] Smith, TL; Wong-Gibbons, D; Maultsby, J. Microcirculatory effects of pulsed electromagnetic fields. *J Orthop Res*, 2004 22, 80-84.

[460] Smith, C; Hancock, H; Blake-Mortimer, J; Eckert, K. A randomized comparative trial of yoga and relaxation to reduce stress and anxiety. *Compl Ther Med*, 2007 15, 77-83.

[461] Somer, E. Hypnotherapy in the treatment of the chronic nocturnal use of a dental splint prescribed for bruxism. *Int J Clin Exp Hypn*, 1991 39, 145-154.

[462] Somer, E. Hypnobehavioral and hypnodynamic interventions in temporomandibular disorders. *Hypn Int Monographs*, 1997 3, 87-98.

[463] Souil, E; Capon, A; Mordon, S; Dinh-Xuan, AT; Polla, BS. Bachelet, M. Treatment with 815-nm diode laser induces long-lasting expression of 72-kDa heat shock protein in normal rat skin. *Brit J Dermatol*, 2001 144, 260-266.

[464] Staats, J. & Krause, WR. *Hypnotherapie in der zahnärztlichen Praxis*. Heidelberg: Hüthig; 1995; 87-104.

[465] Stark, TM. & Sinclair, PM. Effect of pulsed electromagnetic fields on orthodontic tooth movement. *Am J Orthod Dentofacial Orthop*, 1987 91, 91-104.

[466] Staudenmayer, H. Psychological treatment of psychogenic idiopathic environmental intolerance. *Occup Med*, 2000 15, 627-646.

[467] Stetter, F. Chronobiological aspects of autogenic training. Thermometric findings of autogenic training in relation to diurnal periodicity in autonomic dystonia patients. *Z Psychosom Med Psychoanal*, 1985 31, 172-186.

[468] Stiller, MJ; Pak, GH; Shupack, JL; Thaler, S; Kenny, C; Jondreau, L. A portable pulsed electromagnetic field (PEMF) device to enhance healing of recalcitrant venous ulcers: a double-blind, placebo-controlled clinical trial. *Br J Dermatol*, 1992 127, 147-154.

[469] Sugimoto, K; Theoharides, TC; Kempuraj, D; Conti, P. Response of spinal myoclonus to a combination therapy of autogenic training and biofeedback. *BioPsychoSoc Med* 2007 1, 18.

[470] Svensson, P; Romaniello, A; Arendt, NL; Sessle, BJ. Plasticity in corticomotor control of the human tongue musculature induced by tongue-task training. *Exp Brain Res*, 2003 152, 42-51.

[471] Tabrah, F; Hoffmeier, M; Gilbert Jr., F; Batkin, S; Bassett, CA. Bone density changes in osteoporosis-prone women exposed to pulsed electromagnetic fields (PEMFs). *J Bone Miner Res*, 1990 5, 437- 442.

[472] Takahashi, T; Murata, T; Hamada, T; Omori, M; Kosaka, H; Kikuchi, M; Yoshida, H; Wada, Y. Changes in EEG and autonomic nervous activity during meditation and their association with personality traits. *Int J Psychphysiol*, 2005 55, 199-207.

[473] Takano-Yamamoto, T; Kawakami, M; Sakuda, M. Effect of a pulsing electromagnetic field on demineralized bone-matrix-induced bone formation in a bony defect in the premaxilla of rats. *J Dent Res*, 1992 71, 1920-1925.

[474] Tart, CT. Self-report scales of hypnotic depth. *Int J Clin Exp Hypn*. 1970 18, 105-125.

[475] Taylor, D. Extracting patients' fears of dentistry with hypnosis. Eur J Clin Hypn, 1995/a 2(4), 17-19.

[476] Taylor, DN. Effects of a behavioral stress-management program on anxiety, mood, self-esteem, and T-cell count in HIV positive men. Psychol Rep, 1995/b 76, 451-457.

[477] Teasdale, JD; Segal, ZV; Williams, JMG; Ridgway, VA; Soulsby, JM; Lau, MA. Prevention of relapse/recurrence in major depression by mindfulness-based cognitive therapy. *J Consult Clin Psychol*, 2000 68, 615-623.

[478] Tebécis AK. A controlled study of the EEG during transcendental meditation: comparison with hypnosis. *Folia Psychiatr Neurol Jpn*, 1975 29, 305-313.

[479] Tepper, OM; Callaghan, MJ; Chang, EI; Galiano, RD; Bhatt, KA; Baharestani, S; Gan, J; Simon, B; Hopper, RA; Levine, JP; Gurtner, GC. Electromagnetic fields increase in vitro and in vivo angiogenesis through endothelial release of FGF-2. *FASEB J*, 2004 18, 1231-1233.

[480] Teshima, H; Kubo, C; Kihara, H; Imada, Y; Nagata, S; Ikemi, Y. Psychosomatic aspects of skin diseases from the standpoint of immunology. *Psychother Psychosom*, 1982 37, 165-175.

[481] Toyofuku, A. & Kikuta, T. Treatment of phantom bite syndrome with milnacipran - a case series. *Neuropsych Dis Treatment*, 2006 2, 387-390.

[482] Tóth, Zs. & Fábián, TK. Relaxation techniques in dentistry. *Fogorv Szle*, 2006 99, 15-20.

[483] Tönnies, S. Entspannung für Tinnitusbetroffene durch Photostimulation. *HNO*, 2006 54, 481-486.

[484] Travis, F. & Wallace, RK. Autonomic and EEG patterns during eye-closed rest and transcendental meditation (TM) practice: The basis for a neural model of TM practice. *Consciousness Cogn*, 1999 8; 302-318.

[485] Travis, TA; Kondo, CY; Knott, JR. Heart rate, muscle tension, and alpha production of transcendental meditators and relaxation controls. 1976 1, 387-394.

[486] Trock, DH; Bollet, AJ; Dyer Jr., RH; Fielding, LP; Miner, WK; Markoll, R. A double-blind trial of the clinical effects of pulsed electromagnetic fields in osteoarthritis. *J Rheumatol*, 1993 20, 456-460.

[487] Trock, DH; Bollet, AJ; Markoll, R. The effect of pulsed electromagnetic fields in the treatment of osteoarthritis of the knee and cervical spine. Report of randomized, double blind, placebo controlled trials. *J Rheumatol*, 1994 21, 1903-1911.

[488] Tucker, K. Micronutrient status and aging. *Nutr Rev*, 1995 53, S9-S15

[489] Turner, JA; Mancl, L; Aaron, LA. Brief cognitive-behavioral therapy for temporomandibular disorder pain: effects on daily electronic outcome and process measures. *Pain*, 2005 117, 377-387.

[490] Turner, JA; Mancl, L; Aaron, LA. Short- and long-term efficacy of brief cognitive-behavioral therapy for patients with chronic temporomandibular disorder pain: A randomized, controlled trial. *Pain*, 2006 121, 181-194.

[491] Vanhaudenhuyse, A; Boly, M; Laureys, S; Faymonville, ME. Neurophysiological correlates of hypnotic analgesia. *Contemp Hypnosis*, 2009 26, 15-23.

[492] Varani, K; Gessi, S; Merighi, S; Iannotta, V; Cattabriga, E; Spisani, S; Cadossi, R; Borea, PA. Effect of low frequency electromagnetic fields on A_{2A} adenosine receptors in human neutrophils. *Brit J Pharmachol*, 2002 136, 57-66.

[493] Varani, K; Gessi, S; Merighi, S; Iannota, V; Cattabriga, E; Pancaldi, C; Cadossi, R; Borea, PA. Alteration of A3 adenosine receptors in human neutrophils and low frequency electromagnetic fields. *Biochem Pharmachol*, 2003 66, 1897-1906.

[494] Varga, K; Józsa, E; Bányai, ÉI; Gösi-Greguss, AC. Phenomenological experiences associated with hypnotic susceptibility. *Int J Clin Exp Hypn*, 2001 49, 19-29.

[495] Vescovi, P; Merigo, E; Manfredi, M; Meleti, M; Fornaini, C; Bonanini, M; Rocca, JP; Nammour, S. Nd:YAG laser biostimulation in the treatment of bisphosphonate-associated osteonecrosis of the jaw: clinical experience in 28 cases. *Photomed Laser Surg*, 2008 26, 37-46.

[496] Violon, A. The onset of facial pain. A psychological study. *Psychother Psychosom*, 1980 34, 11-16.

[497] von Brück, M. *Ich-Auflösung im Unendlichen? Meditation und Hirnforschung im Disput*. Ulm: Haus der Begegnung; 2003. 23.

[498] Von Korff, M; Balderson BHK; Saunders, K; Miglioretti, DL; Lin, EHB; Berry, S; Moore, J; Turner, JA. A trial of an activating intervention for chronic back pain in primary care and physical therapy settings. *Pain*, 2005 113, 323-330.

[499] Wallace, RK. Physiological effects of transcendental meditation. *Science*, 1970 167, 1751-1754.

[500] Walsh, R. & Roche, L. Precipitation of acute psychotic episodes by intensive meditation in individuals with a history of schizophrenia. *Am J Psychiatry*, 1979 136, 1085-1086.

[501] Walter, WG; Dovey, VJ; Shipton, H. Analysis of the electrical responses of human cortex to photic stimulation. *Nature*, 1946 158, 540-541.

[502] Walton, KG; Pugh, ND; Gelderloos, P; Macrae, P. Stress reduction and preventing hypertension: preliminary support for a psychoneuroendocrine mechanism. *J Altern Complement Med*, 1995 1, 263-283.

[503] Walton, Kg; Fields, JZ; Levitsky, DK; Harris, DA; Pugh, ND; Schneider, RH. Lowering cortisol and CVD risk in postmenopausal women: a pilot study using the Transcendental Meditation program. *Ann NY Acad Sci*, 2004 1032, 211-215.

[504] Wang, MH; Grossmann, ME; Young, CYF. Forced expression of heat-shock protein 70 increases the secretion of Hsp70 and provides protection against tumor growth. *British J Cancer*, 2004 90, 926-931.

[505] Warrenburg, S; Pagano, RR; Woods, M; Hlastala, M. A comparison of somatic relaxation and EEG activity in classical progressive relaxation and transcendental meditation. *J Behav Med*, 1980 3, 73-93.

[506] Watson, JB. & Rayner, R. Conditioned emotional reactions. *J Exp Psychol*, 1920 3, 1-14.

[507] Watt, DM. Clinical application of gnathosonics. *J Prosthet Dent*, 1966/a 16, 83-95.

[508] Watt, DM. Gnathosonics - A study of sounds produced by the masticatory mechanism. *J Prosthet Dent*, 1966/b 16, 73-82.

[509] Weber, C; Arck, P; Mazurek, B; Klapp, BF. Impact of a relaxation training on psychometric and immunologic parameters in tinnitus sufferers. *J Psychosom Res*, 2002 52, 29-33.

[510] Weintraub, MI. & Cole, SP. Pulsed magnetic field therapy in refractory neuropathic pain secondary to peripheral neuropathy: Electrodiagnostic parameters - Pilot study. *Neurorehab Neural Repair*, 2004 18, 42-46.

[511] Wentz, FM. Patient motivation: a new challenge to the dental profession for effective control of plaque. *JADA*, 1972 85, 887-891.

[512] White, TP; Hoffmann, SR; Gale, EN. Psychophysiological therapy for tinnitus. *Ear Hear*, 1986 7, 397-399.

[513] Whitehouse, WG; Dinges, DF; Orne, EC; Keller, SE; Bates, BL; Bauer, NK; Morahan, P; Haupt, BA; Carlin, MM; Bloom, PB; Zaugg, L; Orne, MT. Psychosocial and immune effects of self-hypnosis training for stress management throughout the first semester of medical school. *Psychosom Med*, 1996 58, 249-263.

[514] Widmalm, SE. Use and abuse of bite splints. *Compendium of Continuing Education in Dentistry*, 1999 20, 249-254.

[515] Wilder-Smith, P; Zimmermann, M. Analgesie mittels Transkutaner Elektrischer Nervenstimulation (TENS). *Schweiz Montsschr Zahnmed*, 1989 99, 653-657.

[516] Wilder-Smith, P. Untersuchungen zur Schmerzunterdrückung mittels transkutaner elektrischer Nervenstimulation (TENS). *DZZ*, 1990 45, 356-359.

[517] Williams, P. & West, M. EEG response to photic stimulation in persons experienced at meditation. *Electroencephal Clin Neurophysiol*, 1975 39, 519-522.

[518] Winkler, G. & Krause, WR. Autogenes Training und thermales Feedback unter Kurbedingungen. *Z ärztl Fortbild*, 1989 83, 1187-1188.

[519] Winnicott, DW. Transitional objects and transitional phenomena: a study of the first not-me possession. *Int J Psycho-Anal*, 1953 34, 89-97.

[520] Woelfel, JB. Denture base materials and their effects on oral tissues. In: Laney WR, Gibilisco JA editors. *Diagnosis and treatment in prosthodontics*. Philadelphia: Lea & Febiger; 1983; 235-252.

[521] Wolpe, J. *Psychotherapy by reciprocal inhibition*. Stanford University Press; 1958.

[522] Wöstmann, B. Psychogene Zahnersatzunverträglichkeit. In: Sergl HG, editor. *Psychologie und Psychosomatik in der* Zahnheilkunde. München - Wien - Baltimore: Urban & Schwarzenberg; 1996; 187-213.

[523] Wyler-Harper, J; Bircher, AJ; Langewitz, W; Kiss, A. Hypnosis and the allergic response. *Schweiz Med Wochenschr Suppl*, 1994 62, 67-76.

[524] Yalom, I. *Existential Psychotherapy*. New York: Basic Books; 1980.

[525] Yalom, I. *The therapy and practice of group psychotherapy*. New York: Basic Books; 1995.

[526] Young, SN. The use of diet and dietary components in the study of factors controlling affect in humans: A review. *J Psychiatr Neurosci*, 1993 18, 235-244.

[527] Zachariae, R; Kristensen, JS; Hokland, P; Ellegaard, J; Metze, E; Hokland, M. Effect of psychological intervention in the form of relaxation and guided imagery on cellular immune function in normal healthy subjects. An overview. *Psychother Psychosom*, 1990 54, 32-29.

[528] Zaichkowsky LD. & Kamen, R. Biofeedback and meditation: effects on muscle tension and locus of control. *Percept Mot Skills*, 1978 46, 955-958.

[529] Zeltner, L. & LeBaron, S. Hypnosis and nonhypnotic techniques for reduction of pain and anxiety during painful procedures in children and adolescents with cancer. *J Pediatrics*, 1982 101, 1032-1035.

[530] Zienowicz, RJ; Thomas, BA; Kurtz, WH; Orgel, MG. A multivariate approach to the treatment of peripheral nerve transection injury: the role of electromagnetic field therapy. *Plast Reconstr Surg*, 1991 87, 122-129.

[531] Zittermann, A; Vitamin D in preventive medicine: are we ignoring the evidence? *Br J Nutr*, 2003 89, 552-572.

[532] Zuccolotto, MC; Vitti, M; Nóbilo, KA; Regalo, SC; Siéssere, S; Bataglion, C. Electromiographic evaluation of masseter and anterior temporalis muscles in rest

position of edentulous patients with temporomandibular disorders, before and after complete dentures with sliding plates. *Gerodontology*, 2007 24, 105-110.

Chapter 7

MEDICINAL HERB AND DIET THERAPY

ABSTRACT

Medicinal herb and diet therapy are important supplemental modalities of psychosomatic dental therapy. Maintenance of a proper nutritional status and proper use of medicinal herbs seems to be highly important to maintain oral health and/or to prevent several oral manifestations. Proper alterations of patients' diet and administration of medicinal herbs may also be used for therapeutic purposes efficiently. However, to avoid potential health hazards, great care should be taken especially in the case of patients with severe systemic diseases, during pregnancy and lactation as well as if long run administration of medicinal herbs and/or long run modification of the patient's diet that incorporates patient's total health needs is needed. In such cases consultation with (or referral to) a registered dietitian and/or internist and/or family doctor is highly recommended before starting diet therapy or medicinal herb therapy. It should be also considered that, medicinal herb and diet therapy are frequently used for health enhancement by patients without any professional control; and unfortunately, they also use them during pregnancy and lactation or under severe systemic diseases, which may cause significant health hazards. Concurrent use of medicinal herbs and pharmaceutical drugs without any control of medical or dental professionals is also relatively common and the majority of herbal medicine users are not aware of potential adverse effects. Therefore, dentist should carefully collect information about the patients' medicinal herb related usage. Since dentists may exert significant influence on their patients' decisions about herbal medicine use, proper up-to-date knowledge related to medicinal herb therapy is highly important also for those dentists not preferring the use of medicinal herb therapy in their practice.

7.1. INTRODUCTION

Medicinal herb and diet therapy are important supplemental modalities of psychosomatic dental therapy. Maintenance of a proper nutritional status and proper use of medicinal herbs seems to be highly important to maintain oral health and to prevent several oral manifestations [*Touger-Decker 1998, 2003, Touger-Decker et al. 2007*]. Further, they may be utilized also for therapeutic purposes efficiently. However, potential health hazards should be avoided. Therefore, great care should be taken especially in the case of patients with severe systemic diseases as well as during pregnancy and lactation [*Palmer 2003, Touger-Decker 2003, Touger-Decker et al. 2007, Zhang et al. 2008*]. Similarly, great care should also be taken, when long run modification of the patient's diet and/or long run administration of medicinal herbs is needed [*Palmer 2003, Touger-Decker 2003, Touger-Decker et al. 2007, Zhang et al. 2008*].

7.2. MEDICINAL HERB THERAPY

7.2.1. Aloe-Vera

Aloe vera (Aloe barbadensis) is a native plant of the Mediterranean region and Africa. Aloe vera leaf pulp extract (inner gel of leaves) exerts anti-bacterial [*Habeeb et al. 2007/a, Pandey & Mishra in press*] anti-fungal [*Rosca-Casian et al. 2007*] and anti-protozoan [*Dutta et al. 2007, 2008*] activity. It also exerts anti-inflammatory properties [*Reuter et al. 2008, Habeeb et al. 2007/b*]. Aloe vera inner gel seems to be highly effective as a topical treatment of oral lichen planus including also erosive and ulcerative forms [*Choonhakarn et al. 2008*]. Systemic administration of Aloe vera inner gel may prevent tumor formation and may inhibit tumor growth in certain cases as indicated in an animal study [*Akev et al. 2007*]. Certain hepatoprotective potential of internally used Aloe vera was also reported [*Chandan et al. 2007*]; however, severe acute hepatitis associated with the intake of Aloe vera products may also occur in certain cases [*Bottenberg et al. 2007, Curciarello et al. 2008*]. Therefore, intake (systemic use) of Aloe vera products for patients with liver pathologies, and concurrent intake of Aloe vera with pharmaceutical drugs (metabolized in the liver) should be avoided. In contrast, there is no adverse effect reported in the case of topical administration of Aloe vera inner gels.

7.2.2. Black Cohosh

Black cohosh (Cimicifuga racemosa) is a native plant of North America containing triterpine glycosides, flavonoids aromatic acids and numerous other constituents [*Geller & Studee 2005*]. Although the exact mechanism of action of this botanical is not yet clearly understood it is likely that, black cohosh acts on serotonin receptors and may relieve hot flashes of women and improve mood through a serotoninergic effect [*Burdette et al. 2003, Geller & Studee 2005*]. Improvement of sleeping, fatigue and abnormal sweating [*Pockaj et al. 2004*] could also be based on premised serotoninergic (antidepressant) effect. It is also likely that, black cohosh exerts bone-protective effects [*Wuttke et al. 2003*], although this effect is not yet characterized in details. The combination of black cohosh with St John's wort (see below) was found efficient also in psychovegetative disorders, likely via a synergistic effect [*Liske 1998*]. Besides promising effects above, there are some contraindications of the use of black cohosh including pregnancy, lactation, failured liver function and may be breast cancer [*Geller & Studee 2005, Low Dog 2005*]

7.2.3. Cocoa

Cocoa is derived from fermented and roasted seeds of *Theobroma cacao* [*McShea et al. 2008*] a native plant of Middle and South America and West Africa. Cocoa contains a variety of active substances. *N-acyletahanolamines* (*N-oleoylethanolamine* and *N-linoleoyethanolamine*) are fatty acids chemically and pharmacologically related to *Anandamide* [*Bruinsma & Taren 1999*] and act at the same site in the brain like cannabis [*DiTomaso et al. 1996*]. *Phenylethylamine* is another active substance of cocoa acting in a similar manner to amphetamine [*Benton & Donohoe 1999*]. There are also several *other biogenic amines* in cocoa exerting similar "drug-like" neurophysiological effects such as tyramine, normethanephrine, synephrine, ethylamine, isobutylamine, isoamylamine, tryptamine, methylamine, dimethylamine, trimethylamine and octopamine [*Bruinsma & Taren 1999*]. Although the level of these "drug like" substances is much less than that needed to produce a pharmacological action [*Benton & Donohoe 1999*], a slight effect of such constituents may not be excluded [*Bruinsma & Taren 1999*].

Besides "drug-like" constituents, cocoa also contains relatively high amount of stimulants like *theobromine* and *caffeine* [*Bruinsma & Taren 1999, Benton & Donohoe 1999*]. Cocoa powder also provide a relatively high amount of *magnesium* [*Bruinsma & Taren 1999*], which improves mood [*Poleszak et al. 2005*] and may improve coping ability with stress [*Peeters et al. 2005*]. Cocoa also contains *flavonols*, from which particularly abundant in cocoa are the flavan-3-ol monomers, epicatechin and catechin and their related oligomers the procyanidins [*Mao et al. 2003*]. Cocoa flavonols are likely to exert beneficial effects on blood pressure, insulin resistance, vascular damage and oxidative stress [*Martín et al. in press, Grassi et al. 2005, Selmi et al. 2008*]. Cocoa flavonols also exert anti-inflammatory properties [*Selmi et al. 2006*]. Cocoa based products (see also chocolate in *paragraph 7.3.13.*) may be used to improve mood (for a short time [*Parker et al. 2006; Macht & Mueller 2007*]), and the anti-inflammatory properties of cocoa flavonols [*Selmi et al. 2006*] seem to be another promising possibility for psychosomatic therapy.

7.2.4. Coffee

Coffee is derived from fermented and roasted seeds (coffee beans) of *Coffea arabica* a native plant of Africa and Near East. Coffee is a complex mixture of chemicals that provides significant amounts of *caffeine, chlorogenic acid, cinnamic acid* (*caffeic acid*), *cafestol, kahveol,* and *micronutrients* like magnesium, potassium, niacin and vitamin E [*Higdon & Frei 2006*]. *Caffeine* is a purine alkaloid, exerting several physiological effects including central nervous system stimulation, acute elevation of blood pressure, increased metabolic rate and diuresis. *Chlorogenic acid* and *cinnamic acid* also exert rather significant antioxidant activity [*Higdon & Frei 2006, Koren et al. in press/a,b*]. *Cafestol* and *kahweol* are agents raising serum level of total and LDL cholesterol [*Urgert & Katan 1997*]. Importantly, boiled "Scandinavian" "Turkish" or "French" coffee contain high levels, while filtered coffee, percolated coffee and instant coffee contain only very low levels of cafestol and kahveol; therefore care should be taken of choosing of brewing method [*Urgert et al. 1995*].

Moderate coffee consumption (up to 3-4 cups in a day) may help to prevent several chronic diseases, including type 2 diabetes mellitus, Parkinson's disease and liver diseases (cirrhosis and hepatocellular carcinoma); whereas most prospective cohort studies have not found coffee consumption to be associated with significantly increased risk of cardiovascular or other diseases [*Higdon & Frei 2006, Lopez-Garcia et al. 2008*]. Caffeine consumption is associated with a reduced risk of depression [*Smith 2009*], improved cognitive functioning [*Smith 2009*], improved mood [*Robelin & Rogers 1998*], improved psychomotor performance [*Robelin & Rogers 1998*] and decreased fatigue [*Smith 2002*] all of which are rather advantageous also for psychosomatic therapies. However, concomitant intake of coffee (and consumption with meals) should be avoided, because several polyphenols and zinc chelating compounds of coffee significantly inhibit intestinal absorption of iron and zinc respectively [*Higdon & Frei 2006*]. High doses of caffeine may also influence bone metabolism and may lead to increased bone loss in periodontitis [*Bezerra et al. 2008*] and decrease of bone density in elderly women [*Rapuri et al. 2001*]. It should be also considered that, consumption of very large amounts of coffee ("overdosage" of caffeine) may increase anxiety and impair sleep [*Smith 2002*].

7.2.5. Chastetree

Chastetree (Vitex Agnus Castus) is a *progesterone*-like substance containing [*Brown 1997, Geller & Studee 2005*] native plant of South Europe, West Asia and East Africa. Chastetree is approved for the treatment of premenstrual syndrome (PMS), breast tenderness and irregularities of menstrual cycle [*Geller & Studee 2005*]. Similarly, chastetree may improve peri- and postmenopausal symptoms including emotional problems and hot flashes [*Lucks 2003*]. The use of this plant should be avoided during pregnancy and lactation [*Daniele et al. 2005*]. Although no drug interaction was reported so far, interference of chastetree with dopaminergic antagonists was expected [*Daniele et al. 2005*].

7.2.6. Ginko

Ginkgo (Ginkgo biloba) is a native plant of South-East Asia having significant vascular effect increasing blood flow especially to the brain [*Geller & Studee 2005*]. Further, ginkgo increases uptake of glucose by brain cells and improve transmission of nerve signals [*Geller & Studee 2005*]. Ginco is approved for use of cerebral insufficiency, vertigo, tinnitus and also for peripheral vascular diseases like Raynaud's syndrome [*Kleinen & Knipschild 1992, Geller & Studee 2005*]. Ginco can also be used to improve memory function [*Subhan & Hindmarch 1984, Gessner et al. 1985, Hofferberth 1989*] and may be also to improve dementia [*Geller & Studee 2005*].

7.2.7. Ginseng

Ginseng (Panax ginseng) is a native plant of South-East Asia used as a tonic for invigoration and fortification in times of fatigue, for improvement of declining capacity for work or concentration, and for coping with psychosocial stress [*Geller & Studee 2005*]. It may also be used to improve depression and insomnia, and to improve well being [*Tode et al. 1999, Wiklund et al. 1999*]. Ginseng was also found effective for the treatment of unexplained chronic fatigue [*Bentler et al. 2005*]. Ginseng also enhances the anti-allergic effect of green tea [*Maeda-Yamamoto et al. 2007*]. Ginseng also induces molecular chaperones including the major chaperone family of HSP70/HSPA type stress proteins in both animal and human cell culture models [*Yeo et al. 2008, Papamichael & Tiligada 2008*] indicating that, ginseng may influence numerous stress related (concretely: stress protein related) pathways. Besides its advantageous effects, care should be taken with the use of ginseng in the case of malignancies (especially breast cancer), because in such cases use of ginseng could be contraindicated [*Geller & Studee 2005*].

7.2.8. Red Clover

Red clover (Trifolium pratense) is a native plant of Europe containing hormone-like phytoestrogen isoflavones (i.e. genistein, daidzein, biochanin-A and formononetin) [Geller & Studee 2005, Low Dog 2005] similarly to soy (see in paragraph 7.3.8.). Premised phytoestrogens likely act like selective estrogen receptor modulators (SERMs) [Teede et al. 2004, Geller & Studee 2005], acting primarily on beta type estrogen receptors [Kuiper et al. 1998, Carlsson et al. 2008]. Therefore, it is likely that red clover has minimal or no effects on menopausal hot flashes similarly to soy products [Geller & Studee 2005]; however, selectivity minimizes risk of adverse effects on endometrial and breast tissue [Geller & Studee 2005, Carlsson et al. 2008]. Similarly to soy, red clover likely exerts bone-protective effects [Clifton-Bligh et al. 2001, Atkinson et al. 2004], improves lipid profile [Clifton-Bligh et al. 2001] and possibly cognition [Geller & Studee 2005] although the evidence is limited. Since red clover and soy share similar chemical profiles (including premised phytoestrogen isoflavones), most known effects of soy may also be assigned to red clover (see also soy in paragraph 7.3.8.). Since red clover isoflavones can inhibit cytochrome P-450 dependent drug metabolism [Unger & Frank 2004, Low Dog 2005], possible herb-drug interaction should be considered before use [Low Dog 2005] (even if no such interaction has been reported yet).

7.2.9. Scutellaria Radix

Scutellaria radix (Scutellaria baicalensis) is a native plant of North America and East Asia, containing naturally occurring polyphenolic flavonid *wogonin* (5,7-dihydroxy-8-methoxyflavonate). Wogonin exerts anti-inflammatory effects in macrophages via inhibition of inducible nitric oxide synthase (iNOS) [*Chi et al. 2001, Shen et al. 2002*]; and also through influencing arachidonic acid (AA) metabolism via selective inhibition of cycloxigenase-2

(COX-2) [*Chi et al. 2001*] and consequent inhibition of prostaglandin E_2 (PGE_2) synthesis [*Chi et al. 2001 Shen et al. 2002*]. Wogonin also inhibits inflammatory activation of cultured brain microglia by diminishing lipopolysaccharide-induced production of tumor necrosis factor alpha (TNF-α), interleukin 1-beta (IL-1β) and nitric oxide (NO) [*Lee et al. 2003*]. Wogonin also exerts neuroprotective properties under transient global ischemia and excitotoxic injuries of the brain in animal models, by inhibiting inflammatory activation of microglia [*Lee et al. 2003*] (which is a critical component of pathogenic inflammatory responses in neurodegenerative diseases [*Lee et al. 2003*]).

7.2.10. St John's Wort

St John's wort (Hypericum perforatum) is a native plant of Europe and Asia containing numerous possible (but not yet clearly identified) active constituents [*Hostettmann & Wolfender 2005*]. St John's wort seems to be effective to improve mild to moderate depressive symptoms (but not major depression) [*Linde et al. 1996, 2005, Volz 2005*], as well as fatigue [*Volz 2005*], atypical depression [*Volz 2005*], several somatoform disorders [*Volz 2005*] and likely also anxiety [*Volz 2005*]. A synergistic effect of St John's wort with black cohosh (see above) in the case of psychovegetative disorders is also very likely [*Liske 1998, Geller & Studee 2005*]. Climacteric symptoms including several psychological and psychosomatic symptoms and sexual well-being may also be improved efficiently with the use of St John's wort [*Grube et al. 1999*].

Using St John's wort great care should be taken with *herb-drug interactions*. St John's wort is a potent ligand for pregnane X receptor [*Moore et al. 2000, Carlson et al. 2008*] and consequently increases cytochrome P450 [*Moore et al. 2000, Staudinger et al. 2006, Carlson et al. 2008*] dependent hepatic drug metabolism; therefore decreases blood concentration of several drugs including anticoagulants, oral contraceptives, cyclosporin, digoxin and protease inhibitors used for HIV treatment [*Moore et al. 2000, Geller & Studee 2005*]. In relation with oral contraceptives it should be considered that, St John's wort may cause breakthrough bleeding and in some cases unplanned pregnancies [*Geller & Studee 2005*]. St. John's wort administration may also interact with psychiatric antidepressant medication.

7.2.11. Tea

Tea (Camellia sinensis) is a native plant of South Asia. *Black tea* is made *via* post-harvest "fermentation" prior to drying, which is an auto-oxidation process catalyzed by a polyphenol oxidase present in the plant. *Green tea* is steamed to inactivate polyphenol oxidase prior to drying, therefore green tee is not "fermented". *Oolong tea* is produced by a partial oxidation of the leaves intermediate between the process of black tea and green tea [*McKay et al. 2002*]. Since *oolong tea* is a partially "fermented" tea, therefore the composition of its constituents and their expectable therapeutic effects are likely intermediate between black and green tee (which are detailed below). In general, the flavonoid content decreases, whereas the caffeine content increases with "fermentation"; however geographical location and growing conditions also influence the composition of constituents [*McKay et al. 2002*].

Black tea is rich in caffeine but, the total content of flavonoids are usually lower, and *polymerized catechins* such as *theaflavines* and *thearubigens* are predominate [*McKay et al. 2002*]. Primarily because of caffeine effects, consumption of black tea is associated with a reduced risk of depression [*Smith 2009*], improved cognitive functioning [*Smith 2009*], improved mood [*Robelin & Rogers 1998*], improved psychomotor performance [*Robelin & Rogers 1998*] and decreased fatigue [*Smith 2002*]. The antioxidant capacity of black tea is also rather high [*McKay et al. 2002*]; the plasma antioxidant potential following consumption of black tea is similar to that following consumption of green tea [*Gardner et al. 2007*].

Green tea is rich in *L-theanine* and several *flavonoids*, but the caffeine content is much lower than in black tee (2-4% versus 8-11% dry weight of green and black tea respectively [*Kakuda 2002, Gardner et al. 2007*]). *L-theanine* (γ-glutamylethilamide) is a compound similar to the excitatory neurotransmitter glutamic acid [*Kakuda 2002*]. Although the binding capacity of L-theanine to glutamate receptors is markedly less than that of glutamic acid, there is a significant neuroprotective effect of L-theanine on glutamate toxicity [*Kakuda 2002*]. There is also evidence that, administration of L-theanine could be associated with relaxation of the central nervous system and consequent increase of alpha brainwave activity [*Bryan 2008*]. The major *flavonoids* present in green tea include *catechins* such as *epicatechin* (EC), *epicatechin-3-gallate* (ECG), *epigallocatechin* (EGC) and *epigallocatechin-3-gallate* (EGCG) [*McKay et al. 2002*].

Research activities have focused primarily on EGCG, because it is likely to exert the strongest biological activity. EGCG induces immunosuppressive alterations on human dendritic cells, *via* induction of apoptosis and suppression of antigen presentation [*Yoneyama et al. 2008*]. EGCG also decreases the adhesiveness and migration of mast cells, and decrease their potential to produce signals eliciting monocyte recruitment [*Melgarejo et al. 2007*]. EGCG is likely to inhibit T-cell activation as well [*Shim et al. 2008*]. EGCG has inhibitory effects on the activity and expression of matrix metalloproteinases (MMPs) which are agents causing alveolar bone loss as well [*Yun et al. 2004*]. EGCG also inhibits osteoclast formation [*Yun et al. 2004*] and induce apoptotic cell death of osteoclasts through a caspase-mediated pathway [*Yun et al. 2007*]. Interestingly, EGCG also exerts significant anxiolytic, sedative and psychological stress reducing properties [*Adachi et al. 2006, Vignes et al. 2006*]. The antioxidant capacity of green tea flavonoids is also rather high [*McKay et al. 2002, Emara & El-Bahrawy 2008, Koren et al. in press/a,b*], and they also exert anti-allergic properties [*Maeda-Yamamoto et al. 2007*]. Green tea flavonoids are also likely to protect against autoimmune arthritis [*Kim et al. 2008*].

Taking together all above data it may be concluded that, tea consumption could be rather advantageous also for psychosomatic therapies, to improve psychological functions and to modulate several inflammatory and oxidative processes. Tea polyphenols also inhibit bacterial growth including several oral bacteria (i.e. *E. coli, S. salivarus* and *S. mutans*) [*McKay et al. 2002, Stoicov et al. in press*] and may improve oral leukoplakia [*McKay et al. 2002*]. Tea flavonoids may also stimulate B cell proliferation [*Yang et al. 2000, McKay et al. 2002*], however this immune stimulatory properties are likely not the principal health benefits of tea flavonoids [*McKay et al. 2002*]. It should be also noted that, consumption of tea (especially green tea but also black and oolong tea) likely decreases the risk of cancer [*McKay et al. 2002, Zhang et al. 2009*] and cardiovascular diseases [*McKay et al. 2002, Gardner et al. 2007*]. However, concomitant intake (and consumption with meals) of tea should be avoided, because it appears to inhibit intestinal absorption of iron [*McKay et al. 2002*]. Since tea flavonoids inhibit hepatic cytochrome P450-dependent enzymes [*Yang et al. 2000, McKay et al. 2002*], possible herb-drug interactions should also be considered. A *very large* amount of black tea may also increase anxiety and impair sleep, because of "overdosage" of caffeine [*Smith 2002*].

7.2.12. Contraindication of Medicinal Herb Therapy

Concurrent use of medicinal herbs and pharmaceutical drugs without any control of medical or dental professionals is relatively common and the majority of herbal medicine users are not aware of potential adverse effects [*Zhang et al. 2008*]. Therefore, dentist should carefully collect information about the patients' medicinal herb related usage. Besides specific contraindications, potential health hazards including possible interactions with medications [*Segelman et al. 1976*], risk of abuse of medicinal herbs [*Siegel 1979*] and risk of herbal intoxication [*Siegel 1976*] should also be considered very carefully before starting medicinal herb therapy.

Notwithstanding that, a *principled* multi-target strategy of medicinal herb therapy may be advantageously used [*Ginsburg et al. 2008*]; the use of an *unprincipled* combination of medicinal herbs should be strictly avoided. To avoid any potential adverse effects, dentist should administer medicinal herb therapy for a limited time span (few months) only. Following this period the *therapeutic* administration (*at least* two cups per day and/or use of medicinal herb extracts) of medicinal herbs should be either terminated or surrendered to the family doctor (or other professionals like internist, psychiatrist etc.). In the case of pregnancy, lactation, and any severe compromised health conditions, a consultation with the family doctor (or any other professionals responsible for the treatment of the condition at issue) is highly recommended *before* starting any medicinal herb therapy.

7.3. DIET THERAPY

7.3.1. Nutritional Status

Nutritional status seems to be highly important to maintain oral health and to prevent several oral manifestations [*Touger-Decker 1998, 2003, Touger-Decker et al. 2007*]. Further, there is a synergistic bidirectional interrelatationship between nutritional status and oral health [*Touger-Decker 1998, 2003, Touger-Decker et al. 2007*]. *On the one hand*, dental status, masticatory function, lubricating effect of saliva, food perception and taste influence nutritional status significantly [*Rhodus & Brown 1990, Raphael et al. 2002, Borges-Yañez et al. 2004, Soini et al. 2006, Nowjack-Raymer & Sheiham 2007*]. *On the other hand* nutritional intake also influences oral health status and incidence of several oral symptoms significantly

[*Touger-Decker 1998, 2003, Borges-Yañez et al. 2004, Soini et al. 2006, Touger-Decker et al. 2007*]. Moreover, several nutritional compounds may also be used for therapeutic purposes as detailed below. (Please note that, therapeutic use of some dietary compounds like vitamins and medicinal herbs are discussed in previous paragraphs such as paragraphs *6.6.7. and 7.2.*)

It should be also considered that, dental patient may have significantly lower intake of dietary fibers, certain vitamins (vitamin A and beta-carotene, vitamin B_1, vitamin B_2, vitamin B_6, folate, vitamin C, vitamin E) and certain ions (calcium, potassium, iron, zinc, phosphorus). Premised alterations may occur primarily because of lower intake of raw vegetables, fresh fruits and salads [*Laurin et al. 1994, Krall et al. 1998, Suzuki et al 2005, Nowjack-Raymer & Sheiham 2003, 2007*]. There is a high risk of such alterations especially in five groups of patients: (1) patients with missing teeth but wearing no dentures [*Nowjack-Raymer & Sheiham 2007*] especially if fewer than 21 natural teeth are present [*Budtz-Jørgensen et al. 2001, Borges-Yañez et al. 2004*]; (2) patients wearing RPDs but having fewer than 5 natural teeth [*Kwok et al. 2004, Suzuki et al 2005*]; (3) edentulous patients, even if wearing complete dentures [*Brodeur et al. 1993, Nowjack-Rajmer & Sheiham 2003*]; (4) patients with xerostomia [*Rhodus & Brown 1990*]; (5) and patients with severe orofacial pain [*Raphael et al. 2002*].

7.3.2. Dietary Protein Intake

Dietary protein intake (as a unique source of essential amino acids and nitrogen) is one of the most important parameter of nutrition, because of the highly important and far-reaching functions of amino acids, synthesized proteins and other nitrogen-containing compounds in the body. Great care should be taken to ensure adequate intake of *essential amino acids* (which are not synthesized in the body) such as *isoleucine, leucine, lysine, methionine, phenylalanine, threonine, tryptophan* and *valine* (and also histidine and may be arginine for growth of infants and children) [*Nestle 1985*]. In case of patients consuming *vegetarian diets* (avoiding meat, fish, milk and eggs) *complementary amino acid composition* of consumed vegetable foods should be controlled and ensured [*Nestle 1985*]. Besides general importance of adequate protein intake, significant effects of protein ingestion on hard tissues may command special interest in relation with oral/orofacial symptoms.

Protein intake increases serum levels of known bone formation markers such as insulin-like growth factor-I (IGF-I), bone specific alkaline phosphatase (BSAP) and osteocalcin of postmenopausal women [*Arjmani et al. 2005*]. Similarly protein intake significantly improve bone mineral content (BMC) and bone mineral density (BMD) of growing female rats in animal model [*Chen et al. 2008*]. Further, protein intake significantly improves quality of hard dental tissues in animal studies as well [*Fábián & Fejérdy 1975, Fábián et al. 1972, 1975, 1979, Tóth et al. 1988*]. Besides general importance of adequate protein intake in most kind of disorders; above findings indicate that, increased protein ingestion seems to be especially reasonable during healing processes of several bone and hard dental tissue pathologies including idiopathic pain (or another idiopathic symptoms) of bone and/or teeth.

Tryptophan intake may also be of particular interest in relation with psychosomatic disorders, because tryptophan is the precursor of serotonin, and can cross from the blood into the brain via specific transporters [*Bourre 2006/b*]. Dietary tryptophan has a significant antidepressive effect [*Köhler 2005, Bourre 2006/b*], and it is likely to be involved in other important psychological functions like coping with stress [*Peeters et al. 2005, Firk & Markus 2008*], regulation of sleep and pain sensation [*Bourre 2006/b*]. Preliminary results indicated significant psychological effects of *tyrosine* as well [*Avraham et al. 2001, Bourre 2006/b*]. However, tyrosine competes with tryptophan for passage into the brain (i.e. for the transporter molecule) [*Benton & Donohoe 1999, Bourre 2006/b*], therefore, specific serotonin precursor effects of tryptophane may be decreased with high intake of tyrosine. Intake of *pre-germinated grain* (especially brown rice) containing surprisingly high amount of the amino acid derivative *GABA* (gamma-aminobutyrate, a decarboxyled form of L-glutamate) also improve mood and stress tolerance significantly [*Sakamoto et al. 2007*].

7.3.3. Digestible Carbohydrates

Digestible carbohydrates like *sugars* (mono- and disaccharides) and *starch* accounts for a large proportion of the daily intake. Prior to digestion and absorption from the intestine, a proportion of dietary carbohydrates are fermented and utilized by several bacteria of the gastrointestinal tract. Bacterial fermentation of sugars also occur in bacterial biofilm (dental plaque) attached to tooth surfaces in the oral cavity, which leads to formation of dental caries [*Sreebny 1982*]. Digestion and absorption result in three *principal* monosaccharides namely *glucose fructose* and *galactose*, although some other monosaccharides (like several pentoses) are also absorbed [*Mayes 1985/d*]. Since both fructose and galactose are readily converted to glucose by the liver, therefore carbohydrate are utilized by cells mainly in the form of glucose [*Mayes 1985/d*]. Glucose function as fuel to be oxidized and provide energy for other metabolic processes [*Mayes 1985/d*]. Besides functioning as a fuel, absorbed carbohydrates are also incorporated into highly important molecules like nucleotides, glycoproteins, glycosaminoglycans, proteoglycans, and glycolipids. An amount of absorbed dietary carbohydrate is converted to fat.

Besides premised highly important functions, sugar ingestion and blood glucose have been related to the regulation of mood as well. There is good evidence that a meal that is *almost exclusively* carbohydrate will increase the ratio of tryptophan to large neutral amino acids; therefore, relatively more tryptophan (the precursor of serotonin) is transported into the brain [*Wurtman 1984, Wurtman & Wurtman 1989*]. However, it should be also noted that, as little as 5% of the *caloric intake* as protein will prevent this increased provision of tryptophan [*Benton & Donohoe 1999, Benton 2002/b*]. Another psychological effect of carbohydrates (especially sugars) can be based on the fact that palatable foods induce a release of endorphins in the brain [*Dum et al. 1983, Benton 2002/b*], which would be expected to reduce stress as endogenous opiates modulate the bodily response to pain and pleasure [*Benton 2002/b*]. (Please consider that, many of palatable foods are sweet, like fruits, candies, ice cream, cake, chocolate etc..) Finally, it is also known that, increased blood glucose prevents the decrease in arousal (weariness) that occurs when individuals perform cognitively demanding tasks [*Owens et al. 1997*].

Although there is a need in future research to recognize the real impact of carbohydrates on mood and other psychological functions; it may be concluded that: *transiently* and *moderately* increased consumption of sweets (sugars) may be advantageous under several psychosocial stress conditions and may be also used for initial psychosomatic therapy. However, contraindications including diabetes, obesity, carbohydrate abuse, pathological experience of guilt after eating sweets, level of oral hygiene and risk of caries etc. should also be considered carefully. Since the expected mood benefits of sweets are at best ephemeral, sugars when consumed as a comfort eating or emotional (stress associated) "eating strategy" are more likely to be associated with prolongation rather than cessation of a dysphoric mood.

7.3.4. Dietary Fibers

Dietary fibers (also called *prebiotics*) are nondigestible carbohydrates originating *primarily* from plant sources. Dietary fibers are incompletely absorbed (or not absorbed) in the small intestine but are at least partly fermented by bacteria in the large intestine [*Scholz-Ahrens et al. 2001, Grabitschke & Slavin 2008*]. Besides advantageous decreasing effects of adequate fiber intake on the risk for obesity, coronary hard diseases, colon cancer and diabetes [*Nestle 1985, Grabitschke & Slavin 2008*], adequate dietary fiber intake advantageously improve oral health as well [*Petti et al. 2000, Borges-Yañez et al. 2004*]. From this point of view, especially specific effects of certain decomposition products of dietary fibers (namely fructooligosaccharides) are of particular interest.

Fructooligosaccharides (FOS) are low molecular weight nondigestible (but fermentable) oligosaccharides found in many foods such as wheat, onions, bananas, honey, garlic or leeks [*Chow 2002*]. They are usually obtained by partial enzymatic hydrolysis of chicory inuline [*Raschka & Daniel 2005*], or manufactured from sucrose using fructosyltransferase [*Hidaka et al. 1988, Morohashi et al. 1998*]. FOS are fermented by the microflora (primarily bifidobacteria [*Hikada et al. 1991, Bouhnik et al. 1999*]) in the large intestine (and may be already in the ileum) resulted in production of short chain fatty acids (SCFA) mainly acetate propionate and butyrate [*Campbell 1997, Morohashi et al. 1998*]. Resulted SCFAs decrease luminal pH leading to increased calcium solubility and transepithelial calcium gradient [*Raschka & Daniel 2005*]. Further, SCFAs (especially butyrate) stimulate mucosal cell proliferation, which in turn may increase the absorptive surface area of ileum (via increase of villus height) [*Morohashi et al. 1998; Raschka & Daniel 2005*]. In addition, FOS likely alter transcript level of several mucosal genes that can be linked to transcellular and paracellular transport processes [*Raschka & Daniel 2005*].

Likely based on premised mechanisms FOS are known to maximize absorption of several minerals, including calcium [*Ohta et al. 1995, Morohashi et al. 1998*] being highly important for bone homeostasis. FOS also maximize absorption of other important ions such as magnesium [*Ohta et al. 1995, 1998*] iron [*Ohta et al. 1998, Ohta 2006*] and zinc [*Scholz-Ahrens et al. 2001*]. FOS likely play a role in protein coupled bone regeneration processes as well [*Devareddy et al. 2006, Johnson et al. in press, Morohashi et al. 2005*], enhancing protein related increase of BMC, BMD and BSAP and decrease of urinary deoxypyridinoline (DPD; a specific marker of bone resorption) [*Johnson et al. in press*]. Fructooligosaccharides also enhance protein related improvement of bone biomechanical properties [*Johnson et al. in press*], and maximize bone-protective effects of soy isoflavones (see below) in postmenopausal women [*Mathey et al. 2004*]. Similarly, to bone effects, FOS likely improves *dentine* formation highly efficiently as well [*Morohashi et al. 2005*].

Importantly, fiber content in the US Department of Agriculture food composition database does *not* include inuline and fructooligosaccharides; therefore amount of FOS (and/or inuline) in a food is advantageously indicated in the list of ingredients with terms like "inuline", "fructan", "chicory root", "chicory root extract", "chicory root fiber" or "Jerusalem artichoke" (another plant source of inuline [*Mayes 1985/a*]) helping dentists and patients to recognize available fructooligosaccharides sources [*Grabitschke & Slavin 2008*]. It should also be noted that, not exclusively fructooligosaccharides but several other prebiotics may have similar effects. However, their efficiency seems to be specific to the type of carbohydrate, and it is likely to be related to the rate of fermentation too [*Scholz-Ahrens et al. 2001*].

7.3.5. Dietary Lipids

Dietary lipids are heterogeneous group of compounds related either actually or potentially to the fatty acids [*Mayes 1985/b*]. *Fatty acids* that occur in natural fats and oils (fats in liquid state) are carboxylic acids usually containing an even number of carbon atoms (because they are synthesized from 2-carbon units) and are straight chain derivatives [*Mayes 1985/b*]. The chain may be *saturated* (containing no double bonds), *monounsaturated* (containing one double bounds) or *polyunsaturated* (containing more double bonds) [*Mayes 1985/b, Ross et al. 2007*]. Several saturated fatty acids can be found in the fat of ruminants, in butter, or in fats of other animal origin, whereas others can be found in peanut, nutmeg, palm kernel, coconut, myrtles, laurels, cinnamon [*Mayes 1985/b*]. Monounsaturated fatty acids are subdivided into *omega-9* and *omega-7* series depending on the position of the double bond counting from the end carbon atom (omega atom) of the molecule. Omega-9 and omega-7 series derived from *oleic acid* or *palmitoleic* acid respectively, and these are the most common fatty acids in natural fats [*Mayes 1985/b*]. Polyunsaturated fatty acids (PUFAs) are subdivided into *omega-6* and *omega-3* series, depending on the position of *first* double bond counting from the omega atom of the molecule.

Omega-6 series are derived from *linoleic acid* (LA) which is termed *essential fatty acid*, because mammalian cells are unable to synthesize it [*Mayes 1985/b,c, Ross et al. 2007*]. Although LA can be converted into *arachidonic acid* (AA), the rate of conversion is very slow; therefore, AA is also termed *essential* [*Mayes 1985/c Ross et al. 2007*]. Similarly, *gamma*-linolenic acid (GLA) and dihomogammalinolenic acids (DGLA) also belongs to omega-6 group. Although GLA and DGLA is not termed essential, however rate of conversion is rather slow also in their cases [*Ross et al. 2007*]. *Omega-3 series* are derived from *alpha-linolenic acid* (ALA), which also belongs to *essential fatty acids* [*Mayes 1985/b,c, Ross et al. 2007*]. ALA is converted into longer chain omega-3 PUFAs such as *eicosapentaeoic acid* (EPA) and *docosahexaenoic acid* (DHA), however the rate of conversion is rather slow in humans [*Ross et al. 2007*].

Although intake of most lipids is abundant under normal nutrition, adequate intake of premised essential and other omega-3 and omega-6 type PUFAs should be controlled and ensured; either because they are not synthesized at all or because their synthesis is rather limited in human [*Ross et al. 2007*]. Especially omega-3 type PUFAs are of particular interest, since the intake of these fatty acids is considered to be low in western diets [*Ross et al. 2007*]. Main sources of omega-6 PUFAs are corn, peanut, cottonseed, soybean, plant oils and evening primrose. Main sources of omega-3 PUFAs are linseed, fish oils, and cod liver oil [*Mayes 1985/b*]. PUFAs are participating in various highly important biological functions including prostaglandin-, leukotriene- and structural lipid formation, growing and reproduction, maintenance of the health of skin and kidney [*Mayes 1985/c*] and coping with stress [*Lucas et al. 2009, Mayes 1985/c*].

In certain cases essential and other omega-3 type polyunsaturated fatty acids may also be used for therapeutic purposes, especially for several mental illnesses [*Peet and Stokes 2005, Kidd 2007, Lucas et al. 2009*]. Phospholipid attached forms of omega-3 PUFAs seems to be especially promising for such purposes [*Kidd 2007*]. Supplementation of the diet with omega-3 PUFAs (especially with EPA [*Peet & Stokes 2005, Kidd 2007*]) significantly reduces depression [*Lin & Su 2007, Ross et al. 2007, Lucas et al. 2009*], and likely also reduces anxiety [*Ross et al. 2007*]. Omega-3 PUFAs may also improve attention deficit hyperactivity disorder [*Ross et al. 2007*]. Improvement in mental, emotional and social well-being [*Lucas et al. 2009, Rubin et al. 2008*] was also reported. Omega-3 PUFAs may also be used advantageously to support the treatment of schizophrenia [*Peet & Stokes 2005, Kidd 2007*] and borderline personality disorder [*Kidd 2007*]. Due to their expected anti-inflammatory and neuroprotective effects, omega-3 PUFAs could also be used for the treatment of neurodegenerative diseases [*Song & Zhao 2007*] and psychosomatic inflammatory symptoms (i.e. acne vulgaris) [*Rubin et al. 2008*]. Although further research is needed to reach clear clinical conclusion, omega-3 PUFA supplementation is recommended for use as an adjunct to the therapy of orofacial psychosomatic disorders as well.

7.3.6. Minerals and Trace Elements

Minerals and *trace elements* (which are needed in much smaller amounts) perform a great variety of essential physiologic functions [*Martin 1985/c*]. Body composition studies demonstrated that, nearly all of the chemical elements can be found in the human body [*Nestle 1985*]. Minerals and trace elements are widely distributed in whole-grain cereals, fruits and vegetables, dairy products, meats, and seafood [*Nestle 1985*]; however, they are usually present in these foods in relatively small quantities [*Nestle 1985*]. Certain types of industrial food processing (i.e. refinement, extraction rate of flour [*Martin 1985/c, Nestle 1985*]) and also home food processing (i.e. pouring out the cooking water in which minerals are dissolved) may also decrease their amounts strongly. Further, their absorption in human is rather inefficient, and usually greater quantities remain in the intestines than are absorbed [*Nestle 1985*]. Therefore, a sufficient quantity and variety of food must be consumed to meet daily requirements. Consumption of mineral water is also highly recommended. It should be also considered that, various nutritional factors (i.e. presence of chelating agents, protein, fat, other minerals, dietary fiber) may also either improve or decrease their absorption [*Martin 1985/c, Nestle 1985*].

Besides their various essential functions [*Martin 1985/c*], minerals and trace elements seem to be important tools for the prevention and treatment of oral disorders as well. *Calcium* and *phosphorus* are major constituents of bone and hard tissues of the teeth. Although their *intake* is usually adequate under normal nutrition, facilitation of calcium *absorption* with the help of other nutriments (i.e. fructooligosaccharides, see above) seems to be needed especially under several bone pathologies [*Morohashi et al. 2005, Ohta 2006*]. Further, proper dietary *zinc* intake can be rather effective for treatment of several dysgeusias [*Sato & Mikami 2002*] and salivary hypofunctions [*Sato & Mikami 2003*] especially when combined with advice to improve mastication activity, slightly increased weekly physical activity and other modalities of psychosomatic treatment [*Sato & Mikami 2002, 2003*]. Zinc intake can also be considered as a significant chaperone (HSP70/HSPA) inducer of human CD3+ and CD3- lymphocytes [*Putics et al. 2008/b*], which may influence immune-inflammatory reactions also in the orofacial region. Significant antidepressive [*Levenson 2006*] and stress reducing [*Marcellini et al. 2008*] effect of zinc was also reported.

Similarly, intake of *magnesium* also improves mood [*Poleszak et al. 2005*] and may improve coping ability with stress [*Peeters et al. 2005*]. *Selenium* [*Benton 2002/a*] and *chromium* [*Davidson et al. 2003*] also improves mood and depressive symptoms. Proper dietary intake of *iron* is also highly important, because many symptoms including depression, anxiety, apathy, somnolence, irritability, decrease of attention, inability to concentrate and memory loss may also occur because of deficient iron intake (even in the absence of anemia) [*Benton & Donohoe 1999, Bourre 2006/a*]. A closer relationship between iron status and cognitive performance was also expected [*Brown 2001, Bourre 2006/a*].

7.3.7. Vitamins

Vitamins are organic molecules in food that are required for normal metabolism but cannot be synthesized in adequate amounts by the human body. Vitamins were given alphabetic designations in the order of their discovery, and named when they were isolated and their chemical structures were identified [*Nestle 1985*]. Although they are exceedingly heterogeneous in chemical structure and biochemical function, they can be grouped conveniently into two classes that share common characteristics: fat-soluble vitamins and water-soluble vitamins [*Martin 1985/a,b, Nestle 1985*]. The *fat-soluble vitamins* include vitamins A, D, E, and K. These vitamins are present in food fats such as fatty meats, liver, dairy fats, egg yolks, vegetable seed oils and also in leafy green vegetables [*Martin 1985/a, Nestle 1985*]. Importantly, fat-soluble vitamins are not excreted in urine, therefore, they can be accumulated in storage tissues to toxic level [*Nestle 1985*].

The *water-soluble vitamins* include members of vitamin B group, and vitamin C. They are excreted in urine when their serum levels exceed tissue saturation, thus water-soluble vitamins must be supplied continually in the diet. Most water-soluble vitamins (except vitamin C and vitamin B_{12}) are found in whole-grain cereals, pre-germinated grain, legumes, leafy green vegetables, meat, and dairy products. Vitamin C (ascorbic acid) is found in fresh fruits and vegetables but especially in citrus fruits. Vitamin B_{12} (cobalamin) is synthesized by microorganisms; it is incorporated into animal tissues and is present in liver, meat, and dairy foods (thus strict vegetarians may be at risk for deficiency) [*Martin 1985/b, Nestle 1985*].

For optimal food processing it should be considered that, water-soluble vitamins are somewhat unstable to heat (especially vitamin C); and they dissolve in cooking water which therefore should be utilized (or at least kept to a minimum) to prevent vitamin losses [*Nestle 1985*]. It should be also considered that, fat-soluble vitamins can be accumulated in the body; therefore, megadose ingestion of fat-soluble vitamins is potentially dangerous [*Nestle 1985*]. Administration of vitamins could also be useful in the treatment of orofacial psychosomatic disorders. Adequate intake of vitamins should be controlled and ensured via optimal diet and/or adequate use of multivitamin products. *Therapeutic use* of vitamins in somewhat higher dosages may be also useful (as described in *paragraph 6.6.7.*).

7.3.8. Soy

Soy may also be used efficiently in diet therapy of several oral symptoms, because of its hormone-like phytoestrogen isoflavones (i.e. *genistein, daidzein, biochanin-A and formononetin*) [*Geller & Studee 2005, Chen et al. 2008, Tanaka et al. 2008*]. Soy phytoestrogens likely act like *selective estrogen receptor modulators* (SERMs) [*Teede et al. 2004, Geller & Studee 2005*], acting primarily on *beta type* estrogen receptors [*Kuiper et al. 1998, Carlsson et al. 2008*]. Therefore, it is likely that, soy has at best only minimal effects on menopausal hot flashes [*Geller & Studee 2005*], however premised selectivity minimizes risk of estrogen-related adverse effects on endometrial and breast tissue [*Geller & Studee 2005, Carlsson et al. 2008*]. Accordingly, there is no evidence that, soy would have any effect on certain pain symptoms induced by changes of estrogen level [*Woda & Pionchon 2000, 2001*]; although in the absence of data this expectation should not be excluded yet.

However, soy may be used effectively to improve bone mineral content (BMC) and/or bone mineral density (BMD) of postmenopausal women [*Potter et al. 1998, Alekel et al. 2000, Mei et al. 2001, Chen et al. 2008*]. Premised bone effect of soy phytoestrogens is based on inhibition of osteoclastogenesis and bone resorbing capacity of osteoclasts via downregulation of RANKL (receptor activator of nuclear factor-κβ ligand, a member of tumor necrosis factor superfamily) [*Chen et al. 2008*], which is essential for final differentiation steps of osteoclasts as well as for their bone resorbing capacity. Further, soy increases serum levels of bone formation markers such as insulin-like growth factor-I (IGF-I) [*Arjmani et al. 2005*], bone specific alkaline phosphatase (BSAP) [*Arjmani et al. 2005, Chen et al. 2008*], osteocalcin [*Arjmani et al. 2005, Chen et al. 2008*] and insulin-like growth factor binding protein-3 (IGFBP-3) [*Arjmani et al. 2005*]. Moreover, soy decreases bone resorption marker RatLaps values in serum (measure of rat type I collagen fragment) in animal model [*Chen et al. 2008*]. Beside phytoestrogens, soy-proteins seem to play important role in bone related effects of soy as well [*Chen et al. 2008, Johnson et al in press*], especially in the presence of several bioactive compounds like fructooligosaccharides (see also *paragraph 7.3.4.*) [*Johnson et al. in press*].

Besides above, soy isoflavones improve lipid profile reducing low density lipoproteins (LDL), triglycerides and LDL-cholesterol level, and increasing high density lipoproteins (HDL) and HDL-cholesterol level; which leads to atherosclerosis decreasing and cardioprotective effects [*Anderson et al. 1995, Knight et al. 1999, Kerckhoffs et al. 2002,*

Pereira & Abdala 2006]. Soy isoflavones also suppress heat shock proteins in aortic tissues (i.e. Hsp60, Hsp70 and Hsc70) improving premised atherosclerosis decreasing effect [*Pereira & Abdala 2006*]. Soy isoflavones suppress heat shock proteins in tumor cells (i.e. Hsp70 and Grp78) as well, leading to significant carcinoprotective effect [*Zhou & Lee 1998*] especially against breast cancer, endometrial cancer [*Foth & Kline 1998*] and leukemia [*Zhou & Lee 1998*]. In contrast, soy isoflavones *increases* the expression of HSP70/HSPA type heat shock proteins in peripheral blood mononuclear cells [*Fuchs et al. 2007*], which may lead to immune-activating and/or immune-modulator effects [*Miyake et al 2005, Cooke et al. 2006, Tanaka et al. 2008*] and may be used to prevent or improve several periodontal inflammations [*Tanaka et al. 2008*] and periodontal/mucosal allergic reactions [*Miyake et al 2005*]. Further, some improvement of cognitive functions including verbal memory, tracking and attention may also be expected following intake of soy isoflavones [*Kritz-Silverstein et al. 2003, Monteiro et al. 2008*], although data are still somewhat contradictory [*Hogervorst et al. 2008*].

Specific effect of soy reach diet on the exocrine glands including exocrine pancreas and salivary glands should also be mentioned. Soy induces hypertrophy and hyperplasia of both exocrine pancreas [*McGuinnes et al. 1980, 1981, McGuinnes & Wormsley 1986*] and salivary glands (concretely: parotid gland) [*Zelles et al. 2005, Szőke et al. in press*]. Premised effects could be advantageous for the treatment of xerostomia; however, it should also be considered that, soy intake may sensitize pancreas to carcinogens which might produce neoplastic changes [*McGuinnes et al. 1980, 1981, McGuinnes & Wormsley 1986*]. Consequently, despite anticarcinogenic effects of soy in numerous tissues (mentioned above), soy intake should be avoided in patients suffering from exocrine gland tumors or any other exocrine gland disorders with increased risk of malignancies. Blood pressure decreasing effect of soy in both hypertensive and normotensive patients [*Carlson et al. 2008*] should also be considered before use. Isoflavones similar to those of soy (red clover isoflavones, see *paragraph 7.2.8.*) were reported to inhibit cytochrome P-450 dependent drug metabolism [*Unger & Frank 2004*]. Therefore, possible soy-drug interactions should be considered before use, even if no such interaction has been reported yet.

7.3.9. Dried Plum

Dried plum (prune, Prunus domestica) is particularly rich in *polyphenols* and have one of the highest *oxygen radical absorbance capacity* (ORAC) among the most frequent fruits and vegetables [*Nakatani et al. 2000, Kayano et al. 2004*]. Besides many kind of polyphenol containing *fruits* and *vegetables* [*New et al. 2000, Mulhauer et al. 2003*], and also *green tee* [*Yun et al. 2004, 2007*] *especially dried plum* seems to be highly efficient tool for diet therapy aimed at improvement of BMC and/or BMD values of postmenopausal women [*Arjmani et al. 2002, Deyhim et al. 2005*], as well as of androgen deficit induced osteopenia of males [*Franklin et al 2006, Bu et al. 2007*]. Bone effect of dried plum polyphenols seems to be additive to that of soy [*Johnson et al. in press*] indicating at least partly different pathways comparing to those induced by soy. Dried plum consumption significantly increases serum levels of insulin-like growth factor-I (IGF-I) [*Arjmani et al. 2002, Franklin et al 2006*] and bone specific alkaline phosphatase (BSAP) [*Arjmani et al. 2002*] both of which are associated with greater rates of bone formation [*Arjmani et al. 2002, Franklin et al 2006*]. Further, dry plum polyphenols significantly inhibit osteoclastogenesis [*Bu et al. in press*] and bone resorbing capacity of osteoclasts via three major pathways: (1) downregulation of RANKL, which is a receptor activator of nuclear factor-κβ ligand [*Franklin et al 2006*]; (2) decrease of nitric oxide (NO) and tumor necrosis factor alpha (TNF-α) production which continues downregulation of RANKL-mediated osteoclastogenesis [*Bu et al. in press*]; (3) downregulation of NFATc1 which is a nuclear factor of activated T cells, and a key transcription factor in the regulation of osteogenesis [*Bu et al. in press*]. Considering all premised data, dried plum consumption may have beneficial effect on the healing of several bone related pathologies including idiopathic pain (or another idiopathic symptoms) of bone.

7.3.10. Grapes

Grapes (*Vitis infera*) and related products like dried grapes (raisins), and wines (especially red wines or other special wines produced in the presence of grape skin) are the most important sources of resveratrol. *Resveratrol* (3,4',5-trihydroxystilbene) is a naturally occurring phytoalexin compound, which may act as an antioxidant, promote nitric oxide production, inhibit platelet aggregation, improve blood lipoprotein profile and thereby serve as a cardioprotective agent [*Caimi et al. 2003, Bhat et al. 2001, Leifert & Abeywardena 2008*]. Resveratrol is likely to function as a cancer chemopreventive agent as well [*Bhat et al. 2001*]. Resveratrol also exhibits anti-inflammatory, neuroportective and antiviral properties [*Bhat et al. 2001, Das & Das 2007, Vingtdeux et al. 2008*]. Resveratrol may also improve muscular function, and may protect skeletal muscle from oxidative injury and catabolic protein degradation [*Naylor in press*]. Resveratrol was recently recognized as a significant inducer of major chaperone HSP70/HSPA proteins in human cell lines and freshly prepared peripheral lymphocytes too [*Putics et al. 2008/a*]. Based on above, it is very likely that consumption of grapes and raisins may also be used advantageously for the therapy of psychosomatic dental patients. A *few amount* of fine wines (especially red wines or other special wines produced in the presence of grape skin) may also be used advantageously [*Caimi et al. 2003, Vingtdeux et al. 2008, Walzem 2008*], however *use of wine (even if small amount) should be strictly avoided if any risk of alcohol dependency comes to hand*. Use of red wine vinegar or balsam vinegar for salads may also be advantageous.

7.3.11. Garlic

Garlic (*Allium sativum*) is a native plant of Middle Asia. Garlic contains high amount of *flavonoids* and nonprotein *sulfur amino acid secondary metabolites*, most prominently *alliin* (*S-allyl-L-cysteine S-oxide*). Alliin is cleaved by alliinase (an enzyme of most *Allium* species like garlic and onion) to form *ammonium pyruvate* and *2-propenesulfenic acid* [*Vaidya et al. 2009*]. The latter compound (*2-propenesulfenic acid*) as *sulfenic acid* exerts highly potent antioxidant capacity [*Vaidya et al. 2009*]. Premised *2-propenesulfenic acid* also undergoes

self-condensation to yield *allicin* that provides garlic with its odor and flavor [*Vaidya et al.*
2009].

Since garlic is able to accumulate the selenium from soil (similarly to onion see below),
there are high amount of selenium-enriched compounds in it, including *Se-methyl*
selenocysteine and *γ-glutamyl-Se-methyl selenocysteine* [*Arnault & Auger 2006*]. Premised
seleno-compounds may exert certain anticarcinogenic properties [*Arnault & Auger 2006*].
Raw garlic also exerts significant antibacterial [*Elnima et al. 1983, Ruddock et al. 2005,*
Groppo et al. 2007] and antifungal [*Elnima et al. 1983, Low et al. 2008*] properties that may
be utilized topically in the oral cavity [*Groppo et al. 2007*]. Garlic was also shown to have
various effects on the immune functions including increase of NK cell activity [*Kyo et al.*
1999, Kyo et al. 2001], and decrease of IgE mediated allergic reactions [*Kyo et al. 2001*] in
animal models. Consumption of garlic also increased brain serotonin level [*Haider et al.*
2008] and prevented the psychological stress induced decrease of immune functions [*Kyo et*
al. 1999, Kyo et al. 2001] in animal models. Raw garlic may also have a modest but
significant effect on platelet aggregation that may prevent platelet mediated cardiovascular
disorders [*Tattelman 2005*]. Because of premised antiplatelet activity, patients taking
anticoagulants should be cautious [*Tattelman 2005*]; and it seems also prudent to stop taking
high amount of *raw* garlic seven to 10 days before surgery [*Tattelman 2005*] (because it may
prolong bleeding time).

7.3.12. Onion

Onion (*Allium cepa*) is a native plant of Middle Asia. Onions are rich in two chemical
groups such as flavonoids (including *anthocyanins*, *quercetin* and its derivatives), and
alk(en)yl cystein sulphoxides (ACSOs), which, when cleaved by alliinase (an enzyme of most
Allium species like garlic and onion) generate the characteristic odor and taste of onion
[*Griffiths et al. 2002*]. The downstream products of ACSOs are a complex mixture of
compounds, which include *thiosulphinates, thiosulphonates, mono-, di-* and *trisulphides*
[*Griffiths et al. 2002*]. The decomposition of *thiosulphinates* results in *sulfenic acids*, which
are highly potent antioxidants [*Vaidya et al. 2009*]. Since onion have the ability to accumulate
the selenium from soil (similarly to garlic see above), there are also high amount of selenium-
enriched compounds in onion including *Se-methyl selenocysteine* and *γ-glutamyl-Se-methyl*
selenocysteine [*Arnault & Auger 2006*]. Several compounds from raw onion (including
premised seleno-compounds) may have certain anticarcinogenic properties [*Griffiths et al.*
2002, Arnault & Auger 2006]; whereas others inhibit platelet aggregation and may prevent
platelet mediated cardiovascular disorders [*Briggs et al. 2001, Griffiths et al. 2002*]. Because
of premised antiplatelet activity, patients taking anticoagulants should be cautious; and it
seems also reasonable to stop taking *high* amount of *raw* onion seven to 10 days before
surgery. Raw onion also exerts significant antibacterial [*Elnima et al. 1983, Griffiths et al.*
2002] and antifungal [*Elnima et al. 1983, Griffiths et al. 2002*] properties that may be utilized
topically in the oral cavity.

7.3.13. Chocolate

Chocolate is described as a high sugar and high fat (cocoa butter) containing food [*Benton & Donohoe 1999*] that also contains significant amount (roughly 4-8 %) of proteins [*Bruinsma & Taren 1999*]. Chocolate contains a variety of cocoa originated "drug-like" constituents as well. *N-acyletahanolamines* (*N-oleoylethanolamine* and *N-linoleoyethanolamine*) are fatty acids chemically and pharmacologically related to *Anandamide* [*Bruinsma & Taren 1999*] and act at the same site in the brain like cannabis [*DiTomaso et al. 1996*]. *Phenylethylamine* acts in a similar manner to amphetamine and is also found in chocolate [*Benton & Donohoe 1999*]. Several *other biogenic amines* exerting similar "drug-like" neurophysiological effects were also found in chocolate [*Bruinsma & Taren 1999*]. Although the level of these "drug like" substances provided by a bar of chocolate is much less than that needed to produce a pharmacological action [*Benton & Donohoe 1999*], a slight effect of such constituents on mood and other psychological functions may not be excluded [*Bruinsma & Taren 1999*]. Besides "drug-like" constituents, chocolate contains relatively high amount of stimulants like *theobromine* and a *caffeine* too [*Bruinsma & Taren 1999, Benton & Donohoe 1999*].

Chocolate also contains a relatively high amount of *magnesium* [*Bruinsma & Taren 1999, Benton & Donohoe 1999*], which improves mood [*Poleszak et al. 2005*] and may improve coping ability with stress [*Peeters et al. 2005*]. Chocolate (especially that of low amount of protein [*Benton & Donohoe 1999*]) as a source of sugar may also increase tryptophan transport into the brain [*Wurtman 1984, Wurtman & Wurtman 1989*] that increase brain serotonin synthesis and enhance mood. Chocolate also contains *cocoa flavonols* (see in *paragraph 7.2.3.*) likely to exert beneficial effects on blood pressure, insulin resistance, vascular damage and oxidative stress [*Martín et al. in press, Grassi et al. 2005, Selmi et al. 2008*]. Cocoa flavonols also exert significant anti-inflammatory properties [*Selmi et al. 2006*]. Finally, it should be also considered that, chocolate is rich in flavor and contains both sugar and fat, therefore it is a *highly palatable food* [*Bruinsma & Taren 1999, Benton & Donohoe 1999, Benton 2002/b*]. (Please note that, not only flavour but constitutes like sugar and fat are also *highly* characteristic of many palatable foods [*Desor et al. 1977, Drewnowski & Greenwood 1983, Drewnowski et al. 1989, Drewnowski 1997*]). Importantly, palatable foods like chocolate are known to induce release of *endorphins* in the brain [*Dum et al. 1983, Benton & Donohoe 1999, Benton 2002/b, Macht & Mueller 2007*], which probably modulates responses to pain, increases pleasure, and reduces stress [*Benton 2002/b*].

Taking together all above data, it is likely that, chocolate have several beneficial effects which may also be utilized for *initial* psychosomatic therapy. Chocolate may be used to improve mood for a short time [*Parker et al. 2006; Macht & Mueller 2007*], however it is more likely to be associated with prolongation rather than cessation of a dysphoric mood when consumed as a comfort eating or emotional (stress associated) eating strategy [*Parker et al. 2006, Macht & Mueller 2007*]. Further, the anti-inflammatory properties of cocoa flavonols [*Selmi et al. 2006*] seem to be another promising possibility for psychosomatic therapy of certain chronic inflammatory disorders [*Selmi et al. 2006*]. However, contraindications like obesity, diabetes, chocolate abuse, pathological experience of guilt following eating chocolate, as well as level of oral hygiene and risk of caries should be considered carefully before therapeutical use.

There are three principal type of chocolate may be offered. High-cocoa-content *dark chocolate* contains the highest amount of psychologically and biologically active substances including "drug-like" constituents, stimulants, flavonols and magnesium [*McShea et al. 2008, Bruinsma & Taren 1999*]. However, its taste is usually not as favorable as of other chocolates (even if sugar is added); because of the high amount of cocoa flavonols which impart a bitter astringent flavor to dark chocolate [*McShea et al. 2008*]. (Premised bitter astringent flavour may be masked by aggressive processing, however such processes may decrease the biological activity of cocoa substances too [*McShea et al. 2008*].) *Milk chocolate* contains less, but still significant amount of active substances, and there is also higher amount of sugar and milk in it, leading to a delicious taste [*McShea et al. 2008*]. *White chocolate* usually contains cocoa *butter,* milk and sugar but *not* the cocoa *solids* (i.e. cocoa powder, the main source of active substances). Therefore, white chocolate may be rather tasty, but the level of active substances is the lowest comparing to other chocolates.

7.3.14. Contraindication of Diet Therapy

Besides the specific contraindications mentioned above, any other possible contraindications of diet therapy should also be considered. Great care should be taken especially in the case of patients with severe systemic diseases, during pregnancy and lactation as well as if long run modification of the patient's diet that incorporates patient's total health needs (including oral health) is needed [*Palmer 2003, Touger-Decker 2003, Touger-Decker et al. 2007*]. Therefore consultation with (or referral to) a registered dietitian and/or internist and/or family doctor is highly recommended before starting diet therapy in such cases [*Palmer 2003, Touger-Decker 2003, Touger-Decker et al. 2007*].

7.4. CONCLUSION

Medicinal herb and diet therapy are important supplemental modalities of psychosomatic dental therapy. However, medicinal herb and diet therapy are frequently used for health enhancement by patients without any professional control; and unfortunately, they also use them during pregnancy and lactation or under severe systemic diseases, which may cause significant health hazards [*Segelman et al. 1976, Siegel 1976, 1979, Zhang et al. 2008*]. Concurrent use of medicinal herbs and pharmaceutical drugs without any control of medical or dental professionals is also relatively common and the majority of herbal medicine users are not aware of potential adverse effects [*Zhang et al. 2008*]. Therefore, dentist should carefully collect information about the patients' medicinal herb related usage. Since dentists may exert significant influence on their patients' decisions about herbal medicine use, proper up-to-date knowledge related to medicinal herb therapy is highly important also for those dentists not preferring the use of medicinal herb therapy in their practice.

REFERENCES

[1] Adachi, N; Tomonaga, S; Tachibana, T; Denbow, DM; Furuse, M. (-)-Epigallocatechin gallate attenuates acute stress response through GABAergic system in the brain. *Eur J Pharmachol*, 2006 531, 1717-175.

[2] Akev, N; Turkay, G; Can, A; Gurel, A; Yildiz, F; Yardibi, H; Ekiz, EE; Uzun, H. Effect of Aloe vera leaf pulp extract on Ehrlich ascites tumors in mice. *Eur J Cancer Prev*, 2007 16, 151-157.

[3] Alekel, DL; Germain, AS; Peterson, CT; Hanson, KB; Stewart JW; Toda T. Isoflavone-rich soy protein isolate attenuates bone loss in the lumbar spine of perimenopausal women. *Am J Clin Nutr*, 2000 72, 844-852.

[4] Anderson, JW; Johnstone, BM; Cook-Newell, ME. Meta- analysis of the effects of soy protein intake on serum lipids. *N Engl J Med*, 1995 333, 276-282.

[5] Arjmani, BH; Khalil, DA; Lucas, EA; Georgis, A; Stoecker, BJ; Hardin, C; Payton, ME; Wild, RA. Dried plums improve indices of bone formation in postmenopausal women. *J Women's Health Gend-Based Med*, 2002 11, 61-68.

[6] Arjmani, BH; Lucas, EA; Khalil, DA; Devareddy, L; Smith, BJ; McDonald, J; Arquitt, AB; Payton, ME; Mason, C. One-year soy protein supplementation has positive effects on bone formation markers but not bone density in postmenopausal women. *Nutr J*, 2005 4, 8.

[7] Arnault, I. & Auger, J. Seleno-compounds in garlic and onion. *J Chromatography A*, 2006 1112, 23-30.

[8] Atkinson, C; Compston, JE; Day, NE; Dowsett, M; Bingham, SA. The effects of phytoestrogen isoflavones on bone density in women: a double-blind, randomized, placebo-controlled trial. *Am J Clin Nutr*, 2004 79, 326-333.

[9] Avraham, Y; Hao, S; Mendelson, S; Berry, F. Tyrosine improve appetite, cognition, and exercise tolerance in activity anorexia. *Med Sci Sprot Exerc*, 2001 33, 2104-2110.

[10] Bentler, SE; Hartz, AJ; Kuhn, EM. Prospective observational study of treatments for unexplained chronic fatigue. *J Clin Psychiatry*, 2005 66, 625-631.

[11] Benton, D. Selenium intake, mood and other aspects of psychological functioning. *Nutr Neurosci*, 2002/a 5, 363-374.

[12] Benton D. Carbohydrate ingestion, blood glucose and mood. *Neurosci Behav Rev*, 2002/b 26, 293-308.

[13] Benton, D. & Donohoe, RT. The effects of nutrients on mood. *Public Health Nutr*, 1999 2, 403-409.

[14] Bezerra, JP; da Silva, LRF; de Alvarenga Lemos; VA; Duarte, PM; Bastos, MF. Administration of high doses of caffeine increases alveolar bone loss in ligature-induced periodontitis in rats. *J Periodontol*, 2008 79, 2356-2360.

[15] Bhat, KPL; Kosmeder, JW 2nd; Pezzuto, JM. Biological effects of resveratrol. *Antioxid Redox Signal*, 2001 3, 1041-1064.

[16] Borges-Yañez, SA; Maupomé, G; Martinez-Gonzalez, M; Cervantez-Turrubiante, L; Guitérrez-Robledo, LM. Dietary fiber intake and dental health status in urban-marginal, and rural communities in central Mexico. *J Nutr Health Aging*, 2004 8, 333-339.

[17] Bottenberg, MM; Wall, GC; Harvey, RL; Habib, S. Oral aloe vera-induced hepatitis. *Ann Pharmacoter*, 2007 41, 1740-1743.

[18] Bouhnik, Y; Vahedi, K; Achour, L; Attar, A; Salfati, J; Pochart, P; Marteau, P; Flourie B; Bornet, F; Rambaud, JC. Short-chain fructo-oligosaccharide administration dose-dependently increases fecal bifidobacteria in healthy humans. *J Nutr*, 1999 129, 113-116.

[19] Bourre, JM. Effects of nutrients (in food) on the structure and function of the nervous system: update on dietary requirements for brain. Part 1: Micronutrients. *J Nutr Health Aging*, 2006/a 10, 377-385.

[20] Bourre, JM. Effects of nutrients (in food) on the structure and function of the nervous system: update on dietary requirements for brain. Part 2: Macronutrients. *J Nutr Health Aging*, 2006/b 10, 386-399.

[21] Briggs, WH; Folts, JD; Osman, HE; Goldman, IL. Administration of raw onion inhibits platelet-mediated thrombosis in dogs. *J Nutr*, 2001 131, 2619-2622.

[22] Bryan, J. Psychlogical effects of dietary components of tea: caffeine and L-theanine. *Nutr Rev*, 2008 66, 82-90.

[23] Brodeur, JM; Laurin, D; Vallee, R; Lachapelle, D. Nutrient intake and gastrointestinal disorders related to masticatory performance in the edentulous elderly. *J Prosthet Dent*, 1993 70, 468-473.

[24] Brown, D. The use of Vitex agnus castus for hyperprolactinemia. *Quarterly Rev Nat Med*, 1997 (SPRING), 19-21.

[25] Brown, D. Link between iron and youth cognitive skills? *J Am Diet Assoc*, 2001 101, 1308-1309.

[26] Bruinsma, K. & Taren, DL. Chocolate: Food or drug? *J Am Diet Assoc*, 1999 99, 1249-1256.

[27] Bu, SY; Lucas, EA; Franklin, M; Marlow, D; Brackett, DJ; Boldrin, EA; Devareddy, L; Arjmani, BH; Smith, BJ. Comparison of dried plum supplementation and intermittent PTH in restoring bone in osteopenic orchidectomized rats. *Osteoporos Int*, 2007 18, 931-942.

[28] Bu, SY; Lerner, M; Stoecker, BJ; Boldrin, E; Brackett, DJ; Lucas, EA; Smith, BJ. Dried plum polyphenols inhibit osteoclastogenesis by downregulating NFATc1 and inflammatory mediators. *Calcif Tissue Int*, in press; DOI: 10.1007/s00223-008-9139-0

[29] Budtz-Jørgensen, E; Chung, JP; Rapin, CH. Nutrition and oral health. *Best Practice & Research Clinical Gastroenterology*, 2001 15, 885-896.

[30] Burdette, JE; Liu, J; Chen, SN; Fabricants, DS; Piersen, CE; Barker, EL; Pezzuto, JM; Mesecar, A; Van Breemen, RB; Farnsworth, NR; Bolton, JL. Black cohosh acts as a mixed competitive ligand and partial agonist of the serotonin receptor. *J Agric Food Chem*, 2003 51, 5661-5670.

[31] Caimi, G; Carollo, C; Lo Presti, R. Wine and endothelial function. *Drugs Exp Clin Res*, 2003 29, 235-242.

[32] Campbell, JM; Fahey Jr., GC; Wolf, BF. Selected indigestible oligosaccharides affect large bowel mass, cecal and fecal short-chain fatty acids, pH and microflora in rats. *J Nutr*, 1997 127, 130-136.

[33] Carlson, S; Peng, N; Prasain, JK; Wyss, JM; Effects of botanical dietary supplements on cardiovascular, cognitive, and metabolic function in males and females. *Gender Med*, 2008 5 (Suppl.A), S76-S90.

[34] Chandan, BK; Saxena, AK; Shukla, S; Sharma, N; Gupta, DK; Suri, KA; Suri, J; Bhadauria, M; Singh, B. Hepatoprotective potential of *Aloe barbadensis* Mill. against carbon terachloride induced hepatotoxicity. *J Ethnopharmacology*, 2007 111, 560-566.

[35] Chen, JR; Singhal, R; Lazarenko, OP; Liu, X; Hogue, WR; Badger, TM; Ronis, MJJ. Short term effects on bone quality associated with consumption of soy protein isolate and other dietary protein sources in rapidly growing female rats. *Exp Biol Med*, 2008 233, 1348-1358.

[36] Chi, YS; Cheon, BS; Kim, HP. Effect of wogonin, a plant flavone from Scutellaria radix, on the supression of cyclooxygenase-2, and the induction of inducible nitric oxide synthase in lipopolysaccharide-treated RAW 264.7 cells. *Biochem Pharmacol*, 2001 61, 1195-1203.

[37] Choonhakarn, C; Busaracome, P; Sripanidkulchai, B; Sarakarn, P. The efficacy of aloe vera gel in the treatment of oral lichen planus: a randomized controlled trial. *Brit J Dermatol*, 2008 158, 573-577.

[38] Chow, J. Probiotics and prebiotics: A brief overview. *J Ren Nutr*, 2002 12, 76-86.

[39] Clifton-Bligh, PB; Baber, RJ; Fulcher, GR; Nery, ML; Moreton, T. The effect of isoflavones extracted from red clover (Rimostil) on lipid and bone metabolism. *Menopause*, 2001 8, 259-265.

[40] Cooke, PS; Selvaraj, V; Yellayi, S. Genistein, estrogen receptors, and the acquired immune response. *J Nutr*, 2006 136, 704-708.

[41] Curciarello, J; De Ortúzar, S; Borzi, S; Bosia, D. Severe acute hepatitis associated with intake of Aloe vera tea. *Gastroenterol Hepatol*, 2008 31, 436-438.

[42] Daniele, C; Coon, JT; Pittler, MH; Ernst, E. Vitex agnus castus: A systematic review of adverse events. *Drug Safety*, 2005 28, 319-332.

[43] Das, S. & Das, DK. Anti-inflammatory responses of resveratrol. *Inflamm Allergy Drug Targets*, 2007 6, 168-173.

[44] Davidson, JR; Abraham, K; Connor, KM; McLeod, MN. Effectiveness of chromium in atypical depression: a placebo-controlled trial. *Biol Psychiatry*, 2003 53, 261-264.

[45] Desor, JA; Maller, O; Green, LS. Preferences for sweet in humans: infants, children, and adoults. In: Weiffenbach J, editor. *Taste and development. The genesis of sweet preference.* Washington DC: US Dept of Health Education and Welfare; 1977; Publication No: NIH 77-1068.

[46] Devareddy, L; Khalil, DA; Korlagunta, K; Hooshmand, S; Bellmer, DD; Arjmandi, BH. The effects of fructo-oligosaccharides in combination with soy protein on bone in osteopenic ovariectomized rats. *Menopause*, 2006 13, 692-699.

[47] Deyhim, F; Stoecker, BJ; Brusewitz, GH; Devareddy, L; Arjmani, BH. Dried plum reverses bone loss in an osteopenic rat model of osteoporosis. *Menopause*, 2005 12, 755-762.

[48] DiTomaso, E; Beltramo, M; Piomelli, D. Brain cannabinoids in chocolate. *Nature*, 1996 382, 677-678.

[49] Drewnowski, A. Why do we like fat? *J Am Diet Assoc*, 1997 97, S58-62

[50] Drewnowski, A. & Greenwood, MRC. Cream and sugar: human preferences for high-fat foods. *Physiol Behav*, 1983 30, 629-633.

[51] Drewnowski, A; Gossnell, B; Krahn, DD; Canum, K. Sensory preferences for sugar and fat: evidence for opioid involvement. *Appetite*, 1989 12, 206.

[52] Dum, J; Gramsch CH; Herz, A. Activation of hypothalamic beta-endorphin pools by reward induced by highly palatable food. *Pharmachol Biochem Behav*, 1983 18, 443-447.

[53] Dutta, A; Bandyopadhyay, S; Mandal, C; Chatterjee, M. *Aloe vera* leaf exsudate induces a caspase-independent cell death in *Leishmania donovani* promastigotes. *J Med Microbiol*, 2007 56, 629-636.

[54] Dutta, A; Sarkar, D; Gurib-Fakim, A. In vitro and in vivo activity of *Aloe vera* leaf exsudate in experimental visceral leishmaniasis. *Parasitol Res*, 2008 102, 1235-1242.

[55] Elnima, EI; Ahmed, SA; Mekkawi, AG; Mossa, JS. The antimicrobial activity of garlic and onion extracts. *Pharmazie*, 1983 38, 747-748.

[56] Emara, AM. & El-Bahrawy, H. Green tea attenuates benzene-induced oxidative stress in pump workers. *J Immunotoxicol*, 2008 5, 69-80.

[57] Fábián, T. & Fejérdy, P. The effect of low-protein diet on hard dental tissues in rats. *Fogorv Szle*, 1975 68, 113-115.

[58] Fábián, T; Szelényi, T; Zelles, T., Fejérdy P. Influence of dietary protein intake on the incisors of rats. *Acta Medica Academiae Scientiarum Hungaricae*, 1972 29, 339-345.

[59] Fábián, T; Fejérdy, P; Zelles, T. The effect of low protein diet on the calcium content and solubility of dental hard tissues in the molars of rats at different ages. *Fogorv Szle*, 1975 68, 161-163.

[60] Fábián, T; Bidló, G; Fejérdy, P. Roentgen diffraction study of hard dental tissue in white rats kept on low-protein diet. *Fogorv Szle*, 1979 72, 175-178.

[61] Firk, C. & Markus, R. Effects of acute tryptophan depletion on affective processing in first-degree relatives of depressive patients and controls after exposure to uncontrollable stress. *Psychopharmacology*, 2008 199, 151-160.

[62] Foth, D. & Cline, JM. effects of mammalian and plant estrogens on mammary glands and uteri of macaques. *Am J Clin Nutr Dec*, 1998 68, 1413S-1417S.

[63] Franklin, M; Bu, SY; Lerner, MR; Lancaster, EA; Bellmer, D; Marlow, D; Lightfoot, SA; Arjmani, BH; Brackett, DJ; Lucas, EA; Smith, BJ. Dried plum prevents bone loss in a male osteoporosis model via IGF-I and the RANK pathway. *Bone*, 2006 39, 1331-1342.

[64] Fuchs, D; Vafeidou, K; Hall, WL; Daniel, H; Williams, CM; Schroot, JH; Wenzel, U. Proteomic biomarkers of peripheral blood mononuclear cells obtained from postmenopausal women undergoing an intervention with soy isoflavones. *Am J Clin Nutr*, 2007 86, 1369-1375.

[65] Gardner, EJ; Ruxton, CHS; Leeds, AR. Black tea - helpful or harmful? A review of the evidence. *European J Clin Nutr*, 2007 61, 3-18.

[66] Geller, SE. & Studee, L. Botanical and dietary supplements for menopausal symptoms: What works, what doesn't. *J Womens Health (Larchmt)*, 2005 14, 634-649.

[67] Gessner, B; Voelp, A; Klasser, M. Study of the long-term action of a Ginkgo biloba extract on vigilance and mental performance as determined by means of quantitative pharmaco-EEG and psychometric measurements. *Arzneimittelforschung*, 1985 35, 1459-1464.

[68] Ginsburg, I; Vennos, C; Koren, E. Inflammaging - Altern als Konsequenz chronischer Entzündungen: Das Beispiel Padma 28. *Schweiz Zschr GanzheitsMedizin*, 2008 20, 412-417.

[69] Grabitske, HA. & Slavin, JL. Low-digestible carbohydrates in practice. *J AM Diet Assoc*, 2008 108, 1677-1681.

[70] Grassi, D; Necozione, S; Lippi, C; Croce, G; Valeri, L; Pasqualetti, P; Desideri, G; Blumberg, JB; Ferri, C. Cocoa reduces blood pressure and insulin resistance and improves endothelium-dependent vasodilatation in hypertensives. *Hypertension*, 2005 46, 398-405.

[71] Griffiths, G; Trueman, L; Crowther, T; Thomas, B; Smith, B. Onions -- a global benefith to healt. *Phytother Res*, 2002 16, 603-615.

[72] Groppo, FC; Ramacciato, JC; Motta, RH; Ferraresi, PM; Sartoratto, A. Antimicrobial activity of garlic against oral streptococci. *Int J Dent Hyg*, 2007 5, 109-115.

[73] Grube, B; Walper, A; Wheatley, D. St John's wort extract: efficacy for menopausal symptoms of psyhological origin. *Adv Ther*, 1999 16; 177-186.

[74] Habeeb, F; Shakir, E; Bradbury, F; Cameron, P; Taravati, MR; Drummond, AJ; Gray, AI; Ferro, VA. Screening methods used to determine the anti-microbial properties of Aloe vera inner gel. *Methods*, 2007/a 42, 315-320.

[75] Habeeb, F; Stables, G; Bradbury, F; Nong, S; Cameron, P; Plevin, R; Ferro, VA. The inner gel component of Aloe vera suppresses bacterial-induced pro-inflammatory cytokines from human immune cells. *Methods*, 2007/b 42, 388-393.

[76] Haider, S; Naz, N; Khaliq, S; Perveen, T; Haleem, DJ. Repeated administration of fresh garlic increases memory retention in rats. *J Med Food*, 2008 11, 675-679.

[77] Hidaka, H; Hirayama, M; Sumi, N. A fructooligosaccharide-producing enzyme from *Aspergillus niger* ATCC 20611. *Agric Biol Chem*, 1988 52, 1181-1187.

[78] Higdon, JV. & Frei, B. Coffee and health: A review of recent human research. *Crit Rev Food Sci Res*, 2006 46, 101-123.

[79] Hikada, H; Tashiro, T; Eida, T. Proliferation of bifidobacteria by oligosaccharides and their useful effect on human health. *Bifidobacteria Microflora*, 1991 10, 65-79.

[80] Hofferberth, B. The effect of Ginko biloba extract on neurophysiological and psychometric measurement results in patients with psychotic organic brain syndrome. A double-blind study against placebo. *Arzneimittelforschung*, 1989 39, 918-922.

[81] Hogervorst, E; Sadjimim, T; Yesufu, A; Kreager, P; Rahardjo, TB. High tofu intake is associated with worse memory in elderly Indonesian Men and Women. *Dement Geriatr Cogn Disord*, 2008 26, 50-57.

[82] Hostettmann, K. & Wolfender, JL. Phytochemistry. In: Müller WE, editor. *St. John's worth and its active principles in depression and anxiety*. Basel-Boston-Berlin: Birkhäuser Verlag; 2005; 5-20.

[83] Johnson, CD; Lucas, EA; Hooshmand, S; Campbell, S; Akhter, MP; Arjmandi, BH. Addition of fructooligosaccharides and dried plum to soy-based diets reverse bone loss in the ovarectomized rat. *eCAM*, in press. DOI: 10.1093/ecam/nen050

[84] Kakuda, T. Neuroprotective effects of green tea components theanine and catechins. *Biol Pharm Bull*, 2002 25, 1513-1518.

[85] Kayano, S; Kikuzaki, H; Ikami, T; Suzuki, T; Mitani, T; Nakatani, N. A new bipyrrole and some phenolic constituents in prunes (*Prunus Domestica* L.) and their oxygen radical absorbance capacity (ORAC) *Biosci Biotechnol Biochem*, 2004 68, 942-944.

[86] Kerckhoffs, DAJM; Brouns, F; Hornstra, G; Mensink, RP. Effects on the human serum lipoprotein profile of β-Glucan, soy protein and isoflavones, plant sterols and stanols, garlic and tocotrienols. *J Nutr*, 2002 132, 2494-2505.

[87]   Kidd, PM. Omega-3 DHA and EPA for cognition, behavioral, and mood: clinical findings and structural-functional synergies with cell membrane phospholids. *Altern Med Rev*, 2007 12, 207-227.

[88]   Kim, HR; Rajaiah, R; Wu, QL; Satpute, SR; Tan, MT; Simon, JE; Berman, BM; Moudgil, KD. Green tea protects rats against autoimmune arthritis by modulating disease-related immune events. *J Nutr*, 2008 138, 2111-2116.

[89]   Kleinen, J. & Knipschild, P. Ginkgo biloba. *Lancet*, 1992 340, 1136-1139.

[90]   Knight, DC; Howes, JB; Eden, JA. The effect of Promensil, an isoflavone extract, on menopausal symptoms. *Climacteric*, 1999 2, 79-84.

[91]   Koren, E; Kohen, R., Ginsburg, I. A cobalt-based tetrazolium salts reduction test to assay polyphenols. *J Agric Food Chem*, in press/a. DOI: 10.1021/jf9006449

[92]   Koren, E; Kohen, R; Ovadia, H; Ginsburg, I. Bacteria coated by polyphenols acquire potent oxidant-scaveging capacities. *Exp Biol Med*, in press/b. DOI: 10.3181/0901-RM-22

[93]   Köhler, T. Fortbildung: Psychopharmakotherapie (2. Teil). *Verhaltenstherapie & Verhaltensmedizin*, 2005 26, 141-168.

[94]   Krall, E; Hayes, C; Garcia, R. How dentition status and masticatory function affect nutrient intake. *JADA*, 1998 129, 1261-1269.

[95]   Kritz-Silverstein, D; Von Muhlen, D; Barrett-Connor, E; Bressel, MA. Isoflavones and cognitive function in older women: the Soy and Postmenopausal Health in Aging (SOPHIA) Study. *Menopause*, 2003 10, 196-202.

[96]   Kuiper, GG; Lemmen, JG; Carlsson, B; Corton, JC; Safe, HS; van der Saag, PT, van der Burg, B; Gustafsson, JA. Interaction of estrogenic chemicals and phytoestrogens with estrogen receptor beta. *Endocrinology*, 1998 139, 4252-4263.

[97]   Kwok, T; Yu, CN; Hui, HW; Kwan, M; Chan, V. Association between functional dental state and dietary intake of Chinese vegetarian old age home residents. *Gerodontology*, 2004 21, 161-166.

[98]   Kyo, E; Uda, N; Ushijima, M; Kasuga, S; Itakura, Y. Prevention of psychological stress-induced immune supression by aged garlic extracts. *Phytomedicine*, 1999 6, 325-330.

[99]   Kyo, E; Uda, N; Kasuga, S; Itakura, Y. Immunomodulatory effects of aged garlic extracts. *J Nutr*, 2001 131, 1075S-1079S.

[100]   Laurin, D; Brodeur, JM; Bourdages, J; Vallée, R; Lachapelle, D. Fibre intake in elderly individuals with poor masticatory performance. *J Can Dent Assoc*, 1994 60, 443-446, 449.

[101]   Lee, H; Kim, YO; Kim, H; Kim, SY; Noh, HS; Kang, SS; Cho, GJ; Choi, WS; Suk, K. Flavonoid wogonin from medicinal herb is neuroprotective by inhibiting inflammatory activation of microglia. *FASEB J*, 2003 17, 1943-1944.

[102]   Leifert, WR. & Abeywardena, MY. Cardioprotective actions of grape polyphenols. *Nutr Res*, 2008 28, 729-737.

[103]   Levenson, CW. Zinc: the new antidepressant? *Nutr Rev*, 2006 64, 39-42.

[104]   Lin, PY. & Su, KP. A meta-analytic review of double-blind, placebo-controlled trials of antidepressant efficacy of omega-3 fatty acids. *J Clin Psychiatry*, 2007 68, 1056-1061.

[105]   Linde, K; Ramirez, G; Mulrow, CD; Pauls, A; Weidenhammer, W; Melchart, D. St John's wort for depression -- an overview and meta-analysis of randomized clinical trials. *Brit Med J*, 1996 313, 253-258.

[106] Linde, K; Ramirez, G; Mulrow, CD; Pauls, A; Weidenhammer, W; Melchart, D. St John's wort for depression: meta-analysis of randomized controlled trials. *Brit J Psychiatry*, 2005 186, 99-107.

[107] Liske, E. Therapeutic efficacy and safety of Cimifuga racemosa for gynecologic disorders. *Adv Ther*, 1998 15, 45-53.

[108] Lopez-Garcia, E; van Dam, RM; Li, TY; Rodriguez-Artalejo, F; Hu, FB. The relationship of coffee consumption with mortality. *Ann Intern Med*, 2008 148, 904-914.

[109] Low, CF; Chong, PP; Yong, PVC; Lim, CSY; Ahmad, Z; Othman, F. Inhibition of hyphae formation and *SIR2* expression in *Candida albicans* treated with fresh *Allium sativum* (garlic) extract. *J Appl Microbiol*, 2008 105, 2169-2177.

[110] Low Dog, T. Menopause: a review of botanical dietary supplements. *Am J Med*, 2005 118, 98S-108S.

[111] Lucks, BC. Vitex agnus castus essential oil and menopausal balance: a research update. *Compl Ther Nurs Midwifery*, 2003 9, 157-160.

[112] Lucas, M; Asselin, G; Mérette, C; Poulin, MJ; Dodin, S. Ethyl-eicosapentaenoic acid for the treatment of psychological distress and depressive symptoms in middle-aged women: a double-blind, placebo-controlled randomized clinical trial. *Am J Clin Nutr*, 2009 89, 641-651.

[113] Macht, M. & Mueller, J. Immediate effects of chocolate on experimentally induced mood states. *Appetite*, 2007 49, 667-674.

[114] Maeda-Yamamoto, M; Ema, K; Shibuichi, I. In vitro and in vivo anti-allergic effects of "benifuuki" green tea containing *O*-methylated catechin and ginger extract. *Cytotechnology*, 2007 55, 135-142.

[115] Mao, TK; Van De Water, J; Keen, CL; Schmitz, HH; Gershwin, ME. Cocoa flavonols and procyanidins promote transforming growth factor-ß₁ homeostasis in peripheral blood mononuclear cells. *Exp Biol Med*, 2003 228, 93-99.

[116] Marcellini, F; Giuli, C; Papa, R; Gagliardi, C; Dedoussis, G; Monti, D; Jajte, J; Giacconi, R; Malavolta, M; Mocchegiani, E. Zinc in elderly people: effects of zinc supplementation on psychological dimensions in dependence of IL-6-174 polymorphysm: a Zinkage study. *Rejuvenation Res*, 2008 11, 479-483.

[117] Martin Jr., DW. Fat-soluble vitamins. In: Martin DW, Mayes PA, Rodwell VW, Granner DK editors. *Harper's review of biochemistry*. Twentieth edition. Los Altos, California: Lange Medical Publications; 1985/a; 118-127.

[118] Martin Jr., DW. Water-soluble vitamins. In: Martin DW, Mayes PA, Rodwell VW, Granner DK editors. *Harper's review of biochemistry*. Twentieth edition. Los Altos, California: Lange Medical Publications; 1985/b; 101-117.

[119] Martin Jr., DW. Water & minerals. In: Martin DW, Mayes PA, Rodwell VW, Granner DK editors. *Harper's review of biochemistry*. Twentieth edition. Los Altos, California: Lange Medical Publications; 1985/c; 649-660.

[120] Martín, MÁ; Serrano, ABG; Ramos, S; Pulido, MI; Bravo, L; Goya, L. Cocoa flavonoids up-regulate antioxidant enzyme activity via the ERK1/2 pathway to protect against oxidative stress-induced apoptosis in HepG2 cells. *J Nutr Biochem*, in press. DOI: 10.1016/j.jnutbio.2008.10.009

[121] Mathey, J; Puel, C; Kati-Coulibaly, S; Bennetau-Pelissero, C; Davicco, MJ; Lebecque P; Horcajada, MN; Coxam, V. Fructooligosaccharides maximize bone-sparing effects

of soy isoflavone-enriched diet in the ovarectomized rat. *Calcif Tissue Int*, 2004 75, 169-179.

[122] Mayes, PA. Carbohydrates. In: Martin DW, Mayes PA, Rodwell VW, Granner DK editors. *Harper's review of biochemistry*. Twentieth edition. Los Altos, California: Lange Medical Publications; 1985/a; 147-157.

[123] Mayes, PA. Lipids. In: Martin DW, Mayes PA, Rodwell VW, Granner DK editors. *Harper's review of biochemistry*. Twentieth edition. Los Altos, California: Lange Medical Publications; 1985/b; 194-207.

[124] Mayes, PA. Metabolism of lipids: I. Fatty acids. In: Martin DW, Mayes PA, Rodwell VW, Granner DK editors. *Harper's review of biochemistry*. Twentieth edition. Los Altos, California: Lange Medical Publications; 1985/c; 208-231.

[125] Mayes, PA. Metabolism of carbohydrate. In: Martin DW, Mayes PA, Rodwell VW, Granner DK editors. *Harper's review of biochemistry*. Twentieth edition. Los Altos, California: Lange Medical Publications; 1985/d; 166-193.

[126] McGuinnes, EE; Morgan, RGH; Levison, DA; Frape, DL; Hopwood, D; Wormsley, KG. The effects of long-term feeding of soya flour on the rat pancreas. *Scand J Gastroenterol*, 1980 15, 497-502.

[127] McGuinnes, EE; Morgan, RGH; Levison, DA; Hopwood, D; Wormsley, KG. Interaction of azaserine and raw soya flour on the rat pancreas. *Scand J Gastroenterol*, 1981 16, 49-56.

[128] McGuinnes, EE & Wormsley, KG. Effects of feeding partial and intermittent raw soya flour diets on the rat pancreas. *Cancer Letters*, 1986 32, 73-81.

[129] McKay, DL. & Blumberg, JB. The role of tea in human health: An update. *J Am Coll Nutr*, 2002 21, 1-13.

[130] McShea, A; Ramiro-Puig, E; Munro, SB; Casadesus, G; Castell, M; Smith, MA. Clinical benefit and preservation of flavonols in dark chocolate manufacturing. *Nutr Rev*, 2008 66, 630-641.

[131] Mei, J; Yeung, SS; Kung, AW. High dietary phytoestrogen intake is associated with higher bone mineral density in postmenopausal but not premenopausal women. *J Clin Endocrinol Metab*, 2001 86, 5217-5221.

[132] Melgarejo, E; Medina, MA; Sánches-Jiménez, F; Botana, LM; Domínguez, M; Escribano, L; Orfao, A; Urdiales, JL. (-)-Epigallocatechin-3-gallate interferes with mast cell adhesiveness, migration and its potential to recruit monocytes. *Cell Mol Life Sci*, 2007 64, 2690-2701.

[133] Miyake, Y; Sasaki, S; Ohya, Y; Miyamoto, S; Matsunaga, I; Yoshida, T; Hirota, Y; Oda, H. Soy, isoflavones, and prevalence of allergic rhinitis in Japanese women: the Osaka Maternal and Child Health Study. *J Allergy Clin Immunol*, 2005 115, 1176-1183.

[134] Monteiro, SC; de Mattos, CB; Ben, J; Netto, CA; Wyse, ATS. Ovariectomy impairs spatial memory: prevention and reversal by a soy isoflavone diet. *Metab Brain Dis*, 2008 23, 243-253.

[135] Moore, LB; Goodwin, B; Jones, SA; Wisely, GB; Serabjit-Singh, CJ; Willson, TM; Collins, JL; Kliewer, SA. St John's wort induced hepatic drug metabolism through activation of the pregnane X receptor. *Proc Natl Acad Sci USA*, 2000 97, 7500-7502.

[136] Morohashi, T; Sano, T; Ohta, A; Yamada, S. True calcium absorption in the intestine is enhanced by fructooligosaccharide feeding in rats. *J Nutr*, 1998 128, 1815-1818.

[137] Morohashi, T; Sano, T; Sakai, N; Yamada, S. Fructooligosaccharide consumption improves the decreased dentine formation and mandibular defects following gastrectomy in rats. *Oral Dis*, 2005 11, 360-364.

[138] Mulhauer, RC; Lozano, A; Reinli, A; Wetli, H. Various selected vegetables, fruits, mushrooms and red wine residue inhibit bone resorption in rats. *J Nutr*, 2003 133, 3592-3597.

[139] Nakatani, N; Kayano, S; Kikuzaki, H; Sumino, K; Katagiri, K; Mitani, T. Identification, quantitative determination, and antioxidative activities of chlorogenic acid isomers in prune (*Prunus Domestica* L.). *J Agric Food Chem*, 2000 48, 5512-5516.

[140] Naylor, AJD. Cellular effects of resveratrol in skeletal muscle. *Life Sciences*, in press. DOI: 10.1016/j.lfs.2009.02.011

[141] Nestle, M. Nutrition. In: Martin DW, Mayes PA, Rodwell VW, Granner DK editors. *Harper's review of biochemistry*. Twentieth edition. Los Altos, California: Lange Medical Publications; 1985; 661-680.

[142] New, SA; Robins, SP; Campbell, MK; Martin, JC; Garton, MJ; Bolton-Smith, C; Grubb, DA; Lee, SJ; Reid, DM. Dietaryinfluences on bone mass and bone metabolism: further evidence of a positive link between fruit and vegetable consumption and bone health? *Am J Clin Nutr*, 2000 71, 142-151.

[143] Nowjack-Raymer, RE. & Sheiham, A. Association of edentulism and diet and nutrition in US adults. *J Dent Res*, 2003 82, 123-126.

[144] Nowjack-Raymer, RE. & Sheiham, A. Numbers of natural teeth, diet, and nutritional status in US adults. *J Dent Res*, 2007 86, 1171-1175.

[145] Ohta, A. Prevention of osteoporosis by foods and dietary supplements. The effect of fructooligosaccharides (FOS) on the calcium absorption and bone. *Clin Calcium*, 2006 16, 1639-1645.

[146] Ohta, A; Ohtsuki, M; Baba, S; Adachi, T; Sakata, T; Sakaguchi, E. Calcium and magnesium absorption from the colon and rectum are increased in rats fed fructooligosaccharides. *J Nutr*, 1995 125, 2417-2424.

[147] Ohta, A; Ohtsuki, M; Uehara, M; Hosono, S; Hirayama, M; Adachi, T; Hara, H. Dietary fructooligosaccharides prevent postgastrectomy anemia and osteopenia in rats. *J Nutr*, 1998 128, 485-490.

[148] Owens, DS; Parker, PY; Benton, D. Blood glucose and subjective energy following demanding cognitive tasks. *Physiol Behav*, 1997 62, 471-478.

[149] Palmer, CA. Gerodontic nutrition and dietary counseling for prosthodontic patients. *Dent Clin North Am*, 2003 47, 355-371.

[150] Pandey, R. & Mishra, A. Antibacterial activities of crude extract of *Aloe barbadensis* to clinically isolated bacterial pathogens. *Appl Biochem Biotechnol*, in press, DOI: 10.1007/s12010-009-8577-0

[151] Papamichael, K. & Tiligada, E. Heat shock proteins in adaptive and protective physiology and pathophysiology of the gastrointestinal mucosa. In: Morel E, Vincent C editors. *Heat shock proteins: New research*. New York: Nova Science Publishers, Inc.; 2008; 299-319.

[152] Parker, G; Parker, I; Brotchie, H. Mood state effects of chocolate. *J Affective Dis*, 2006 92, 149-159.

[153] Peet, M. & Stokes, C. Omega-3 fatty acids in the treatment of psychiatric disorders. *Drugs*, 2005 65, 1051-1059.

[154] Peeters, E; Neyt, A; Beckers, F; De Smet, S; Aubert, AE; Geers, R. Influence of supplemental magnesium, tryptophan, vitamin C, and vitamin E on stress responses of pigs to vibration. *J Anim Sci*, 2005 83, 1568-1580.

[155] Pereira, IRO. & Abdalla, DSP. Soy isoflavones reduce heat shock proteins in experimental atherosclerosis. *Eur J Nutr*, 2006 45, 178-186.

[156] Petti, S; Cairella, G; Tarsitani, G. Nutritional variables related to gingival health in adolescent girls. *Community Dent Oral Epidemiol*, 2000 28, 407-413.

[157] Pockaj, BA; Loprinzi, CL, Sloan, JA; Novotny, PJ; Barton, DL; Hagenmaier, A; Zhang, H; Lambert, GH; Reeser, KA; Wisbey, JA. Pilot evaluation of black cohosh for the treatment of hot flashes in women. *Cancer Invest*, 2004 22, 515-521.

[158] Poleszak, E; Wlaź, P; Szewczyk, B; Kędzierska, E; Wyska, E; Librowski, T; Szymura-Oleksiak, J; Fidecka, S; Pilz, A; Nowak, G. Enhancement of antidepressant-like activity by joint administration of imipramine and magnesium in the forced swim test: Behavioral and pharmacokinetic studies in mice. *Pharmachol Biochem Behav*, 2005 81, 524-529.

[159] Potter, SM; Baum, JA; Teng, H; Stillman, RJ; Shay, NF; Erdman, JW. Soy proteins and isoflavones: their effects on blood lipids and bone density in postmenopausal women. *Am J Clin Nutr*, 1998 68, 1375S-1379S.

[160] Putics, A; Végh, EM; Csermely, P; Sőti, Cs. Resveratrol induces the heat-shock response and protects human cells from severe heat stress. *Antioxid Redox Signal*, 2008/a 10, 65-75.

[161] Putics, Á; Vödrös, D; Malavolta, M; Mocchegiani, E; Csermely, P; Sőti, Cs. Zinc supplementation boots the stress response in the elderly: Hsp70 status is linked to zinc availability in peripheral lymphocytes. *Exp Gerontol*, 2008/b 43, 452-461.

[162] Raphael, KG; Marbach, JJ; Touger-Decker, R. Dietary fiber intake in patients with myofascial face pain. *J Orofac Pain*, 2002 16, 39-47.

[163] Rapuri, PB; Gallagher, JC; Kinyamu, HK; Ryschon, KL. Caffeine intake increases the rate of bone loss in elderly women and interacts with vitamin D receptor genotypes. *Am J Clin Nutr*, 2001 74, 694-700.

[164] Raschka, L. & Daniel, H. Mechanisms underlying the effects of inuline-type fructans on calcium absorption in the large intestine of rats. *Bone*, 2005 37, 728-735.

[165] Reuter, J; Jocher, A; Stump, J; Grossjohann, B; Franke, G; Schempp, CM. Investigation of the anti-inflammatory potential of Aloe vera gel (97,5%) in the ultraviolet erythema test. *Skin Pharmacol Physiol*, 2008 21, 106-110.

[166] Rhodus, NL. & Brown, J. The association of xerostomia and inadequate intake in older adults. *J Am Diet Assoc*, 1990 90, 1688-1692.

[167] Robelin, M. & Rogers, PJ. Mood and psychomotor performance effects of the first, but not of subsequent, cup-of-coffee equivalent doses of caffeine consumed after overnight caffeine abstinence. *Behav Pharmacol*, 1998 9, 611-618.

[168] Rosca-Casian, O; Parvu, M; Vlase, L; Tamas, M. Antifungal activity of *Aloe vera* leaves. *Fitoterapia*, 2007 78, 219-222.

[169] Ross, BM; Seguin, J; Sieswerda, LE. Omega-3 fatty acids as treatments for mental illness: which disorder and which fatty acid? *Lipids in Health and Disease*, 2007 6, 21.

[170] Rubin, MG; Kim, K; Logan, AC. Acne vulgaris, mental health and omega-3 fatty acids: a report of cases. *Lipids in Health and Disease*, 2008 7, 36.

[171] Ruddock, PS; Liao, M; Foster, BC; Lawson, L; Arnason, JT; Dillon, JA. Garlic natural health products exhibit variable constituent levels and antimicrobial activity against Neisseria gonorrhoeae, Staphilococcus aureus and Enterococcus faecalis. *Phytoter Res*, 2005 19, 327-334.

[172] Sakamoto, S; Hayashi, T; Hayashi, K; Murai, F; Hori, M; Kimoto, K; Murakami, K. Pre-germinated brown rice could enhance maternal mental health and immunity during lactation. *Eur J Nutr*, 2007 46, 391-396.

[173] Sato, TP. & Mikami, K. Recovery of a patient with a recurrent dysgeusia monitored by salivary variables and serum zinc content. *Pathophysiology*, 2002 8, 275-281.

[174] Sato, TP. & Mikami, K. Retrospective investigation on management of salivary hypofunction concerning with serum zinc content. *Pathophysiology*, 2003 9, 75-80.

[175] Scholz-Ahrens, KE; Schaafsma, G; van den Heuvel, EGHM; Schrezenmeier, J. Effects of prebiotics on mineral metabolism. *Am J Clin Nutr*, 2001 73 (suppl), 459S-464S.

[176] Segelman, AB; Segelman, FP; Karliner, J; Sofia, D. Sassafras and herb tea. Potential health hazards. *JAMA*, 1976 236, 477.

[177] Selmi, C; Mao, TK; Keen, CL; Schmitz, HH; Gershwin, ME. The anti-inflammatory properties of cocoa flavanols. *J Cardiovasc Pharmacol*, 2006 47 (suppl.2), S163-S171.

[178] Selmi, C; Cocchi, CA; Lanfredini, M; Keen, CL; Gershwin, ME. Chocolate at heart: the anti-inflammatory impact of cocoa flavonols. *Mol Nutr Food Res*, 2008 52, 1340-1348.

[179] Shen, SC; Lee, WR; Lin, HY; Huang, HC; Ko, CH; Yang, LL; Chen, YC. *In vitro* and *in vivo* inhibitory activities of rutin, wogonin, and quercetin on lipopolysacharide-induced nitric oxide and prostaglandin E2 production. *Eur J Pharmachol*, 2002 446, 187-194.

[180] Shim, JH; Choi, HS; Pugliese, A; Lee, SY; Chae, JI; Choi, BY; Bode, AM; Dong, Z. (-)-Epigallocatechin gallate regulates CD3-mediated T cell receptor signaling in leukemia through the inhibition of ZAP-70 kinase. *J Biol Chem*, 2008 283, 28370-28379.

[181] Siegel, RK. Herbal intoxication. Psychoactive effects from herbal cigarettes, tea, and capsules. *JAMA*, 1976 236, 473-476.

[182] Siegel, RK. Ginseng abuse syndrome. Problems with the panacea. *JAMA*, 1979 241, 1614-1615.

[183] Smith, A. Effects of caffeine on human behavior. *Food Chem Toxicol*, 2002 40, 1243-1255.

[184] Smith, AP. Caffeine, cognitive failures and health in a non-working community sample. *Hum Psychopharmachol Clin Exp*, 2009 24, 29-34.

[185] Soini, H; Muurinen, S; Routasalo, P; Sandelin, E; Savikko, N; Suominen, M; Ainamo, A; Pitkala, KH. Oral and nutritional status -- Is the MNA a useful tool for dental clinics. *J Nutr Health Aging*, 2006 10, 495-499.

[186] Song, C. & Zhao, S. Omega-3 fatty acid eicosapentaenoic acid. A new treatment for psychiatric and neurodegenerative diseases: a review of clinical investigations. *Expert Opin Investig Drugs*, 2007 16, 1627-1638.

[187] Sreebny, LM. Sugar availability, sugar consumption and dental caries. *Com Dent Oral Epidemiol*, 1982 10, 1-7.

[188] Staudinger, JL; Ding, X; Lichti, K. Pregnane X receptor and natural products: Beyond drug-drug interactions. *Expert Opin Drug Metab Toxicol*, 2006 2, 847- 857.

[189] Stoicov, C; Saffari, R; Houghton, J. Green tea inhibits Helicobacter growth in vivo and in vitro. *Int J Antimicrob Agents*, in press.

[190] Subhan, Z. & Hindmarch, I. The psychopharmacological effects of Ginkgo biloba extract in normal healthy volunteers. *Int J Clin Pharmacol Res*, 1984 4, 89-93.

[191] Suzuki, K; Nomura, T; Sakurai, M; Sugihara, N; Yamanaka, S; Matsukubo, T. Relationship between number of present teeth and nutritional intake in institutionalized elderly. *Bull Tokyo Dent Coll*, 2005 46, 135-143.

[192] Szőke, E; Zelles, T; Boros, I; Fehér, E. Effects of raw soy diet on the parotid gland. *Acta Alimentaria*, in press, DOI: 10.1556/AAlim.2008.0037

[193] Tanaka, K; Sasaki, S; Murakami, K; Okubo, H; Takahashi, Y; Miyake, Y; Relationship between soy and isoflavone intake and periodontal disease: the Freshmen in Dietetic Courses Study II. *BMC Public Health*, 2008 8, 39.

[194] Tattelman, E. Health effects of garlic. *Am Fam Physician*, 2005 72, 103-106.

[195] Teede, HJ; Dalais, FS; McGrath, BP. Dietary soy containing phytoestrogens does not have detectable estrogenic effects on hepatic protein synthesis in postmenopausal women. *Am J Clin Nutr*, 2004 79, 396-401.

[196] Tode, T; Kikuchi, Y; Hirata, J; Kita, T; Nakata, H; Nagata, I. Effect of Korean red ginseng on psychological functions in patients with severe climacteric syndromes. *Int J Ginecol Obstet*, 1999 67, 169-174.

[197] Tóth Jr., P; Fejérdy, P; Zelles, T; Kóbor, A. The effect of selenium, fluoride and normal or protein deficient diet on the microhardness of the rat incisors and the breaking strength of femurs. *J Int Assoc Dent Child*, 1988 19, 36-40.

[198] Touger-Decker, R. Oral manifestations of nutrient deficiencies. *Mt Sinai J Med*, 1998 65, 355-361.

[199] Touger-Decker, R. Clinical and laboratory assessment of nutrition status in dental practice. *Dent Clin North Am*, 2003 47, 259-278.

[200] Touger-Decker, R; Mobley, CC; & American Dietetic Association; Position of the American Dietetic Association: oral health and nutrition. *J Am Diet Assoc*, 2007 107, 1418-1428.

[201] Unger, M. & Frank, A. Simultaneous determination of the inhibitory potency of herbal extracts on the activity of six major cytochrome P450 enzymes using liquid chromatography/mass spectrometry and automated online extraction. *Rapid Commun Mass Spectrom*, 2004 18, 2273-2281.

[202] Urgert, R. & Katan, MB. The cholesterol-raising factor from coffee beans. *Annu Rev Nutr*, 1997 17, 305-324.

[203] Urgert, R; van der Weg, G; Kosmeijer-Schuil, TG; van de Bovenkamp, P; Hovenier, R; Katan, MB. Levels of the cholesterol-elevating diterpenes cafestol and kahweol in various coffee brews. *J Agric Food Chem*, 1995 43, 2167-2172.

[204] Vaidya, V; Ingold, KU; Pratt, DA. Garlic: Source of the ultimate antioxidants - sulfenic acids. *Angew Chem Int Ed*, 2009 48, 157-160.

[205] Vignes, M; Maurice, T; Lante, F; Nedjar, M; Thethi, K; Guiramand, J; Recasens, M. Anxiolytic properties of green tea polyphenol (-)-epigallocatechin gallatae (EGCG). *Brain Res*, 2006 1110, 102-115.

[206] Vingtdeux, V; Dreses-Werringloer, U; Zhao, H; Davies, P; Marambaud, P. Therapeutic potential of resveratrol in Alzheimer's disease. *BMC Neuroscience*, 2008 9 (Suppl. 2.), S6.

[207] Volz, HP. Clinical efficacy of St. John's wort in psychiatric disorders other than depression. In: Müller WE, editor. *St. John's worth and its active principles in depression and anxiety*. Basel-Boston-Berlin: Birkhäuser Verlag; 2005; 133-143.

[208] Walzem, RL. Wine and health: state of proofs and research needs. *Inflammopharmacology*, 2008 16, 265-271.

[209] Wiklund, IK; Mattsson, LA; Lindgren, R; Limoni, C; Effects of a standardized ginseng extract on quality of life and physiological parameters in symptomatic postmenopausal women: a double-blind, placebo-controlled trial. (Swedish Alternative Medicine Group). *Int J Clin Pharmacol Res*, 1999 19, 89-99.

[210] Woda, A, & Pionchon, P. A unified concept of idiopathic orofacial pain: pathophysiologic features, *J Orofac Pain*, 2000 14, 196-212.

[211] Woda, A. & Pionchon, P. Orofacial idiopathic pain: clinical signs, causes and mechanisms. *Rev Neurol (Paris)*, 2001 157, 265-283.

[212] Wurtman, J. The involvement of brain serotonin in excessive carbohydrate snacking by obese carbohydrate cravers. *J Am Dietet Assoc*, 1984 84, 1004-1007.

[213] Wurtman, RJ. & Wurtman, JJ. Carbohydrates and depression. *Sci Am*, 1989 260, 50-57.

[214] Wuttke, W; Seidlowa-Wuttke, D; Gorkow, C. The Cimicifuga preparation BNO 1055 vs. conjugated estrogens in a double-blind placebo-controlled study: effects on menopause symptoms and bone markers. *Mauritas*, 2003 44 (Suppl.1), S67-S77.

[215] Yang, C; Chung, J; Yang, G; Chhabra, S; Lee, M. Tea and tea polyphenols in cancer prevention. *J Nutr*, 2000 130, 472S-478S.

[216] Yeo, M; Kim, DK; Cho, SW; Hong, HD. Ginseng, the root of *Panax ginseng* C.A. Meyer, protects ethanol-induced gastric damages in rat through the induction of cytoprotective heat shock protein 27. *Dig Dis Sci*, 2008 53, 606-613.

[217] Yoneyama, S; Kawai K; Tsuno, NH; Okaji, Y; Asakage, M; Tsuchiya, T; Yamada, J; Sunami, E; Osada, T; Kitayama, J; Takahashi, K; Nagawa, H. Epigallocatechin gallate affects human dendritic cell differentiation and maturation. *J Allergy Clin Immunol*, 2008 121, 209-214.

[218] Yun, JH; Pang, EK; Kim, CS; Yoo, Yj; Cho, KS; Chai, JK; Kim, CK; Choi, SH. Inhibitory effects of green tea polyphenol (-)-epigallocatechin gallate on the expression of matrix metalloproteinase-9 and on the formation of osteoclasts. *J Periodontal Res*, 2004 39, 300-307.

[219] Yun, Jh; Kim, Cs, Cho, KS; Chai, JK; Kim, CK; Choi, SH. (-)-Epigallocatechin gallate induces apoptosis, via caspase activation, in osteoclasts differentiated from RAW 264.7 cells. *J Periodontal Res*, 2007 42, 212-218.

[220] Zelles, T; Boros, I; Nagy, G; Dobó-Nagy, C; Tollas, Ő; Fehér, E. Caspase-3 activity in parotid gland hypertrophy induced by raw soya. In: *7th European Symposium on Saliva (Conference papers)*. Egmond an Zee (the Netherlands); 2005; 117-118.

[221] Zhang, AL; Story, DF; Lin, V; Vitetta, L; Xue, CC. A population survey on the use of 24 common medicinal herbs in Australia. *Pharmacoepidemiol Drug Saf*, 2008 17, 1006-1013.

[222] Zhang, Y; Han, G; Fan, B; Zhou, Y; Zhou, X; Wei, L; Zhang, J. Green tea (-)-epigallocatechin-3-gallate down-regulates VASP expression and inhibits breast cell migration and invasion by attenuating Rac1 activity. *Eur J Pharmachol*, 2009 606, 172-179.

[223] Zhou, Y. & Lee, AS. Mechanism for the supression of the mammalian stress response by genistein, an anticancer phytoestrogens from soy. *J Natl Cancer Inst*, 1998 90, 381-388.

Chapter 8

COMPLEMENTARY AND ALTERNATIVE MEDICINE (CAM)

ABSTRACT

Complementary and alternative medicine (CAM) denotes a wide range of variable therapies, including also treatments with established benefits and few if any side effects. CAM therapies emphasize self-care, which can lead to advantageously decreased load of the much more expensive health care system. No wonder that, complementary and alternative medicine is increasingly accepted and frequently utilized for children and adults also in such highly developed countries like the United States, several countries of the European Union, Canada and Australia. More than the half (roughly 54% - 62%) of normal adult population uses any CAM method. Roughly one third (roughly 20% - 35%) of CAM methods belongs to mind-body type CAM therapies like Tai-Chi therapy, Qigong therapy, breathing exercises, yoga therapy and some similar therapies; and this proportion is at least doubled when prayer is also included. The rest proportion of CAM therapies include several other approaches like acupuncture, sleep deprivation (vigil), fasting therapy, light therapy and several other therapies. Majority of mind-body CAM techniques used by United States adults, European adults and children in the US and Canada are religious. Since lacking a religious sensitivity, medical science will always be woefully incomplete the importance of such religious methods should not be underestimated. Another advantage is that, there are usually only few contraindications of CAM therapies.

8.1. INTRODUCTION

Complementary and alternative medicine (CAM) denotes a wide range of variable therapies, including also treatments with established benefits and few if any side effects [*Wahner-Roedler et al. 2005, Fábián in press*]. CAM therapies emphasize self-care, which can lead to advantageously decreased load of the much more expensive health care system [*Tindle et al. 2005*]. No wonder that, complementary and alternative medicine is increasingly accepted and frequently utilized for children [*Sanders et al. 2003; Losier et al. 2005; Wall 2005*] and adults also in such highly developed countries like the United States [*Cuellar et al. 2003; Barnes et al. 2004; Honda & Jacobson 2005, Tindle et al. 2005*], several countries of the European Union [*Langmead et al. 2002; Menniti-Ippolito et al. 2002; Hanssen et al. 2005, Walach 2006*], Canada [*Losier et al. 2005*] and Australia [*MacLennan et al. 1996*]. More than the half (roughly 54% - 62%) of normal adult population uses any CAM method [*Honda & Jacobson 2005; Goldstein et al. 2005; Barnes et al. 2004*]. Roughly one third (roughly 20% - 35%) of CAM methods belongs to mind-body type CAM therapies [*Barnes et al. 2004; Honda & Jacobson 2005; Upchurch & Chyu 2005; Goldstein et al. 2005*] like Tai-Chi therapy, Qigong therapy, breathing exercises, yoga therapy and some similar therapies; and this proportion is at least doubled when prayer is also included [*Barnes et al. 2004; Honda & Jacobson 2005, Wahner-Roedler et al. 2005, Tindle et al. 2005*]. The rest proportion of CAM therapies include several other approaches like acupuncture, sleep deprivation (vigil), fasting therapy, light therapy and several other therapies.

8.2. PRAYER FOR HEALING

Lacking a religious sensitivity, medical science will always be woefully incomplete, no matter how great its discoveries [*Pollack 1999*]. The importance of religious methods is derived from that, they possess spiritual (sacral, transcendent) surplus, which improves efficiency of these kind of therapies [*Butler et al. 1998, Fábián et al. 2005, Wachholtz & Pargament 2005, Jantos & Kiat 2007, Fábián & Müller 2008, Fábián in press*]. Evidently, religious methods also improve religiosity, which is known to be associated with health promoting attitude and decreased frequency of medical symptoms and diseases [*Kass et al. 1991, Schumacher 1992, Oxman et al. 1995, de Gouw et al. 1995, Benson 1996, Timio et al. 1988, 1997, Timio 1997, Krebs 2000, Packer 2000, Moss 2002, Dedert et al. 2004*]. No wonder that, majority of mind-body CAM techniques used by United States adults [*Cuellar et al. 2003, Barnes et al. 2004, Rhee et al. 2004, Honda & Jacobson 2005, Upchurch & Chyu 2005, Mao et al. 2007*], European adults [*Sunter et al. 2006, D'Inca et al. 2007*] and children in the US and Canada [*Sanders et al. 2003, Losier et al. 2005*] are religious. For psychosomatic therapy of *religious patients* at least prayer (the most frequently used religious CAM practice [*Krause 2004, Tindle et al. 2005, Wahner-Roedler et al. 2005*]) should be considered and utilized [*Rajski 2003, Fábián in press*].

Prayer is an active process of communicating with and/or appealing to God or other supernatural being belonging to God. Besides intercessory prayer (petitions on behalf of others) there are three major forms of prayer [*Jantos & Kiat 2007*] including conversational prayer (informal conversation with God), ritual prayer (reciting or reading well known prayers) and meditative prayer (i.e. repetition of short formulas, contemplation, imagery of religious themes etc., see also in *paragraph 6.4.4.*). Despite numerous religious and health related functions of prayer [*Pollack 1999, Harris et al. 2005, Jantos & Kiat 2007, Masters & Spielmans 2007, Mao et al. 2007, Fábián in press*] it is not frequently studied empirically because of its perceived intimacy [*Harris et al. 2005*]; consequently there are only few psychophysiological data in the literature related to this religious practice.

A study indicated brain activations in the dorsolateral prefrontal, dorsomedial frontal, medial parietal and cerebellar areas during recitation prayer [*Azari et al. 2001*]. Spontaneous decrease of respiratory rate (to ≈ 6/min) coupled with increase of heart rate variability and parasympathetic activity was also reported [*Bernardi et al. 2001*]. A rhythmic (respiration synchronized) fluctuation of cerebral blood flow with possible influence on central nervous oscillations was observed too [*Bernardi et al. 2001*]. Prayer also frequently resulted in subjectively experienced relaxation and general well-being [*Masters & Spielmans 2007*]. A prolonged increase of *overall mental health* also occurs following regular practice of prayer [*Meisenhelder & Chandler 2000*] including positive mood [*Wachholtz & Pargament 2005*], decreased level of illness-related depression [*Coleman et al. 2006*], decreased anxiety [*Harris et al. 2005, Wachholtz & Pargament 2005*], higher level of perceived control over emotional reactions [*Harris et al. 2005*] and existential well being [*Wachholtz & Pargament 2005*]. Long-run practice of prayer also *decreases psychophysiological stress reactions* including salivary cortisol stress response [*Tartaro et al. 2005*], and daily rhythm of salivary cortisol level may also be preserved [*Dedert et al. 2004*]. It is also likely that, prayer improves *immunological functions*, and defense against infectious disorders [*Fitzpatrick et al. 2007*]. Regarding *contraindication* it should be mentioned that, in general there is no contraindication of prayer, however practice of *meditative forms* may have similar contraindication like any other mind-body therapies (see in *paragraph 6.4.7.*).

8.3. ACUPUNCTURE

Acupuncture is a traditional Chinese practice that attempts to regulate and restore energy balance by stimulating specific acupoints [*Whittaker 2004*]. Acupuncture can be used efficiently also in dentistry [*Rosted 2000*] for the treatment of myofascial pain [*Dahlström 1992*], temporomandibular disorder [*Schmid-Schwap et al. 2006*], oral and/or dental pain [*Lao et al. 1999, Vachiramon & Wang 2005*], orofacial pain [*Goddard 2005*] gagging [*Vachiramon & Wang 2002*], xerostomia [*Wang et al. 2004*] and drooling (of saliva) [*Wong et al. 2001*]. Although the mechanisms behind acupuncture therapy is not yet clear, it should be considered that traditional needle acupuncture (including its modern derivative electro acupuncture) is frequently coupled with moderately painful stimuli. Similarly, infiltration of intraoral acupoints (used for oral acupuncture) may also induce pain, even if local anesthetic [*Schmid-Schwap et al. 2006*] is injected (i.e. 0.1 – 0.3 ml procaine). Therefore pain induced activation of reticular system, thalamus, periaqueductal gray matter, limbic system and hypothalamus [*Heinze 1993*], as well as increased level of endogenous opioids [*Hiemke 2003*] including encephalin and beta endorphin [*Heinze 1993*] should be considered as a possible pathway of the therapeutic effects. Moreover, stimulation of acupoints with pain free (laser) stimuli clearly indicated a specific (pain independent) effect of acupoints on the cortical function [*Siedentopf et al. 2002*]; indicating that, *absolutely painless forms* of acupuncture (i.e. acupressure, laser- or PEMF acupuncture [*Whittaker 2004, Fábián in press*]) can also be used efficiently.

Acupuncture therapy may be based on the trigger point method, in which painful trigger points are recognized and stimulated with acupuncture needles and/or with any other acupuncture modalities (i.e. electro acupuncture, laser- or PEMF acupuncture, acupressure, moxibustion etc.) [*Baldry 2005*] Similarly, acupuncture treatment of intraoral painful points (i.e. oral acupuncture) may also be used [*Schmid-Schwap et al. 2006*]. In this case most painful points are selected by the "very-point method" [*Gleditsch 1980, 1985*] after palpation of the retromolar areas of maxilla and mandible and the vestibulum [*Gleditsch 1980, 1985,*

Schmid-Schwap et al. 2006]. Besides trigger point (and/or intraoral "very-point") based treatment, acupuncture therapy based on the traditional Chinese conception of vital energy (called "Chi" or "Qi") may also be used [*Veith 1949; Lu & Needham 1980; Baldry 2005*].

Traditional acupoint Hegu (LI-4; located on the dorsum of the hand between the first and second metacarpal bones) may be used for the treatment of oral and/or dental pain [*Lao et al. 1999, Vachiramon & Wang 2005, Zeng et al. 2006*] as well as for the treatment of TMD disorder [*Schmid-Schwap et al. 2006*]. Yifeng (SJ-17; located in a depression anterior and inferior to the mastoid process) may also be used for the treatment of oral and/or dental pain [*Lao et al. 1999*]. Chengjiang (REN-24; located in the horizontal mentolabial groove approximately midway between chin and lower lip) may be used for control gag reflex [*Vachiramon & Wang 2002*] and also for the treatment of xerostomia [*Wang et al. 2004*]. Jiache (ST-6; located one finger breadth anterior and superior to the angle of mandible) and Xiaguan (ST-7; located at the lower border of the zygomatic arch in the depression anterior to the condylar process of the mandible) may be used for the treatment of xerostomia [*Wang et al. 2004*] and also for the treatment of oral and/or dental pain [*Lao et al. 1999*]. Certain other points on the face such as Daying (ST-5; located directly anterior to the angle of the mandible, in a depression at the anterior border of the masseter muscle) and Tinggong (SI-19; located in the depression between the middle of the tragus and condylar process of the mandible) may also be used to treat xerostomia [*Wang et al. 2004*]. Certain acupoints of the tongue may be used for the treatment of drooling of saliva as well [*Wong et al. 2001*].

Regarding *contraindications* it should be noted that, serious adverse effects following acupuncture are rare [*Vachiramon & Wang 2005*]. However acupuncture may be contraindicated in the case of patients with certain psychiatric conditions like paranoid psychosis, hypochondria (etc.). Further, great care should be taken for infection control; and injuries of blood vessels nerves and any other sensitive tissues should also be strictly avoided when needle type acupuncture is used. Specific cautions should also be considered when laser-, electric-, or electromagnetic (PEMF) stimulation are used (see also *paragraph 6.5.*).

8.4. BREATHING EXERCISES

Breathing exercises can be classified primarily by frequency (low ≈6/min; high ≈60-140/min and very low frequency ≤3-4/min) [*Fábián in press*] but also by tidal volume (shallow or deep breathing), by location (abdominal, thoracic) and by specifically modified phases during breathing (shortening or lengthening inhalation, retention, exhalation and apnea) [*Fábián in press*]. Comfortable low frequency breathing decreases heart rate and blood pressure [*Kaushik et al. 2006*] whereas increases heart rate variability [*Lehrer et al. 2003; Peng et al. 2004*] and baroreflex sensitivity [*Bernardi et al. 2002; Lehrer et al. 2003*]. This kind of breathing may lead to decreased muscle activity [*Kaushik et al. 2006*] and drowsiness or light sleep with appearance of theta/delta bands on EEG [*Fumoto et al. 2004*]. High frequency (and/or deep) breathing usually resulted in hyperventilation with consequent alterations of blood CO_2 and oxygen values and appearance of a certain alteration of consciousness [*Mészáros 1984; Heinze 1993; Fábián & Fábián 1998*]. High frequency breathing also coupled with increased sympathetic and decreased vagal activity [*Raghuraj et al. 1998*], increased pulse rate [*Peng et al. 2004*] and decreased heart rate variability [*Peng et al. 2004*]. Further, high frequency breathing increases alpha and beta-1 activity on the EEG [*Stancák et al. 1991*]. Very low frequency breathing induce similar changes on the EEG with increased high frequency alpha- [*Fumoto et al. 2004*], beta- and paroxysmal gamma activity [*Vialatte et al. in press*] and decrease of theta activity [*Vialatte et al. in press*]. Very low frequency breathing exercises also exerts antidepressive and anxiolytic properties may be through serotonergic brain activations [*Fumoto et al 2004*]. Most breathing exercises (including comfortable low frequency breathing of slow exhalation [*Danucalov et al. in press*]) rise metabolic rate (VO_2 and VCO_2), whereas very low frequency breathing may decrease it [*Telles & Desiraju 1991*]. Some breathing exercises may also improve immune function including activation of antiapoptotic and prosurvival genes and also genes encoding antioxidant enzymes in white blood cells [*Sharma et al. 2008*].

Breathing exercises are primarily used to preserve healthiness, however they may also be used efficiently for therapeutic purposes. Breathing techniques can be utilized for mind-body therapies (see in *paragraph 6.4.*) as a self-focus skill or anchor [*Ospina et al. 2007, Fábián & Fábián 1998, Fábián in press*] also in the treatment of orofacial symptoms [*Fábián & Fábián 1998*]. Similarly, combination of abdominal/diaphragmatic breathing with cognitive-behavioral therapy (see in *paragraph 6.3.3.*) and progressive muscle relaxation (see in *paragraphs 6.4.1.*) was highly efficient to reduce pain-activity interference, pain intensity, depression, maladaptive pain beliefs, and catastrophizing as well as to improve masticatory jaw function in a randomized controlled trial (RCT) of TMD related orofacial pain patients [*Turner et al. 2006*]. Regarding *contraindication* it should be mentioned that, breathing exercises coupled with meditation have similar contraindication like mind-body therapies (see in *paragraph 6.4.7.*). Further, breathing exercises may be contraindicated in case of pregnancy, cardiac problems, pacemaker patients and other conditions with strongly compromised health [*Vígh 1972, Fábián in press*].

8.5. TAI-CHI AND QIGONG THERAPIES

Tai-Chi (Tai Chi Chuan) and Qigong (Chi Kung) are traditional Chinese practices of meditation designed to control expected vital energy (called "Chi" or "Qi") of the body to promote health and spiritual development [*Lewis 2000; McCaffrey and Flower 2003*]. Thai-Chi (but not Qigong) may also be considered as a Chinese martial art based on suppleness and evasion [*Cheng 2007*] coupled with control of premised expected vital energy ("Chi"/"Qi"). Besides some static body postures [*Lewis 2000*] and voice training [*McCaffrey and Flower 2003*] there are three *major* components of Tai-Chi and Qigong training including *slow moving* exercises, *breathing* exercises and *meditation* [*Lewis 2000; Jones 2001; McCaffrey and Flower 2003*]. Movement in Qigong usually involve meditative visualizing of internal consequences of flow of the expected vital energy, although in some cases vital energy is expected to be transferred into other persons (patients) on purpose to cure. Movement in Tai-Chi (although usually practiced slowly) may be sped up and might involve meditative visualizing the external consequences of a motion as well (i.e. to provide a self-defense) which is not the case in Qigong.

Tai-Chi and Qigong exercises *promptly* increase heart rate [*Zhou et al. 1984; Lan et al. 2004*], metabolic activity [*Zhou et al 1984; Li et al. 2001; Lan et al. 2004*], catecholamine [*Jin 1989*] growth hormone [*Lee & Ryu 2004*] and melatonin level [*Lee & Ryu 2004*] and decrease plasma level of cortisol [*Lee & Ryu 2004*]. All these changes indicate a *prompt appearance of calm and relaxed* [*Wetterberg 1999, Ray 2003, Solberg et al. 2004*] psychophysiological state *with somewhat increased arousal* level. Tai-Chi and Qigong practice can also be advantageously utilized for the treatment of psychosomatic patients especially when practiced repeatedly for *longer-run*. Prolonged *increase of overall mental health* [*Ko et al. 2006, Esch et al. 2007, Irwin et al. 2007*] can be achieved with long-run practicing regularly, including decrease of perceived stress [*Esch et al. 2007*] and (trait)anxiety [*Tsai et al. 2003*]; a well as improve of mood [*Tsang et al. 2002, 2006, Yeh et al. 2006*], vitality [*Ko et al. 2006, Irwin et al. 2007*] sleep quality [*Lee et al. 2003/b, Yeh et al. in press*] and general social functioning [*Esch et al. 2007*]. Decreased value of *stress hormones* including mean value (24 hours, urine) of norepinephrine [*Skoglund & Jansson 2007*] as well as decreased level of cortisol in saliva [*Esch et al. 2007*] were also reported following *long-run* practicing.

Thai-Chi and Qigong training also significantly influence *immune functions*. There is a *prompt* increase of the number of lymphocytes [*Lee et al. 2003/a*], number of monocytes [*Lee et al. 2003/a*] and superoxide radical (O_2^-) production of neutrophils [*Lee & Ryu 2004; Lee et al. 2005*] as well as decrease of the number of NK cells [*Lee et al. 2003/a*], and alteration of the activation of apoptotic genes in neutrophile PMN cells [*Li et al. 2005*]. Following repeated practicing for a *long run*, there is a *sustained increase* of the number of CD4$^+$ CD25$^+$ regulatory T-cells [*Yeh et al. 2006*], proliferation ability of CD4$^+$ CD45RO$^+$ memory T-cells [*Irwin et al. 2003, 2007*], ability to rise in antibody titers in response to infection [*Yang et al. 2007/b*], production of regulatory cytokine (IL10) of mononuclear cells [*Yeh et al. 2006*] and production of growth factor (TGF-β) of mononuclear cells [*Yeh et al. 2006*]; as well as a *sustained decrease* of the total number of leukocytes [*Manzaneque et al. 2004*] relative number of monocytes [*Yeh et al. 2006*], relative number of eosinophile PMN cells [*Manzaneque et al. 2004*] and complement (C3) concentration [*Manzaneque et al. 2004*].

Rheumatoid arthritis [*Wang et al. 2005*], osteoarthritis [*Song et al. 2003*], *fibromyalgia* [*Taggart et al. 2003*], *tension type headache* [*Abbott et al. 2007*] and several *somatoform symptoms* [*Lee et al. 2003/b*] may be treated efficiently with Tai-Chi and Qigong therapies. There is also a significant effect of Tai-Chi and Qigong on the *musculoskeletal system*. Flexibility [*Hong et al. 2000, Qin et al. 2005*], endurance [*Xu et al. 2006*], muscle strength [*Qin et al. 2005, Xu et al. 2006*], gait [*Yang et al. 2007/a*] and bone mineral density [*Chan et al. 2004, Qin et al. 2005, Woo et al. 2007*] can be improved significantly with long-run practicing. Similarly, complex muscle function [*Yeh et al. 2006, Voukelatos et al. 2007*] as well as joint proprioception [*Tsang & Hui-Chan 2003, Xu et al. 2004*], neuromuscular reaction time [*Xu et al. 2005*], and balance control [*Tsang & Hui-Chan 2003, Thornton et al. 2004, Qin et al. 2005, Voukelatos et al. 2007, Yang et al. 2007/a*] can also be improved significantly. *Wound healing* may also be improved with Tai-Chi and Qigong practice [*Lee et al. 2003/b*]. Regarding *contraindication* it should be mentioned that, meditative form of Tai-Chi and Qigong practices have similar contraindication like mind-body therapies (see in *paragraph 6.4.7.*). Further, slow movement exercises, breathing exercises, and body postures may be contraindicated in case of pregnancy, cardiac problems, pacemaker patients and other conditions with strongly compromised health [*Vigh 1972, Fábián in press*].

8.6. YOGA THERAPY

Yoga is a collective noon of traditional practices developed in India to improve health, and to prepare body and mind for meditation and spiritual development. Classical yoga incorporates moral and ethical observances (yama, niyama), body postures and exercises (i.e. hatha yoga), breathing techniques (pranayama) and meditative techniques (i.e. dhyana, samadhi) [*Joshi 1967; Ospina et al. 2007, Fábián in press*]. There are several major subdivisions of yogic tradition such as hatha yoga, pranajama, kundalini yoga, and raja yoga [*Fábián in press*]. There are also some modern schools of yoga such as Iyengar yoga and Vivekananda yoga [*Fábián in press*].

Hatha yoga includes some dynamic body exercises, but most typically several breathing exercises (pranayama, see below) and body postures like sittings, standing poses, inverted poses, muscle and spine stretching poses, trunk rotating poses, symbolic hand/body gestures, and relaxing poses. *Pranayama* is a collective noon of all breathing exercises of yoga tradition including breathing exercises (see also *paragraph 8.4.*) of hatha yoga and kundalini yoga. *Kundalini yoga* is a yogic practice aimed at control of expected vital-energy of the body (called "prana") via meditation coupled with certain body postures and breathing exercises. *Raja yoga* is a pure meditative form of yogic exercises aimed at self-absorption experience (called "samadhi") [*Fábián in press*]. *Iyengar yoga* is based on hatha yoga traditions (including pranayama and meditation) but employs props that allow to practice body postures despite limited experience and flexibility. *Vivekananda yoga* is also based on hatha yoga traditions (including pranayama and meditation) but aimed at therapeutic utilization of yoga tradition.

Yoga postures usually induce significant changes of local blood (and lymph) circulation leading to several metabolic changes of the targeted tissues including the brain [*Fábián in press*]. Similarly, the circulation of liquor cerebrospinalis may also be changed [*Fábián in press*]. Usually significant elevation of heart rate and metabolic activity is also induced [*Hagins et al. 2007*] Moderate transient pain sensations may also appear practicing postures blocking blood circulation or stretching muscles, tendons and ligaments leading to release of opioids in the brain [*Hiemke 2003*] changing mood and increasing trance-ability [*Heinze 1993*]. Increased level of brain gamma-aminobutiric acid (GABA) under practicing such postures may also occur [*Streeter et al. 2007*] leading to remarkable antidepressive and anxiolytic effects [*Kjellgren et al. 2007; Streeter et al. 2007*]. Similarly to body postures, breathing- and meditative yoga exercises also induce certain significant psychophysiological changes, which can be utilized for therapeutic purposes (see *paragraphs 6.4.4. and 8.4.*).

Long-run practice of yoga induce *prolonged increase of overall mental health* [*Smith et al. 2007*] including increased level of optimism [*Kjellgren et al. 2007*] and decreased level of perceived stress [*Smith et al. 2007, Kjellgren et al. 2007*], neuroticism [*Shapiro et al. 2007*], depression [*Shapiro et al. 2007, Kjellgren et al. 2007*], (trait)anxiety [*Shapiro et al. 2007,*

Smith et al. 2007, Kjellgren et al. 2007], and anger under chronic illness-stress [*Shapiro et al. 2007*]. Yoga was found highly efficient in the treatment of unexplained chronic fatigue as well [*Bentler et al. 2005*]. There is also a significant long-run effect of yoga practices on the *musculoskeletal system*. Flexibility [*Tran et al. 2001, Puymbroeck et al. 2007*], endurance [*Tran et al. 2001, Puymbroeck et al. 2007*], muscle strength [*Tran et al. 2001, Puymbroeck et al. 2007*] and gait [*DiBenedetto et al. 2005, Manjunath & Telles 2008*], as well as balance control [*Bastille & Gill-Body 2004, Puymbroeck et al. 2007, Manjunath & Telles 2008*] and other complex muscle functions [*Manjunath & Telles 2008*] can be improved highly efficiently with long run yoga practices. It is also likely that, there are some *immunological effects* of yoga practices as well [*Rao et al. 2008*]. Regarding *contraindication* it should be mentioned that, yoga practices coupled with meditation have similar contraindication like mind-body therapies (see in *paragraph 6.4.7.*). Further, body postures, breathing exercises and slow movement exercises may be contraindicated in case of pregnancy, cardiac problems, pacemaker patients and other conditions with strongly compromised health [*Vígh 1972, Fábián in press*].

8.7. OTHER CAM THERAPIES

8.7.1. Sleep Deprivation (Vigil)

Sleep deprivation (vigil) positively influences mood having prompt and significant antidepressive effect [*Benedetti et al. 2002, 2003/a,b; Wirz-Justice et al. 2005*]. Vigil was also shown to increase amylase encoding mRNA level [*Seugnet et al. 2006*] and amylase concentration in the saliva [*Seugnet et al. 2006*] indicative of increased sympathetic activity [*Nater et al 2005*]. Vigil decreases anterior cingulate cortex metabolism likely due to an increase in the activity of brain serotonergic [*Wu et al. 2001; Benedetti et al. 2003/a*] and dopaminergic [*Wu et al. 2001; Benedetti et al. 2003/b*] pathways as well. Sleep deprivation coupled increase of the serotonergic neural activity in dorsal raphe nucleus was also demonstrated in an animal study [*Gardner et al. 1997*]. Sleep deprivation also increases the expression of inducible heat shock protein 70 in rat gastrointestinal (concretely: gastric) mucosa and improve mucosal surface defense [*Shen et al. 2001*].

8.7.2. Fasting (Keep Fast)

Keeping fast is frequently used as a practice to preserve healthiness. Calorie restriction is likely to extend lifespan [*Milne et al. 2007, Pearson et al. 2008*], produces advantageous metabolic profile [*Milne et al. 2007*] and protect against carcinogenesis [*Pearson et al. 2008*]. Fasting therapy may also improve chronic pain [*Michalsen et al. 2002*] as well as syndromes of stress and exhaustion [*Michalsen et al. 2002*]. Fasting activates hypothalamic-pituitary-adrenocortical axis (HPA axis) leading to increased serum cortisol level and sympathetic activity [*Fichter & Pirke 1986*]. Altered function of hypothalamic and hippocampal septal systems was also assumed [*Winkelman 1986; Heinze 1993*]. Fasting also activates the immune system (NK cell activity) and alleviates fatigue [*Masuda et al. 2001*], however a complete food restriction for two-three days (or more) may lead to immune suppression [*Chiapelli & Hodgson 2000*]. Premised changes indicate that, numerous biological mechanisms are placed temporarily in a stress state during keeping fast [*Suzuki et al. 1979; Yamamoto et al. 1979*]. In contrast, brain activity is decreased in general because of a shift toward increased alpha EEG activity; likely as a consequence of the ketone nutrition of brain cells [*Yamamoto et al. 1979*].

8.7.3. Light Therapy

Taking delight in the sunrise, sunset, candlelight, glittering surfaces of water and snow as well as sun-bathing is frequently practiced by many people. Besides the rewarding and symbolic meaning of such practices, also neurophysiologic effects of the light should be counted in these cases. Light stimuli influences the function of pineal gland, epithalamus and supraoptic region of hypothalamic medial zone [*Clark et al 2006*]. Further, significant effect of light exposure on mood (i.e. antidepressive effect [*Benedetti et al 2003/a,c, 2005, Wirz-Justice et al. 2005*]) likely based on brain serotonergic pathways and phase changes of biological rhythms [*Benedetti et al 2003/a*] was also reported. Flash-light effects also induce rather unique and significant neurophysiological changes that can be utilized highly efficiently for therapeutic purposes (see *paragraph 6.4.5.*). Besides premised primarily neurophysiological effects, other biological effects of light exposure should also be considered (see *paragraph 6.5.9.*), at least when stronger exposure occurs (like in the case of sun-bathing).

8.8. CONCLUSION

Complementary and alternative medicine (CAM) denotes a wide range of variable therapies, with established benefits and few if any side effects [*Wahner-Roedler et al. 2005, Fábián in press*]. CAM therapies emphasize self-care, which can lead to advantageously decreased load of the much more expensive health care system [*Tindle et al. 2005*]. Majority of mind-body CAM techniques used by United States adults [*Cuellar et al. 2003, Barnes et al. 2004, Rhee et al. 2004, Honda & Jacobson 2005, Upchurch & Chyu 2005, Mao et al. 2007*], European adults [*Sunter et al. 2006, D'Inca et al. 2007*] and children in the US and Canada [*Sanders et al. 2003, Losier et al. 2005*] are religious. Since lacking a religious sensitivity, medical science will always be woefully incomplete, no matter how great its discoveries [*Pollack 1999*] the importance of such religious methods should not be underestimated. Another advantage is that, there are only few contraindications of CAM therapies. These contraindications are usually similar to those of other mind-body therapies, although some specific contraindications of certain CAM techniques should also be considered.

REFERENCES

[1]   Abbott, RB; Hui, KK; Hays, RD; Li, MD; Pan, T. A randomized controlled trial of Tai Chi for tension headaches. *eCAM*, 2007 4, 107-113.

[2]   Azari, NP; Nickel, J; Wunderlich, G; Niedeggen, M; Hefter, H; Tellmann, L; Herzog, H; Stoerig, P; Birnbacher, D; Seitz, RJ. Neural correlates of religious experience. *Eur J Neurosci*, 2001 13, 1649-1652.

[3]   Baldry, PE. *Acupuncture, trigger points and musculoskeletal pain*. Third edition. Edinburgh-London-New York-Philadelphia-San Francisco-Toronto: Elsevier Churchill Livingstone; 2005. 3-13; 29-36.

[4]   Barnes, PM; Powell-Griner, E; McFann, K; Nahin, RL. *Complementary and alternative medicine use among adults: United States, 2002. Advance data from vital and health statistics; no 343*. Hyattsville, Maryland: National Center for Health Statistics; 2004. 1-20.

[5]   Bastille, JV. & Gill-Body, KM. A yoga-based exercise program for people with chronic post stroke hemiparesis. *Phys Ther*, 2004 84, 33-48.

[6]   Benedetti, F; Lucca, A; Brambilla, F; Colombo, C; Smeraldi, E. Interleukine-6 serum levels correlate with response to antidepressant sleep deprivation and sleep phase advance. *Prog Neuropharmacol Biol Psychiatry*, 2002 26, 1167-1170.

[7]   Bendetti, F; Colombo, C; Serretti, A; Lorenzi, C; Pontiggia, A; Barbini, B; Smeraldi, E. Antidepressant effects of light therapy combined with sleep deprivation are influenced by a functional polymorphism within the promoter of the serotonin transporter gene. *Biol Psychiatry*, 2003/a 54, 687-692.

[8]   Benedetti, F; Serretti, A; Colombo, C; Lilli, R; Lorenzi, C; Smeraldi, E. Dopamine receptor D2 and D3 gene variants are not associated with the antidepressant effects of total sleep deprivation in bipolar depression. *Psychiatry Res*, 2003/b 118, 241-247.

[9]   Benedetti, F; Colombo, C; Pontiggia, A; Bernasconi, A; Florita, M; Smeraldi, E. Morning light treatment hastens the antidepressant effect of citalopram: a placebo controlled trial. *J Clin Psychiatry*, 2003/c 64, 648-653.

[10]   Benedetti, F; Barbini, B; Fulgosi, MC; Colombo, C; Dallaspezia, S; Pontiggia, A; Smeraldi, E. Combined total sleep deprivation and light therapy in the treatment of drug-resistant bipolar depression: acute response and long-term remission rates. *J Clin Psychiatry*, 2005 66, 1535-1540.

[11]   Benson, H. *Timeless healing: the power and biology of belief*. New York: Scribner; 1996.

[12]   Bentler, SE; Hartz, AJ; Kuhn, EM. Prospective observational study of treatments for unexplained chronic fatigue. *J Clin Psychiatry*, 2005 66, 625-631.

[13]   Bernardi, L; Sleight, P; Bandinelli, G; Cencetti, S; Fattorini, L; Wdowczyk-Szulc, J; Lagi, A. Effect of rosary prayer and yoga mantras on autonomic cardiovascular rhythms: comparative study. *MBJ*, 2001 323, 1446-1449.

[14]   Bernardi, L; Porta, C; Spicuzza, L; Bellwon, J; Spadacini, G, Frei, AW; Yeung, LYC; Sanderson, JE; Pedretti, R; Tramarin, R. Slow breathing increases arterial baroreflex sensitivity in patients with chronic heart failure. *Circulation*, 2002 105, 143-145.

[15]   Butler, MH; Gardner, BC; Bird, MH. Not just a time-out: change dynamics of prayer for religious couples in conflict situations. *Fam Process*, 1998 37, 451-478.

[16] Chan, K; Qin, L; Lau, M; Woo, J; Au, S; Choy, W; Lee, K; Lee, S. A randomized prospective study of the effects of Tai Chi Chuan exercise on bone mineral density in postmenopausal women. *Arch Phys Med Rehabil*, 2004 85, 717-722.

[17] Cheng, TO. Thai Chi: The Chinese ancient wisdom of an ideal exercise for cardiac patients. *Int J Cardiology*, 2007 117, 293-295.

[18] Chiapelli, F. & Hodgson, D. Immune suppression. In: Fink G, editor in chief. *Encyclopedia of stress. (vol. 2.).* San Diego: Academic Press; 2000; 531-536.

[19] Clark, DL; Boutros, NN; Mendes, MF. *The brain and behavior. An introduction to behavioral neuroanatomy.* Cambridge: Cambridge University Press; 2006. 131, 133, 135.

[20] Coleman, CL; Holzemer, WL; Eller, LS; Corless, I; Reynolds, N; Nokes, KM; Kemppainen, JK; Dole, P; Kirksey, K; Seficik, L; Nicholas, P; Hamilton, MJ. Gender differences in use of prayer as a self-care strategy for managing symptoms in African Americans living with HIV/AIDS. *J Assoc Nurses Aids Care*, 2006 17, 16-23.

[21] Cuellar, N; Aycock, T; Cahill, B; Ford, J. Complementary and alternative medicine (CAM) use by African American (AA) and Caucasian American (CA) older adults in a rural setting: a descriptive comparative study. *BMC Compl Altern Med*, 2003 3, 8.

[22] Dahlström, L. Conservative treatment methods in craniomandibular disorder. *Swed Dent J*, 1992 16, 217-230.

[23] Danucalov, MÁD; Simoes, RS; Kozasa, EH; Leite, JR. Cardiorespiratory and metabolic changes during yoga sessions: The effects of respiratory exercises and meditation practices. *Appl Psychophysiol Biofeedback*, in press, DOI: 10.1007/s10484-008-9053-2.

[24] Dedert, EA; Studts, JL; Weissbecker, I; Salmon, PG; Banis, PL; Sephton, SE. Religiosity may help preserve the cortisol rhythm in women with stress-related illness. *Int J Psychiatry Med*, 2004 34, 61-77.

[25] de Gouw, HW; Westendorp, RG; Kunst, AE; Mackenbach, JP; Vandenbroucke, JP. Decreased mortality among contemplative monks in the Netherlands. *Am J Epidemiol*, 1995 141, 771-775.

[26] DiBenedetto, M; Innes, KE; Taylor, AG. Rodeheaver, PF; Boxer, JA; Wright, HJ; Kerrigan, DC. Effect of a gentle Iyengar yoga program on gait in the elderly: an exploratory study. *Arch Phys Med Rehabil*, 2005 86, 1830-1837.

[27] D'Inca, R; Garribba, AT; Vettorato, MG; Martin, A; Martines, D; Di Leo, V; Buda, A; Sturniolo, GC. Use of alternative and complementary therapies by inflammatory bowel disease patients in an Italian tertiary referral centre. *Digest Liver Disease*, 2007 39, 524-529.

[28] Esch, T; Duckstein, J; Welke, J; Stefano, GB; Braun, V. Mind/body techniques for physiological and psychological stress reduction: Stress management via Tai Chi training - a pilot study. *Med Sci Monit*, 2007 13, CR488-CR497.

[29] Fábián, TK. *Mind-body connections. Pathways of psychosomatic coupling under meditation and other altered states of consciousness.* New York: Nova Science Publishers; in press.

[30] Fábián, TK. & Fábián, G. Stress of life, stress of death: Anxiety in dentistry from the viewpoint of hypnotherapy. *Ann NY Acad Sci*, 1998 851, 495-500.

[31] Fábián, TK. & Müller, O. Prayer, meditation and healing [Ima és meditáció a gyógyításban]. In: Vértes G, Fábián TK editors. *Religion, faith and healing* [*Vallás és hit a gyógyításban*]. Budapest: Medicina; 2008. 118-125.

[32] Fábián, TK; Vértes, G; Fejérdy, P. Pastoral psychology, spiritual counseling in dentistry. Review of the literature. *Fogorv Szle*, 2005 98, 37-42.

[33] Fichter, MM. & Pirke, KM. Effect of experimental and pathological weight loss upon the hypothalamo-pituitary-adrenal axis. *Psychoneuroendocrinology*, 1986 11, 295-305.

[34] Fitzpatrick, AL; Standish, LJ; Berger, J; Kim, JG; Calabrese, C; Polissar, N. Survival in HIV-1-positive adults practicing psychological or spiritual activities for one year. *Altern Ther Health Med*, 2007 13, 18-24.

[35] Fumoto, M; Sato-Suzuki, I; Seki, Y; Mohri, Y; Arita, H. Appearance of high-frequency alpha band with disappearance of low-frequency alpha band in EEG is produced during voluntary abdominal breathing in an eyes-closed condition. *Neurosci Res*, 2004 50, 307-317.

[36] Gardner, JP; Fornal, CA; Jacobs, BL. Effect of sleep deprivation on serotonergic neuronal activity in the dorsal nucleus of the freely moving cat. *Neuropsychopharmacology*, 1997 17, 72-81.

[37] Gleditsch, JM. Punktversuche und Ermittlung von Reaktionsebenen mit Hilfe der Very-Point-Technik. *Akupunktur Theor Prax*, 1980 8, 58-61.

[38] Gleditsch, J. Trigger-Punkt-Therapie bei funktionellen und entzündlichen Erkrankungen im Zahn-, Mund-, Kiefer-Bereich. *Zahnarzt*, 1985 28, 863-869.

[39] Goddard, G. Short term pain reduction with acupuncture treatment for chronic orofacial pain patients. *Med Sci Monit*, 2005 11, CR71-CR74.

[40] Goldstein, MS; Brown, ER; Ballard-Barbash, R; Morgenstern, H; Bastani, R; Lee, J; Gatto, N; Ambs, A. The use of complementary and alternative medicine among California adults with and without cancer. *eCAM*, 2005 2, 557-565.

[41] Hagins, M; Moore, W; Rundle, A. Does practicing hatha yoga satisfy recommendations for intensity of physical activity, which improves and maintains health and cardiovascular fitness? *BMC Compl Altern Med*, 2007 7, 40.

[42] Hanssen, B, Grimsgaard, S; Lauso, L; Fonnebo, V; Falkenberg, T; Rasmussen, NK. Use of complementary and alternative medicine in the Scandinavian countries. *Scand J Prim Health Care*, 2005 23, 57-62.

[43] Harris, JI; Schoneman, SW; Carrera, SR. Preferred prayer styles and anxiety control. *J Religion Health*, 2005 44, 403-412.

[44] Heinze, R-I. Shamanistic states of consciousness: Access to different realities. In: Hoppál M, Howard KD editors. *Shamans and cultures* (ISTOR books 5). Budapest - Los Angeles: Akadémiai Kiadó & International Society of Trans-Oceanic Research; 1993; 169-178.

[45] Hiemke, C. Biochemische Grundlagen des Schmerzes. In: Egle UT, Hoffmann SO, Lehmann KA, Nix WA editors. *Handbuch Chronischer Schmerz. Grundlagen, Pathogenese, Klinik und Therapie aus bio-psycho-sozialer Sicht*. Stuttgart-New York: Schattauer; 2003. 55-61.

[46] Honda, K. & Jacobson, JS. Use of complementary and alternative medicine among United States adults: the influences of personality, coping strategies, and social support. *Preventive Medicine*, 2005 40, 46-53.

[47] Hong, Y; Li, JX; Robinson, PD. Balance control, flexibility, and cardiorespiratory fitness among older Tai Chi practitioners. *Br J Sports Med*, 2000 34, 29-34.

[48] Irwin, MR; Pike, JL; Cole, JC; Oxman, MN. Effects of a behavioral intervention, Tai Chi chih, on varicella-zoster virus specific immunity and health functioning in older adults. *Psychosom Med*, 2003 65: 824-830.

[49] Irwin, MR; Olmstead, R; Oxman, MN. Augmenting immune responses to varizella zoster virus in older adults: A randomized, controlled trial of Tai Chi. *J Am Geriatr Soc*, 2007 55, 511-517.

[50] Jantos, M. & Kiat, H. Prayer as medicine: how much have we learned? *Med J Australia*, 2007 186, S51-S53.

[51] Jin, P. Changes in heart rate, noradrenalin, cortisol and mood during Tai Chi. *J Psychosom Res*, 1989 33, 197-206.

[52] Jones, BM. Change in cytokine production in healthy subjects practicing Guolin Qigong: a pilot study. *BMC Compl Altern Med*, 2001 1, 8.

[53] Joshi, KS. *Yoga and personality*. Allahabad: Udayana Publications, 1967. 16, 98, 127.

[54] Kass, JD; Friedman, R; Leserman, J; Zuttermeister, PC; Benson, H. Health outcomes and a new index of spiritual experience. *J Sci Study Religion*, 1991 30, 203-211.

[55] Kaushik, RM; Kaushik, R; Mahajan, SK; Rajesh, V. Effects of mental relaxation and slow breathing in essential hypertension. *Compl Therapies Med*, 2006 14, 120-126.

[56] Kjellgren, A; Bood, SÅ; Axelsson, K; Norlander, T; Saatcioglu, F. Wellness through a comprehensive yogic breathing program - A controlled pilot trial. *BMC Compl Altern Med*, 2007 7, 43.

[57] Ko, GTC; Tsang, PCC; Chan, HCK. A 10-week Tai-Chi program improved the blood pressure, lipid profile and SF-36 scores in Hong-Kong Chinese women. *Med Sci Monit*, 2006 12, CR196-CR199.

[58] Krause, N. Religion, aging and health: Exploring new frontiers in medical care. *South Med J*, 2004 97, 1215-1222.

[59] Krebs, K. Stress management, CAM approach. In: Fink G, editor-in-chief. *Encyclopedia of stress. (Vol. III.)* San Diego: Academic Press; 2000; 532-537.

[60] Lan, C; Chou, SW; Chen, SY; Lai, JS; Wong, MK. The aerobic capacity and ventilatory efficiency during exercise in Qigong and Tai Chi Chuan practitioners. *Am J Chin Med*. 2004 32, 141-150.

[61] Langmead, L; Chitnis, M; Rampton, DS. Use of complementary therapies by patients with IBD may indicate psychosocial distress. *Inflam Bowel Dis*, 2002 8, 174-179.

[62] Lao, L; Bergman, S; Hamilton, GR; Langenberg, P; Berman, B. Evaluation of acupuncture for pain control after oral surgery. A placebo-controlled trial. *Arch Otolaryngol Head Neck Surg*, 1999 125, 567-572.

[63] Lee, MS. & Ryu, H. Qi-training enhances neutrophile function by increasing growth hormone levels in elderly men. *Int J Neurosci*, 2004 114, 1313-1322.

[64] Lee, MS; Huh, HJ; Jeong, SM; Lee, HS; Ryu, H; Park, JH; Chung, HT; Woo, WH. Effects of Qigong on immune cells. Am J Chin Med, 2003/a 31, 327-335.

[65] Lee, MS; Hong, SS; Lim, HJ; Kim, HJ; Woo, WH; Moon, SR. Retrospective survey on therapeutic efficacy of Qigong in Korea. Am J Chin Med, 2003/b 31, 809-815.

[66] Lee, MS; Kim, MK; Ryu, H. Qi-training (qigong) enhanced immune functions: what is the underlying mechanism? Int J Neurosci, 2005 115, 1099-1104.

[67] Lehrer, PM; Vaschillo, E; Vaschillo, B; Lu, S-E; Eckberg, DL; Edelberg, R; Shih, WJ; Lin, Y; Kuusela, TA; Tahvanainen, KUO; Hamer, RM. Heart rate variability biofeedback increases baroreflex gain and peak expiratory flow. *Psychosom Med*, 2003 65, 796-805.

[68] Lewis, DE. T'ai chi ch'uan. *Comp Ther Nurs Midwifery*, 2000 6, 204-206.

[69] Li, JX; Hong, Y; Chan, KM. Tai chi: physiological characteristics and beneficial effects on health. *Br J Sports Med*, 2001 35, 148-156.

[70] Li, QZ; Li, P; Garcia, GE; Johnson, RJ; Feng, L. Genomic profiling of neutrophile transcripts in Asian Qigong practitioners: a pilot study in gene regulation by mind-body interaction. *J Altern Compl Med*, 2005 11, 29-39.

[71] Losier, A; Taylor, B; Fernandez, CV. Use of alternative therapies by patients presenting to a pediatric emergency department. *J Emergency Med*, 2005 28, 267-271.

[72] Lu, G-D. & Needham, J. *Celestial lancets. A history and rationale of acupuncture and moxa*. Cambridge: Cambridge University Press; 1980.

[73] MacLennan, AH; Wilson, DH; Taylor, AW. Prevalence and cost of alternative medicine in Australia. *Lancet*, 1996 347, 569-573.

[74] Manjunath, NK. & Telles, S. Effects of Yoga and Ayurveda preparation on gait, balance and mobility in older persons. *Med Sci Monit*, 2008 14, LE19-LE20.

[75] Manzaneque, JM; Vera, FM; Maldonado, EF; Carranque, G; Cubero, VM; Morell, M; Blanca, MJ. Assessment of immunological parameters following a qigong training program. *Med Sci Monit*, 2004 10, CR264-CR270.

[76] Mao, JJ; Farrar, JT; Xie, SX; Bowman, MA; Armstrong, K. Use of complementary and alternative medicine and prayer among a national sample of cancer survivors compared to other populations without cancer. *Compl Ther Med*, 2007 15, 21-29.

[77] Masters, KS. & Spielmans, GI. Prayer and health: Review, meta-analysis, and research agenda. *J Behav Med*, 2007 30, 329-338.

[78] Masuda, A; Nakayama, T; Yamanaka, T; Hatsutanmaru, K; Tei, C. Cognitive behavioral therapy and fasting therapy for a patient with chronic fatigue syndrome. *Internal Medicine*, 2001 40, 1158-1161.

[79] McCaffrey, R. & Flower, NL. Qigong practice. A pathway to health and healing. *Holist Nurs Pract*, 2003 17, 110-116.

[80] Meisenhelder, JB. & Chandler, EN. Prayer and health outcomes in church members. *Altern Ther Health Med*, 2000 6, 56-60.

[81] Menniti-Ippolito, F; Gargiulo, L; Bologna, E; Forcella, E; Raschetti, R. Use of unconventional medicine in Italy: a nation-wide survey. *Eur J Clin Pharmacol*, 2002 58, 61-64.

[82] Mészáros, I. *Hypnosis [Hipnózis]*. Budapest: Medicina; 1984. 140.

[83] Michalsen, A; Weidenhammer, W; Melchart, D; Langhorst, J; Saha, J; Dobos, G. Kurzzeitiges therapeutisches Fasten in der Behandlung von chronischen Schmerz- und Erschöpfungssyndromen. Verträglichkeit und Nebenwirkungen mit und ohne begleitende Mineralstoffergänzung. *Forsch Komplementermed Klass Naturheilk*, 2002 9, 221-227.

[84] Milne, JC. Lambert, PD. Schenk, S. et al. (for list of all the 28 authors see publication) Small molecule activators of SIRT1 as therapeutics for the treatment of type 2 diabetes. *Nature*, 2007 450, 712-716.

[85]   Moss, D. The circle of the soul: The role of spirituality in health care. *Appl Psychophysiol Biofeedback*, 2002 27, 283- 297.

[86]   Nater, UM; Rohleder, N; Gaab, J; Simona, B; Andreas, J; Kirschbaum, C; Ehlert, U. Human salivary alpha-amylase reactivity in a psychosocial stress paradigm. *Int J Psychophysiol*, 2005 55, 333-342.

[87]   Ospina, MB; Bond, TK; Karkhaneh, M; Tjosvold, L; Vandermeer, B; Liang, Y; Bialy, L; Hooton, N; Buscemi, N; Dryden, DM; Klassen, TP. *Meditation practices for health: State of research. Evidence Report/Technology Assessment No. 155.* (AHRQ Publication No. 07-E010). Rockville MD: Agency for Healthcare Research and Quality; 2007. 27-53.

[88]   Oxman, TE; Freeman Jr., DH; Manheimer, ED. Lack of social participation or religious strength and comfort as risk factors for death after cardiac surgery in the elderly. *Psychosom Med*, 1995 57, 5-15.

[89]   Packer, S. Religion and Stress. In: Fink G, editor-in-chief. *Encyclopedia of stress. (Vol. III).* San Diego: Academic Press; 2000; 348-355.

[90]   Pearson, KJ; Lewis, KN; Price, NL. et al. (for list of all the 17 authors see publication) Nrf2 mediates cancer protection but not prolongevity induced by caloric restriction. *PNAS*, 2008 105, 2325-2330.

[91]   Peng, CK; Henry, IC; Mietus, JE; Hausdorff, JM; Khalsa, G; Benson, H; Goldberger, AL. Heart rate dynamics during three forms of meditation. *Int J Cardiology*, 2004 95, 19-27.

[92]   Pollack, R. Wisdom versus knowledge: an agenda for a more humane medical science. *FASEB J*, 1999 13, 1477-1480.

[93]   Puymbroeck, MV; Payne, LL; Hsieh, PC. A phase I feasibility study of yoga on the physical health and coping of informal caregivers. *eCAM*, 2007 4, 519-529.

[94]   Qin, L; Choy, W; Leung, K; Leung, PC; Au, S; Hung, W; Dambacher, M; Chan, K. Beneficial effects of regular Tai Chi exercise on musculoskeletal system. *J Bone Miner Metab*, 2005 23, 186-190.

[95]   Raghuraj, P; Ramakrisnah, AG; Nagendra, HR; Telles S. Effect of two selected yogic breathing techniques on heart rate variability. *Indian J Physiol Pharmachol*, 1998 42, 467-472.

[96]   Rajski, P. Finding God in the silence: Contemplative prayer and therapy. *J Religion Health*, 2003 42, 181-190.

[97]   Rao, RM; Telles, S; Nagendra, HR; Nagarathna, R; Gopinath, KS; Srinath, S; Srikantaiah, C. Effects of yoga on natural killer cell counts in early breast cancer patients undergoing conventional treatment. *Med Sci Monit*, 2008 14, LE3-LE4.

[98]   Ray, CA. Melatonin attenuates the sympathetic nerve responses to orthostatic stress in humans. 2003 551, 1043-1048.

[99]   Rhee, SM; Garg, VK; Hershey, CO. Use of complementary and alternative medicines by ambulatory patients. *Arch Intern Med*, 2004 164, 1004-1009.

[100] Rosted, P. Introduction to acupuncture in dentistry. *Brit Dent J*, 2000 189, 136-140.

[101] Sanders, H; Davis, MF; Duncan, B; Meaney, FJ; Haynes, J; Barton, LL. Use of complementary and alternative medical therapies among children with special health care needs in Southern Arizona. *Pediatrics*, 2003 111, 584-587.

[102] Schmid-Schwap, M, Simma-Kletschka, I, Stockner, A; Sengstbratl, M; Gleditsch, J; Kundi, M; Piehslinger, E. Oral acupuncture in the therapy of craniomandibular

dysfunction syndrome - a randomized controlled trial (RCT). *Wien Klin Wochenschr*, 2006 118, 36-42.

[103] Schumacher, JF. *Religion and mental health*. New York: Oxford Univ Press; 1992.

[104] Seugnet, L; Boero, J; Gottschalk, L; Duntley, SP; Shaw, PJ. Identification of a biomarker for sleep drive in flies and humans. *PNAS*, 2006 103, 19913-19918.

[105] Shapiro, D; Cook, IA; Davydov, DM; Ottaviani, C; Leuchter, AF; Abrams, M. Yoga as a complementary treatment of depression: effects of traits and moods on treatment outcome. *eCAM*, 2007 4, 493-502.

[106] Sharma, H; Datta, P; Singh, A; Sen, S; Bhardwaj, NK; Kochupillai, V; Singh, N. Gene expression profiling in practitioners of Sudarshan Kriya. *J Psychosom Res*, 2008 64, 213-218.

[107] Shen, XZ; Koo, MWL; Cho, CH. Sleep deprivation increase the expression of inducible heat shock protein 70 in rat gastric mucosa. *World J Gastroenterol*, 2001 7, 496-499.

[108] Siedentopf, CM; Golaszewski, SM; Mottaghy, FM; Ruff, CC; Felber, S; Schlager, A. Functional magnetic resonance imaging detects activation of the visual association cortex during laser acupuncture of the foot in humans. *Neurosci letters*, 2002 327, 53-56.

[109] Skoglund, L. & Jansson, E. Qigong reduces stress in computer operators. *Compl Ther Clin Practice*, 2007 13, 78-84.

[110] Smith, C; Hancock, H; Blake-Mortimer, J; Eckert, K. A randomized comparative trial of yoga and relaxation to reduce stress and anxiety. *Compl Ther Med*, 2007 15, 77-83.

[111] Solberg, EE; Holen, A; Ekeberg, Ø; Østerud, B; Halvorsen, R; Sandvik, L. The effects of long meditation on plasma melatonin and blood serotonin. *Med Sci Monit*, 2004 10, CR96-101.

[112] Song, R; Lee, EO; Lam, P; Bae, SC. Effects of tai chi exercise on pain, balance, muscle strength, and perceived difficulties in functioning in older women with osteoarthritis: a randomized clinical trial. *J Rheumatol*, 2003 30, 2039-2044.

[113] Stancák Jr., A; Kuna, M; Srinivasan, Dostálek, C; Vishnudevananta S. Kapalabathi - yogic cleansing exercise: II. EEG topography analysis. *Homeost Health Dis*, 1991 33, 182-189.

[114] Streeter, CC; Jensen, JE; Perlmutter, RM; Cabral, HJ; Tian, H; Terhune, DB; Ciraulo, DA; Renshaw, PF. Yoga asana sessions increase brain GABA levels: a pilot study. *J Altern Complement Med*. 2007 13, 419-426.

[115] Sunter, AT; Guz, H; Ozkan, A; Peksen, Y. The search for non-medical treatments by patients with psychiatric disorders. *J Religion Health*, 2006 45, 396-404.

[116] Suzuki, J; Yamauchi, Y; Yamamoto, H; Komuro, U. Fasting therapy for psychosomatic disorders in Japan. *Psychother Psychosom*, 1979 31, 307-314.

[117] Taggart, HM; Arslanian, CL; Bae, S; Singh, K. Effects of T'ai Chi exercise on fibromyalgia symptoms and health-related quality of life. *Orthop Nurs*, 2003 22, 353-360.

[118] Tartaro, J; Luecken, LJ; Gunn, HE. Exploring heart and soul: Effects of religiosity/spirituality and gender on blood pressure and cortisol stress response. *J Health Psychol*, 2005 10, 753-766.

[119] Telles, S. & Desiraju, T. Oxygen consumption during pranayamic type of very slow-rate breathing. *Indian J Med Res*, 1991 94, 357-363.

[120] Thornton, EW; Sykes, KS; Tang, WK. Health benefits of Tai Chi exercise: improved balance and blood pressure in middle-aged women. *Health Promot Intern*, 2004 19, 33-38.

[121] Timio, M. Blood pressure trend and psychosocial factors: the case of the nuns in a secluded order. *Acta Physiol Scand Suppl*, 1997 640, 137-139.

[122] Timio, M; Lippi, G; Venanzi, S; Gentili, S; Quintaliani, G; Verdura, C; Monarca, C; Saronio, P; Timio, F. Blood pressure trend and cardiovascular events in nuns in a secluded order: a 30-year follow-up study. *Blood Press*, 1997 6, 81-87.

[123] Timio, M; Verdecchia, P; Venanzi, S; Gentili, S; Ronconi, M; Francucci, B; Montanari, M; Bichisao, E. Age and blood pressure changes. A 20-year follow-up study in nuns in a secluded order. *Hypertension*, 1988 12, 457-461.

[124] Tindle, HA; Wolsko, P; Davis, RB; Eisenberg, DM; Phillips, RS; McCarthy, EP. Factors associated with the use of mind body therapies among United States adults with musculoskeletal pain. *Compl Ther Med*, 2005 13, 155-164.

[125] Tran, MD; Holly, RG; Lashbrook, J; Amsterdam, EA. Effects of Hatha yoga practice on the health-related aspects of physical fitness. *Prev Cardiol*, 2001 4, 165-170.

[126] Tsai, JC; Wang, WH; Chan, P; Lin, LJ; Wang, CH; Tomlinson, B; Hsieh, MH; Yang, HY; Liu, JC. The beneficial effects of Tai Chi Chuan on blood pressure and lipid profile and anxiety status in a randomized controlled trial. The beneficial effects of Tai Chi Chuan on blood pressure and lipid profile and anxiety status in a randomized controlled trial. *J Altern Complement Med*, 2003 9, 747-754.

[127] Tsang, HWH; Cheung, L; Lak, D. Qigong as a psychosocial intervention for depressed elderly with chronic physical illnesses. *Int J Geriatr Psychiatry*, 2002 17, 1146-1154.

[128] Tsang, HW; Fung, KM; Chan, AS; Lee, G; Chan, F. Effect of qigong exercise on elderly with depression. *Int J Geriatr Psychiatry*, 2006 21, 890-897.

[129] Tsang, WWN. & Hui-Chan, CWY. Effects of Tai Chi on joint proprioception and stability limits in elderly subjects. *Med Sci Sport Exerc*, 2003 35, 1962-1971.

[130] Turner, JA; Mancl, L; Aaron, LA. Short- and long-term efficacy of brief cognitive-behavioral therapy for patients with chronic temporomandibular disorder pain: A randomized, controlled trial. *Pain*, 2006 121, 181-194.

[131] Upchurch, DM. & Chyu, L. Use of complementary and alternative medicine among American women. *Women's Health Issues*, 2005 15, 5-13.

[132] Vachiramon, A. & Wang, WC. Acupressure technique to control gag reflex during maxillary impression procedures. *J Prosthet Dent*, 2002 88, 236.

[133] Vachiramon, A. & Wang, WC. Acupuncture and acupressure techniques for reducing orthodontic post-adjustment pain. *J Contemp Dent Pract*, 2005 1, 163-167.

[134] Veith, I. *Huang Ti Nei Ching Su Wen: The Yellow Emperor's classic of internal medicine.* Berkeley: University of California Press; 1949.

[135] Vialatte, FB; Bakardjian, H; Prasad, R; Cichocki, A. EEG paroxysmal gamma waves during Bhramari Pranayama: A yoga breathing technique. *Consciousness and Cognition*, in press (doi: 10.1016/j.concog.2008.01.004)

[136] Vigh B. *Yoga and science [Jóga és tudomány]*. Budapest: Gondolat; 1972. 447-449.

[137] Voukelatos, A; Cumming, RG; Lord, SR; Rissel C. A randomized, controlled trial of tai chi for the prevention of falls: The central Sydney tai chi trial. *J Am Geriatr Soc*, 2007 55, 1185-1191.

[138] Wachholtz, AB. & Pargament, KI. Is spirituality a critical ingredient of meditation? Comparing the effects of spiritual meditation, secular meditation and relaxation on spiritual, psychological cardiac and pain outcomes. *J Behav Med*, 2005 28, 369-384.

[139] Wahner-Roedler, DL; Elkin, PL; Vincent, A; Thompson, JM; Oh, TH; Loehrer, LL; Mandrekar, JN; Bauer, BA. Use of complementary and alternative medical therapies by patients referred to a fibromyalgia treatment program at a tertiary care center. *Mayo Clin Proc*, 2005 80, 55-60.

[140] Walach, H. Verfahren der Komplementärmedizin. Beispiel: Heilung durch Gebet und Geistiges Heilen. *Bundesgesundheitsbl gesundheitsforsch Gesundheitschutz*, 2006 8, 788-795.

[141] Wall, RB. Tai Chi and Mindfulness-Based Stress Reduction in a Boston public middle school. *J Pediatr Health Care*, 2005 19, 230-237.

[142] Wang, WC; Vachiramon, S; Vachiramon, A; Vachiramon, T. Treatment of xerostomia on prosthetic patients using local acupuncture points of the face. *J Contemp Dent Pract*, 2004 4, 133-138.

[143] Wang, C; Roubenoff, R; Lau, J; Kalish, R; Schmid, CH; Tighiouart, H; Rones, R; Hibberd, PL. Effect of Tai Chi in adults with rheumatoid arthritis. *Rheumatology*, 2005 44, 685-687.

[144] Wetterberg, L. Melatonin and clinical application. *Repr Nutr Dev*, 1999 39, 367-382.

[145] Whittaker, P. Laser acupuncture: past, present, and future. *Lasers Med Sci*, 2004 19, 69-80.

[146] Winkelman, M. Trance states: A theoretical model and cross cultural analysis. *Ethos*, 1986 14, 174-203.

[147] Wirz-Justice, A; Benedetti, F; Berger, M; Lam, RW; Martiny, K; Terman, M; Wu, JC. Chronotherapeutics (light and wake therapy) in affective disorders. *Psychol Med*, 2005 35, 939-944.

[148] Wong, V; Sun, JG; Wong, W. Traditional Chinese medicine (tongue acupuncture) in children with drooling problems. *Pediatr Neurol*, 2001 25, 47-54.

[149] Woo, J; Hong, A; Lau, E; Lynn, H. A randomized controlled trial of Tai Chi and resistance exercise on bone health, muscle strength and balance in community-living elderly people. *Age Aging*, 2007 36, 262-268.

[150] Wu, JC; Buchsbaum, M; Bunney, WE. Clinical neurochemical implications of sleep deprivation's effects on the anterior cingulate of depressed responders. *Neuropsychopharmacology*, 2001 25, 5 Suppl. 1. S74-S78.

[151] Xu, D; Hong, Y; Li, J; Chan, K. Effects of tai chi exercise on proprioception of ankle and knee joints in old people. Br J Sports Med, 2004 38, 50-54.

[152] Xu, DQ; Li, JX; Hong, Y. Effect of regular Tai Chi and jogging exercise on neuromuscular reaction in older people. Age Aging, 2005 34, 439-444.

[153] Xu, DQ; Li, JX; Hong, Y. Effects of long term Tai chi practice and jogging exercise on muscle strength and endurance in older people. Br J Sports Med, 2006 40, 50-54.

[154] Yamamoto, H; Suzuki, J; Yamauchi, Y. Psychophysiological study on fasting therapy. *Psychother Psychosom*, 1979 32, 229-240.

[155] Yang, Y; Verkuilen, JV; Rosengren, KS; Grubisich, SA; Reed, MR; Hsiao-Wecksler ET. Effect of combined Taiji and Qigong training on balance mechanisms: A randomized controlled trial of older adults. Med Sci Monit, 2007/a 13, CR339-CR348.

[156] Yang, Y; Verkuillen, J; Rosengren, KS; Mariani, RA; Reed, M; Grubisich, SA; Woods, JA. Effects of a Taiji and Qigong intervention on the antibody response to influenza vaccine in older adults. Am J Chin Med, 2007/b 35, 597-607.

[157] Yeh, SH; Chuang, H; Lin, LW; Hsiao, CY; Eng, HL. Regular tai chi chuan exercise enhances functional mobility and CD4CD25 regulatory T cells. Br J Sports Med, 2006 40, 239-243.

[158] Yeh, GY; Mietus, Je; Peng, CK; Phillips, RS; Davis, RB; Wayne, PM; Goldberger, AL; Thomas, RJ. Enhancement of sleep stability with Tai Chi exercise in chronic hearth failure: Preliminary findings using an ECG-based spectrogram method. Sleep Med, in press, DOI: 10.1016/j.sleep.2007.06.003

[159] Zeng, Y; Liang, XC; Dai, JP; Wang, Y; Yang, ZL; Li, M; Huang, GY; Shi, J. Electroacupuncture modulates cortical activities evoked by noxious somatosensory stimulations in human. *Brain Res*, 2006 1097, 90-100.

[160] Zhou, D; Shephard, RJ; Plyley, MJ; Davis, GM. Cardiorespiratory and metabolic responses during Tai Chi Chuan exercise. *Can J Appl Sport Sci*, 1984 9, 7-10.

Chapter 9

CONCLUSION

Even though a prosthesis is fabricated conscientiously and properly, there is no assurance that the patient will be comfortable while wearing it or satisfied with the therapy [*Mazurat & Mazurat 2003*]. A normative evaluation by a dentist and a subjective evaluation by the patient related to the denture or to the dental treatment may be rather different [*Lechner & Roessler 2001*]. The factors not related to operative/technological dental skills that contribute to the success of denture wearing are becoming more and more important [*Ma et al. 2008*]. There are various symptoms, which may occur in relation with psychogenic denture intolerance [*Fábián & Fábián 2000, Fábián et al. 2006, 2007*]. Their pathomechanisms may include both somatic and psychogenic mechanisms.

PDI related symptoms are usually multifactorial (multicausal) [*Fábián & Fábián 2000, Fábián et al. 2006, 2007*], therefore both somatic and psychogenic pathways of pathomechanism should be considered carefully for both diagnosis and treatment. Since psychogenic symptoms may mimic a great variety of somatic symptoms; a clear cut diagnosis and proper differential diagnosis of PDI could be rather difficult. Therefore it should be emphasized that, *the diagnosis of PDI is a presumptive one in many cases.* The diagnosis may change later in the course of the disease as the clinical findings change and/or stabilize, therefore continuous monitoring and evaluation of the patient over time is essential [*Sarlani et al. 2005/a.b*]. A detailed differential diagnosis considering possible disorders of the teeth, and/or oral- and maxillofacial tissues should also be carried out, and *any other possible somatic causes behind the symptoms should also be excluded.*

Prevention is likely to be the most important tool for the management of psychogenic denture intolerance related problems at a social level. Cornerstones of prevention are screening of risk patients, proper treatment planning, proper communication with the patient, screening of the patient-nurse-dentist interrelationships, as well as prevention of dental fear, prevention of treatment induced pain and prevention of relapse [*Fábián & Fábián 2000, Fábián et al. 2007, Fejérdy & Orosz 2007*]. It is also crucial for the prevention that, patients must be made aware of their responsibilities in achieving a satisfactory outcome. It is also a matter of considerable significance that the clinician carefully weigh the option of nontreatment in certain cases [*Levin & Landesman 1976, Stein 1983, Fábián & Fábián 2000, Fábián et al. 2007*]. Dental team members should also be able to accept a patient from the bottom of hart as well as to understand and accept own emotions for a proper and successful treatment and to avoid treatment failure. Therefore *dentists and other team members should become a mature, well-disposed and good person on behalf of the patients as well as on behalf of their own interest.* Maintenance of the mental health of dental team is also crucial for the prevention of PDI [*Fejérdy et al. 2004*].

Majority of psychogenic denture intolerance patients refuse to accept psychological background of their symptoms [*Ross et al 1953, Fábián et al. 2005, Schwichtenberg & Doering 2008*]; and instead of psychiatrists or psychotherapists, first they visit dentist and insist on the somatic origin of their symptoms [*Ross et al. 1953, Fábián et al. 2005*]. Therefore a simple referral to psychiatrist and/or psychotherapist would not solve the problem in most cases. Consequently an initial psychosomatic therapy is needed prior to definitive therapy, which is a scope of dental profession's duty [*Moulton et al. 1957, Pomp 1974*]. Initial psychosomatic therapy may utilize several placebo and/or palliative methods (i.e. physiotherapies, medication, medicinal herb therapy, diet therapy, CAM therapy etc.) combined with supportive communication techniques and administration of any mind-body therapies, which are the "basis therapeutics" for psychosomatic disorders [*Iversen 1989, Binder & Bider 1989, Krause 1994*].

Besides obtaining improvement or recovery of symptoms due to the primarily symptom-centered initial psychosomatic treatment, it may also induce changes towards an over-all improvement of psychological abilities, social functioning, and stress resistance, all of which may support the healing process and stabilize treatment outcome. Mind-body therapies may also induce stress related autonomic and hormonal changes, including decrease of sympathetic activity, blood pressure, HPA axis hormones and catecholamine levels and advantageous changes of heart rate variability (HRV) [*Fábián in press*]; all of which can be highly important for the treatment of stress related orofacial symptoms. General improvement of musculoskeletal functions [*Shaw & Dettmar 1990, Egner & Gruzelier 2003, Raymond et al 2005*] as well as improvement of pain tolerance may also occur as highly important results of the psychosomatic treatment. Further, psychosomatic therapies may upregulate immune system and increase immune surveillance [*Gruzelier 2002*] leading to improved defense against several local or systemic infections, oral microbes and tumor formation. Immunomodulatory effects may also occur [*Hall et al. 1996*], indicating that, exaggerated immunological reactions such as allergy [*Teshima et al. 1982, Wyler-Harper et al. 1994, Langewitz et al. 2005*] or autoimmune conditions [*Collins & Dunn 2005*] may also be balanced with such methods. Salivation problems, and pseudoneurological symptoms may also be treated efficiently in many cases.

Medicinal herb and diet therapy are important supplemental modalities of psychosomatic dental therapy. However, medicinal herb and diet therapy are frequently used for health enhancement by patients without any professional control. Unfortunately they also use them during pregnancy and lactation or under severe systemic diseases, which may cause significant health hazards [*Segelman et al. 1976, Siegel 1976, 1979, Zhang et al. 2008*]. Concurrent use of medicinal herbs and pharmaceutical drugs without any control of medical or dental professionals is also relatively common and the majority of herbal medicine users are not aware of potential adverse effects [*Zhang et al. 2008*]. Therefore dentist should carefully collect information about the patients' medicinal herb related usage. Since dentists could exert significant influence on their patients' decisions about herbal medicine use, proper up-to-date knowledge related to medicinal herb therapy is highly important (also for those dentists not preferring the use of medicinal herb therapy in their practice).

Complementary and alternative medicine (CAM) denotes a wide range of variable therapies, with established benefits and few if any side effects [*Wahner-Roedler et al. 2005, Fábián in press*]. CAM therapies emphasize self-care, which can lead to advantageously decreased load of the much more expensive health care system [*Tindle et al. 2005*]. Majority of mind-body CAM techniques used by United States adults [*Cuellar et al. 2003, Barnes et al. 2004, Rhee et al. 2004, Honda & Jacobson 2005, Upchurch & Chyu 2005, Mao et al. 2007*], European adults [*Sunter et al. 2006, D'Inca et al. 2007*] and children in the US and Canada [*Sanders et al. 2003, Losier et al. 2005*] are religious. Since lacking a religious sensitivity, medical science will always be woefully incomplete, no matter how great its discoveries [*Pollack 1999*] the importance of such religious methods should not be underestimated.

REFERENCES

[1]   Barnes, PM; Powell-Griner, E; McFann, K; Nahin, RL. Complementary and alternative medicine use among adults: United States, 2002. Advance data from vital and health statistics; no 343. Hyattsville, Maryland: National Center for Health Statistics; 2004. 1-20.

[2]   Binder, H. & Binder, K. Autogenes Training, Basispsychotherapeutikum. Köln: Deutscher Ärzteverlag; 1989.

[3]   Collins, MP. & Dunn, LF. The effects of meditation and visual imagery on an immune system disorder: dermatomyositis. J Altern Complement Med, 2005 11, 275-284.

[4]   Cuellar, N; Aycock, T; Cahill, B; Ford, J. Complementary and alternative medicine (CAM) use by African American (AA) and Caucasian American (CA) older adults in a rural setting: a descriptive comparative study. BMC Compl Altern Med, 2003 3, 8.

[5]   D'Inca, R; Garribba, AT; Vettorato, MG; Martin, A; Martines, D; Di Leo, V; Buda, A; Sturniolo, GC. Use of alternative and complementary therapies by inflammatory bowel disease patients in an Italian tertiary referral centre. Digest Liver Disease, 2007 39, 524-529.

[6]   Egner, T. & Gruzelier, JH. Ecological validity of neurofeedback: Modulation of slow-wave EEG enhances musical performance. Neuroreport, 2003 14, 1221-1224.

[7]   Fábián, TK. Mind-body connections. Pathways of psychosomatic coupling under meditation and other altered states of consciousness. New York: Nova Science Publishers; in press.

[8]   Fábián, TK. & Fábián, G. Dental stress. In: Fink G, editor in chef. Encyclopedia of Stress. Vol. 1. San Diego: Academic Press; 2000; 657-659.

[9]   Fábián, TK; Krause, WR; Krause, M; Fejérdy, P. Photo-acoustic stimulation and hypnotherapy in the treatment of oral psychosomatic disorders. Hypnos, 2005 32, 198-202.

[10]   Fábián, TK; Mierzwińska-Nastalska, E; Fejérdy P. Photo-acoustic stimulation. A suitable method in the treatment of psychogenic denture intolerance. Protet Stomatol, 2006 56, 335-340.

[11] Fábián, TK; Fábián, G; Fejérdy, P. Dental Stress. In: Fink G, editor in chef.
      Encyclopedia of Stress. 2-nd enlarged edition, Vol. 1. Oxford: Academic Press; 2007;
      733-736.

[12] Fejérdy, P. & Orosz, M. Personality of the dentist and patient-assistant-dentist
      interrelationships [A fogorvos személyisége, a beteg-asszisztens-fogorvos
      kapcsolatrendszer] In: Vértes G, Fábián TK editors. Psychosomatic dentistry
      [Fogorvosi Pszichoszomatika] Budapest: Medicina; 2007; 22-31.

[13] Fejérdy, P; Fábián, TK; Krause, WR. Mentalhygienische Aufgaben von
      Krankenschwestern in der Zahnmedizin. Kommunikation mit den Patienten und dem
      Zahnarzt. Deutsche Z Zahnärztl Hypn, 2004 3, 32-34.

[14] Gruzelier, JH. A review of the impact of hypnosis, relaxation, guided imagery and
      individual differences on aspects of immunity and health. Stress, 2002 5, 147-163.

[15] Hall, H; Papas, A; Tosi, M; Olness, K. Directional changes in neutrophile adherence
      following passive resting versus active imagery. Int J Neurosci, 1996 85, 185-194.

[16] Honda, K. & Jacobson, JS. Use of complementary and alternative medicine among
      United States adults: the influences of personality, coping strategies, and social support.
      Preventive Medicine, 2005 40, 46-53.

[17] Iversen, G. Geleitwort. In: Binder, H, Binder K editors. Autogenes Training,
      Basispsychotherapeutikum. Köln: Deutscher Ärzteverlag; 1989.

[18] Krause, WR. Hypnose und Autogenes Training (Selbsthypnose) in der Rehabilitation.
      Ergänzung in: Schultz, JH. Hypnose-Technik. Praktische Anleitung zum Hypnotisieren
      für Ärzte. 9. Auflage - bearbeitet und ergänzt von G. Iversen und W.-R. Krause.
      Stuttgart - Jena - New York: Gustav Fischer Verlag; 1994. 71-79.

[19] Langewitz, W; Izakovic, J; Wyler, J; Schindler, C; Kiss, A; Bircher, AJ. Effect of self-
      hypnosis on hay fever symptoms - a randomized controlled intervention study.
      Psychoter Psychosom, 2005 74, 165-172.

[20] Lechner, SK. & Roessler, D. Strategies for complete denture success: beyond
      techniqual excellence. Compend Contin Educ Dent, 2001 22, 553-559.

[21] Levin, B. & Landesmann, HM. A practical questionnaire for predicting denture success
      of failure. J Prosthet Dent, 1976 35, 124-130.

[22] Losier, A; Taylor, B; Fernandez, CV. Use of alternative therapies by patients presenting
      to a pediatric emergency department. J Emergency Med, 2005 28, 267-271.

[23] Ma, H; Sun, HQ, Ji, P. How to deal with esthetically overcritical patients who need
      complete dentures: A case report. J Contemp Dent Pract, 2008 9, 22-27.

[24] Mao, JJ; Farrar, JT; Xie, SX; Bowman, MA; Armstrong, K. Use of complementary and
      alternative medicine and prayer among a national sample of cancer survivors compared
      to other populations without cancer. Compl Ther Med, 2007 15, 21-29.

[25] Mazurat, NM. & Mazurat, RD. Discuss before fabricating: Communicating the realities
      of partial denture therapy. Part II: Clinical outcomes. J Can Dent Assoc, 2003 69, 90-
      94.

[26] Moulton, R; Ewen, S; Thieman, W. Emotional factors in periodontal disease. Oral Surg
      Oral Med Oral Pathol, 1957 5, 833-860.

[27] Pollack, R. Wisdom versus knowledge: an agenda for a more humane medical science.
      FASEB J, 1999 13, 1477-1480.

[28] Pomp, AM. Psychotherapy for the myofascial pain-dysfunction syndrome: a study of factors coinciding with symptom remission. JADA, 1974 89, 629-632.

[29] Raymond, J; Sajid, I; Parkinson, LA; Gruzelier, J. Biofeedback and dance performance: A preliminary investigation. Appl Psychophysiol Biofeedback, 2005 30, 65-73.

[30] Rhee, SM; Garg, VK; Hershey, CO. Use of complementary and alternative medicines by ambulatory patients. Arch Intern Med, 2004 164, 1004-1009.

[31] Ross, GL; Bentley, HJ; Greene Jr., GW. The psychosomatic concept in dentistry. Psychosom Med, 1953 15, 168-173.

[32] Sanders, H; Davis, MF; Duncan, B; Meaney, FJ; Haynes, J; Barton, LL. Use of complementary and alternative medical therapies among children with special health care needs in Southern Arizona. Pediatrics, 2003 111, 584-587.

[33] Sarlani, E; Balciunas, BA; Grace, EG. Orofacial pain - Part I. Assessment and management of musculoskeletal and neuropathic causes. AACN Clin Issues, 2005/a 16, 333-346.

[34] Sarlani, E; Balciunas, BA; Grace, EG. Orofacial pain - Part II. Assessment and management of vascular, neurovascular, idiopathic, secondary, and psychogenic causes. AACN Clin Issues, 2005/b 16, 347-358.

[35] Schwichtenberg, J. & Doering, S. Success of referral in a psychosomatic-psychotherapeutic outpatient unit of a dental school. Z Psychosom Med Psychother, 2008 54, 285-292.

[36] Segelman, AB; Segelman, FP; Karliner, J; Sofia, D. Sassafras and herb tea. Potential health hazards. JAMA, 1976 236, 477.

[37] Shaw, RM, & Dettmar, DM. Monitoring behavioral stress control using a craniomandibular index. Aust Dent J, 1990 35, 147-151.

[38] Siegel, RK. Herbal intoxication. Psychoactive effects from herbal cigarettes, tea, and capsules. JAMA, 1976 236, 473-476.

[39] Siegel, RK. Ginseng abuse syndrome. Problems with the panacea. JAMA, 1979 241, 1614-1615.

[40] Stein, RS. Mutual protective complex of dental restorations. In: Laney WR, Gibilisco JA editors. Diagnosis and treatment of prosthodontics. Philadelphia: Lea & Febiger; 1983; 306-326.

[41] Sunter, AT; Guz, H; Ozkan, A; Peksen, Y. The search for non-medical treatments by patients with psychiatric disorders. J Religion Health, 2006 45, 396-404.

[42] Teshima, H; Kubo, C; Kihara, H; Imada, Y; Nagata, S; Ikemi, Y. Psychosomatic aspects of skin diseases from the standpoint of immunology. Psychother Psychosom, 1982 37, 165-175.

[43] Tindle, HA; Wolsko, P; Davis, RB; Eisenberg, DM; Phillips, RS; McCarthy, EP. Factors associated with the use of mind body therapies among United States adults with musculoskeletal pain. Compl Ther Med, 2005 13, 155-164.

[44] Upchurch, DM. & Chyu, L. Use of complementary and alternative medicine among American women. Women's Health Issues, 2005 15, 5-13.

[45] Wahner-Roedler, DL; Elkin, PL; Vincent, A; Thompson, JM; Oh, TH; Loehrer, LL; Mandrekar, JN; Bauer, BA. Use of complementary and alternative medical therapies by patients referred to a fibromyalgia treatment program at a tertiary care center. Mayo Clin Proc, 2005 80, 55-60.

[46] Wyler-Harper, J; Bircher, AJ; Langewitz, W; Kiss, A. Hypnosis and the allergic response. Schweiz Med Wochenschr Suppl, 1994 62, 67-76.

[47] Zhang, AL; Story, DF; Lin, V; Vitetta, L; Xue, CC. A population survey on the use of 24 common medicinal herbs in Australia. Pharmacoepidemiol Drug Saf, 2008 17, 1006-1013.

ABOUT THE AUTHORS

Dr. Tibor Károly Fábián D.M.D., Ph.D.

Associate professor of the Clinic of Prosthetic Dentistry, Semmelweis University Budapest, Hungary, EU. He is a dentist and psychotherapist having more than 15 years experience in clinical research of psychosomatic dentistry. He was also graduated as a teacher of religion.

Prof. Dr. Pál Fejérdy D.M.D., Ph.D.,

Professor and chairman of the Clinic of Prosthetic Dentistry, former dean of the Faculty of Dentistry, and former pro-rector of education of the Semmelweis University Budapest, Hungary, EU. As a chairman, he established the first psychotherapist's consultation for dental patients in Hungary.

GLOSSARY

Acquired immune response: immune response, which is carried out primarily by T and B cells (including plasmacells), and is regulated primarily by lymphocyte derived cytokines. The antigen presenting function of monocytes/macrophages and dendritic cells is highly important in this response too. Primary effector arms are T-killer cells (cell-mediated response) and plasmacells with their products the antibodies (humoral response). This immune response is directed against specific antigens and is often enhanced following repeated exposure to antigen. This response is also referred to as "adaptive" or "specific" immunity.

Acupuncture: traditional Chinese practice that attempts to regulate and restore energy balance by stimulating specific acupoints. Traditional acupuncture is based on the traditional Chinese conception of vital energy ("Chi" or "Qi"). Painful trigger points may also be stimulated with acupuncture needles (or other acupuncture modalities), which is referred to as trigger point acupuncture. Acupuncture treatment may also be carried out intraorally (stimulating intraoral acupoints/trigger points) which is referred to as oral acupuncture.

Adaptive immunity: see acquired immune response

Allergen elimination test: removal of an expected antigen. In dentistry: removal of all dental restorations containing an expected allergen.

Altered state of consciousness: sudden and transient subjective experience significantly different from those of common everyday experiences. It may induce significant changes of most psychological functions including attention, perceptions, sense of time, body image, self-image, imagination, fantasy, cognition, emotions, arousal, memory, self-control, suggestibility, identity etc.

Atypical odontalgia: tooth-located pain of primarily psychogenic origin.

Autogenic Training: self-hypnotic state induced by giving suggestions toward phenomena spontaneously occurring under relaxation to amplify and control them. In high level form of Autogenic Training deep hypnoid trance state develops similarly to that of hypnosis. Basic level of Autogenic Training may be practiced without profound alterations of consciousness.

Behavioral therapy: an operationalized psychotherapeutic approach, which has its roots in classical learning theory and other findings of experimental psychology. It focuses on current determinants of behavior and draws on the principles of learning to develop individual treatment strategies. The focus in behavior therapy is the presenting problem itself; and it is not assumed that the presenting problem is a manifestation of an underlying primary problem. The aim of behavior therapy is to modify the problem behavior at a behavioral level.

Biofeedback: use of devices that amplify physiological processes that are ordinarily difficult to perceive without some type of amplification. Participants alter their physiological processes using as a guide the provided feedback signals. There are various parameters may be used for biofeedback including several EEG and another brain related parameters, muscle tension (EMG), skin temperature, skin conductance level, heart rate variability parameters (etc.).

Brief dynamic psychotherapy: see psychoanalytic psychotherapy

Bruxism: nonfunctional contact of the teeth during grinding, gnashing, tapping or clenching. Grinding, gnashing and tapping most likely occur at night, whereas clenching may occur during both the day and night.

Burning mouth syndrome: distinct clinical entity characterized by a chief complaint of unremitting oral burning concomitant with no oral mucosal clinically observable lesions, or other relevant apparent organic basis.

Cell mediated response: see acquired immune response

Chaperokine: molecule that is able to function as both cytokine and molecular chaperone.

Client centered therapy: psychotherapeutic approach, which emphasizes the autonomy of clients (and thus avoids the use of term "patient") and the healing effect of the encounter during psychotherapy. It also emphasizes the attitudual qualities of the therapist such as warmth, empathy and genuineness (congruence) as well as the ability of therapist to emphatically recognize and reflect ("mirror") the real sense behind the client's communication.

Cognitive therapy: psychotherapeutic approach, which is based on the assumption that, the person's feelings and behavior are determined by the way in which their experiences are processed cognitively. In this approach, irrational determinants of thoughts are assumed as a major cause of several pathopsychological conditions. Cognitive therapy aims to decrease premised maladaptive irrational cognitions and to increase adaptive cognitions of patients. Cognitive therapy can be advantageously combined with behavioral therapy, and these two approaches are often so interwoven with each other that the term cognitive-behavioral therapy is used.

Cognitive-behavioral therapy: see cognitive therapy

Complementary and alternative medicine: collective noon of a wide range of variable therapies, including also treatments with established benefits and few if any side effects. Therapies of complementary and alternative medicine emphasize self-care, which can lead to advantageously decreased load of the much more expensive health care system.

Convergence theory: theory, which hypothesizes that conducing stimuli of more than one afferent fibers via an only ascending fiber may lead to mislocalization of conducted impulses resulting in pain (or other sensory) radiation phenomena.

Cytokines: molecules that are primarily used for communication of several immune cells with each other. Further, cytokines can cross the blood-brain barrier at leaky points and via specific active transport. Therefore, another important function of cytokines is to influence central nervous functions including stress response as well as other psychoemotional functions.

Definitive psychosomatic therapy: highest level care of psychosomatic patients. Definitive psychosomatic therapy utilizes any available dental, medical and psychotherapeutic treatment possibilities in an evidence based manner.

Dept-psychological: related to unconscious psychological processes.

Dermatome: skin area having sensory innervation from the same central nervous segment. Although the "classical" dermatomes typically belong to spinal cord segments, brainstem is also considered as a "segment" of the central nervous system in this relation, and therefore, skin innervations areas of the branches of trigeminal nerve are considered as dermatomes of the facial region.

Dietary fibers: nondigestible carbohydrates originating primarily from plant sources. Dietary fibers are incompletely absorbed (or not absorbed) in the small intestine, but are at least partly fermented by bacteria in the large intestine. Besides advantageous decreasing effects of adequate fiber intake on the risk for obesity, coronary hard diseases, colon cancer and diabetes, adequate dietary fiber intake advantageously improve oral health as well.

Dynamic psychotherapy: see psychoanalytic psychotherapy

Electrostimulation therapy: see transcutaneous electrical nerve stimulation

Equilibrated splint: splint with simultaneous tooth contacts on the complete occlusal coverage of the arch. Equilibrated splints are primarily used for harmonizing muscle function. Equilibrated splints may also be used to determine optimal position of maximal intercuspidation of dentures under preparation for patients with neuromuscular symptoms.

Equilibrated splints may also be used in the case of patients undergoing bite opening procedures. Equilibrated splints may also be used to prevent or limit the attrition of teeth of patients with bruxism.

Epicutan test: see skin test

Gagging: overactivity of the defense reflex, which attempts to eject unwanted, irritating, or toxic materials from the upper gastrointestinal tract. Although gag reflex is a normal defense function of human, overactive gag reflex ("gagging") may be rather disadvantageous for denture wearers, especially for those wearing removable dentures. Gagging may also lead to failure to tolerate making impression and/or other routine dental procedures.

Hapten: metal ion or other small molecule allergen.

Head-zones: small areas of dermatomes, which were recognized based on the observation that radiating visceral pain usually does not cover the whole dermatome but specific smaller areas only (which are referred to as Head-zones). There are also smaller facial skin areas located roughly concentric around the mouth called „trigeminal projection fields" which are considered as facial Head zones.

Humoral immune response: see acquired immune response

Hypnosis: specific altered state of consciousness induced by verbal and/or nonverbal suggestions and through focusing or widening attention. Hypnosis is characterized by increased receptivity to suggestions, capacity for modification of perception and memory, and potential for control usually involuntary physiological functions. Self-hypnosis is self-induced hypnosis achieved by self-suggestions. Hetero hypnosis achieved by suggestions of other person(s).

Idiopathic environmental intolerance: disorder likely to be of primarily psychogenic origin characterized by various somatic symptoms, which cannot be explained organically, but are attributed to the influences of potentially toxic environmental chemicals in low, usually harmless doses.

Imagery: generation of different mental images. Images are usually classified by the modality of their content such as visual, auditory, olfactory, gustatory, tactile or kinesthetic. Self imagery is generated by oneself. Guided imagery is generated by oneself but guided by a therapist.

Imagination: see imagery

Initial psychosomatic therapy: initial part of the psychosomatic treatment of a patient. The most important goals of initial psychosomatic therapy are avoidance of further useless invasive dental treatment as well as obtaining decrease (recovery) of symptoms and motivation of patients to participate in a definitive psychosomatic therapy. Gradual escalation of therapy and avoidance of irreversible forms of treatment are "cornerstones" of the initial psychosomatic therapy; which utilizes several placebo and/or palliative methods combined with supportive communication techniques. Administration of any mind-body therapies as "basic therapeutics" for psychosomatic disorders is also an important goal if initial psychosomatic therapy.

Innate immune response: immune response, which is carried out primarily by monocytes/macrophages, neutrophile granulocytes, NK cells, as well as the complement system and several nonspecific defense molecules. It is regulated primarily by macrophage-derived cytokines. This response represents a "first-line defense" against pathogens, however it does not discriminate against antigens, and it is not enhanced by repeated exposure to a certain antigen. This immune response is also referred to as "nonspecific", "native" or "natural" immunity.

Intracutan test: see skin test

Jaw closing reflex: stretch reflex of the mandibular elevator muscles acting against gravity and with resulting jaw closure. It is also referred to as jaw jerk.

Jaw jerk: see jaw closing reflex

Jaw opening reflex: reflex that operates to protect the masticatory apparatus and to regulate the force and rhythm of chewing.

Low level laser therapy: a highly efficient physiotherapeutic method utilizing athermic low power lasers. It is also frequently referred to as soft laser therapy.

Massage: therapeutic friction, stroking, kneading or shaking of a part of the body.

Meditation: volitional self-induced altered state of consciousness, established by mental faculties, without dominant contribution of other persons, highly intense body exercises or use of drugs. Practices of meditation may be divided into two subgroups such as concentrative type and nonconcentrative type methods. Although concentrative and nonconcentrative approaches differ from each other, the subjective experience of deeper stages seems to be rather similar phenomenologically. Finally both group of meditation techniques, lead to a state of "Being", a state of "Knowing" or "Experiencing" without objectification and discursive thinking. In religious form of meditation, premised deep meditative states and experiences have certain religious overtones.

Mucosa test (oral): Application of test pieces onto the surfaces of palatal or ridge mucosa using individually prepared removable appliances or using fixation onto labial or buccal tooth surfaces. Mucosa test is used for the assessment of irritative and/or delayed type allergic reactions.

Native immunity: see innate immune response

Natural immunity: see innate immune response

Neurofeedback: see biofeedback

Nocebo effect: see placebo effect

Nociceptor sensitization: phenomenon that pain sensitivity of nociceptors can be enhanced by numerous agents of immune/inflammatory processes (i.e. bradikinin, interleukins, prostaglandins, serotonin etc.).

Nonspecific immunity: see innate immune response

Occlusal dysesthesia: collective noon of several uncomfortable feelings of occlusion, despite the absence of any observable occlusal anomaly or discrepancy. Occlusal dysesthesia is frequently referred to as "phantom bite" or "occlusal neurosis" as well.

Occlusal neurosis: see occlusal dysesthesia

Odontophobia: all kinds of phobic reactions related to the dental treatment, to the dentist, or to the dental surgery office.

Omega-3 fatty acids: series of polyunsaturated fatty acids, which belong to essential fatty acids because mammalian cells are unable to synthesize them. Intake of these fatty acids is considered to be low in western diets. They are participating in various highly important biological functions, and may also be used for therapeutic purposes, especially for several mental illnesses.

Oral acupuncture: see acupuncture

Oral corrosion: release of metallic derivatives as a result of several chemical (or electrochemical) reactions of alloys being in touch with saliva, gingival crevicular fluid, immune cells and oral microbes.

Oral galvanic current: appearance of an electric current caused by electric potential differences between several alloys placed into the mouth (and came into contact with saliva).

Oral motor ability: ability to operate the complex oral sensorimotor function (i.e. ability to fit two test pieces of complementary form together in the mouth).

Oral stereognosis: ability to recognize and discriminate form or shape in the oral cavity.

Orofacial: localized in, or related to the hard and soft tissues of the mouth, the tongue, the teeth, or the face.

Pain: unpleasant sensory and emotional experience associated with actual or potential tissue damage, or described in terms of such damage. Pain is a multifaceted and multilevel phenomenon including a specific sensation, a variable emotional state, an aspect of interoception and a specific behavioral motivation.

Palliative treatment: alleviating or relieving without definitive treatment.

Panic disorder: disorder with a symptom of recurrent intensive alarm attacks linked with various body reactions and fear of death.

Patch test: see skin test

Phantom bite: see occlusal dysesthesia

Phantom tooth pain: psychogenic pain of extraction site (alveolar bone) of a previously extracted tooth.

Phonetic: relating to speech sounds.

Photo-acoustic stimulation: altered state of consciousness induced by flash light stimuli through closed eye and rhythmic noise stimuli through the ear at the same time. Usually stimuli of mixed frequency (ca. 5-10 Hz) are administered via glasses with built-in light emitting diodes (LED), and headphones. In some cases lower (1-4 Hz) or higher (10-15 Hz) frequency bands of stimuli are also used.

Placebo effect: effect that follows the administration of an inert treatment (the placebo). Placebo effect is primarily induced due to expectation and conditioning. The placebo effect is additive to any specific treatment; therefore, it is a highly important phenomenon that brings to fullness any treatment modalities. Importantly, patients' beliefs and expectancies may also lead to negative aspects and worsening of symptoms, which is referred to as nocebo effect.

Prosthodontic treatment: diagnosing, planning, making and inserting fixed or removable artificial devices to replace one or more teeth and associated tissues.

Prayer: an active process of communicating with and/or appealing to God or other supernatural being belonging to God. Besides intercessory prayer (petitions on behalf of others), there are three major forms of prayer including conversational prayer (informal conversation with God), ritual prayer (reciting or reading well known prayers) and meditative prayer (i.e. repetition of short formulas, contemplation, imagery of religious themes etc.).

Prick test: see skin test

Progressive Muscle Relaxation: frequently used basic method to induce relaxed states via voluntary flexing and subsequent relaxation of the muscles.

Pseudoneurological symptom: symptom that appears as if it would be caused by any neurological disorder, however without any detectable somatic/neurological background.

Psychoanalysis: dept-psychological theory, focusing on unconscious psychological processes and their interrelationships with conscious psychological function, as well as on their role in pathopsychological phenomena. There are various theoretical streams of psychoanalysis, all of which have been integrated as psychoanalytic theory. Libido-theory, ego-psychology, object-relationships theory and self-theory are the most important such theories. Major therapeutic interventions of psychoanalysis are analysis of free associations, analysis of resistance, analysis of transference, analysis of counter-transference and the related interpretations; whereas interventions that contain suggestions or directions are usually avoided.

Psychoanalytic psychotherapy: collective noon of those psychotherapeutic methods, which are strongly linked derivatives of psychoanalysis but with some significant modifications related to technique and goal. Psychoanalytic psychotherapy is also referred to as dynamic psychotherapy or psychodynamic psychotherapy. These kinds of therapies are usually less intense in frequency and length comparing to psychoanalysis, they can be explicitly supportive, and utilize modified analytic techniques, which may be mixed also with some non-analytic techniques. There are also several short-term forms of psychoanalytic therapy (referred to as brief dynamic psychotherapy) which are explicitly problem focused and focal.

Psychodynamic psychotherapy: see psychoanalytic psychotherapy

Psychogenic denture intolerance: patient's refusal accepting or wearing truly prepared (standard, properly made) fixed and/or removable denture(s) because of appearing psychogenic symptom(s) in relation to the denture(s) or to the treatment procedure.

Psychogenic fever: common psychosomatic disease with acute or persistent body temperature above normal range under psychosocial stress.

Psychosymbolic function: conscious and unconscious psychological function of an organ.

Pulsed electromagnetic field therapy: a highly efficient physiotherapeutic method utilizing low induction level pulsed electromagnetic field stimulation.

Qigong: a traditional Chinese practice of meditation designed to control expected vital energy (called "Chi" or "Qi") of the body to promote health and spiritual development. Beside some static body postures and voice training there are three major components of Qigong including slow moving exercises, breathing exercises and meditation. Movement in Qigong usually involve meditative visualizing of internal consequences of flow of the expected vital energy, although in some cases vital energy is expected to be transferred into other persons (patients) on purpose to cure.

Regression: psychological state with a change from being in an emotionally controlled to a less well-controlled emotional state, which is associated with a change in relationship status. Because of regression, a relationship may show a typical pattern of interaction between a parent and child or any other pattern of emotionally deep-rooted relationships. Regression is frequently coupled with transference phenomena as well.

Reflex splint: splint that trigger mouth opening reflex due to functioning as an "artificial early contact". Reflex splints are primarily used for reducing stress induced muscle spasm and parafunction activity.

Relaxation: elicitation of a hypometabolic psychophysiologic state coupled with muscle relaxation, decreased sympathetic activity, hypoarousal and reduced feeling of tension.

Relaxation response: a set of profound and integrated psychophysiologic changes mainly opposite directed comparing to those of "stress response". Relaxation response is induced by certain forms of meditation using repetition of a neutral word or phrase; preferably a neutral one-syllable word like "one".

Respiratory feedback: certain form of biofeedback without using any feedback-related task. Feedback of breathing occurs spontaneously with light and sound signals leading to a unique form of deeply relaxed meditative state.

Rest position: position, from which all free movements of the jaw start.

Rule of dermatome: observation that visceral pain is frequently radiated into the dermatome of that central nervous segment, which the visceral organ itself belongs to.

Skin test: application of series of test peaces or standardized test solutions onto the skin (epicutan test, patch test) or into the skin (i.e. prick test, scarification test, intracutan test). Epicutan test (patch tests) is a standard method for delayed type allergic reactions, whereas intracutan test (prick test, scarification test) is primarily used for assessment of risk of immediate IgE mediated reactions.

Scarification test: see skin test

Self-hypnosis: see hypnosis

Soft laser therapy: see low level laser therapy

Specific immunity: see acquired immune response

Tai Chi Chuan: a Chinese martial art based on suppleness and evasion coupled with control of expected vital energy (called "Chi" or "Qi") of the body. Beside some static body postures and voice training there are three major components of Tai Chi including slow moving exercises, breathing exercises and meditation. Movement in Tai Chi (although usually practiced slowly) may be sped up and might involve meditative visualizing the external consequences of a motion as well (i.e. to provide a self-defense). Although Tai Chi Chuan was developed as a self-defense system, it is more often practiced today as a healing art.

"Tell-show-do" technique: technique, which is frequently used to reduce dental fear. It includes describing in simple terms what is about to occur ("tell"); than allowing the patient to see, feel, explore and manipulate the tools or instruments ("show"); and than the starting of the procedure ("do").

Temporomandibular disorder: interrelated set of clinical conditions presenting with signs and symptoms in masticatory and related muscles of the head and neck, and the soft tissue and bony components of the temporomandibular joint.

Theory of facilitation: theory, which hypothesizes that subliminal impulses arriving from more than one afferent fibers to an only ascending fiber may increase the excitability of this ascending fibers to such an extent that it begin to fire in an inappropriate manner, which may lead to misdetermination of impulse quality. Consequently, higher brain centers may recognize non-painful sensory stimuli as if they were nociceptive pain stimuli.

Thickness discrimination ability (occlusal): the sensory perceptive ability in relation with occlusal interferences and/or small foreign bodies.

Tinnitus: auditory phantom phenomenon characterized by the sensation of sounds without objectively identifiable sound sources.

Transcutaneous electrical nerve stimulation: physiotherapeutic technique, which utilizes commercially available devices that apply electric impulses to the peripheral nerves via electrodes placed on the skin. Although electrodes of TENS devices were originally placed on the skin, in dentistry "intraoral TENS" (intraoral electrostimulation therapy) utilizing electrodes placed intraorally may also be used.

Transference: re-experience of emotions and psycho-emotional patterns of a previous relation (primarily from the childhood) in a present actual relation.

Trigger point: focal muscle area(s) of maximum tenderness (located within the muscle or its fascia) typically found in taut muscle bands, which elicit(s) severe local pain and/or aggravation of the referred pain with a characteristic pain referral pattern.

Ultrasound treatment: physiotherapeutic use of ultrasound, producing vibrations within the tissue, which cause particle collision and the release of energy resulting in the production of heat. Ultrasonic treatment induces a combined deep effect of vibration ("micromassage") and deep heat effect.

Vitamins: organic molecules that are required for normal metabolism but cannot be synthesized in adequate amounts by the human body. Vitamins were given alphabetic designations in the order of their discovery, and named when they were isolated and their chemical structures were identified. Although they are exceedingly heterogeneous in chemical structure and biochemical function, they can be grouped conveniently into two classes that share common characteristics: fat-soluble vitamins and water-soluble vitamins.

Yoga: traditional practices developed in India to improve health, and to prepare body and mind for meditation and spiritual development. Classical yoga incorporates moral and ethical observances, body postures and exercises, breathing techniques and meditative techniques.

There are several major subdivisions of yogic tradition such as hatha yoga, pranajama, kundalini yoga, and raja yoga. There are also some modern school of yoga such as Iyengar yoga and Vivekananda yoga.

APPENDIX

TREATMENT PLANNING FOR PARTIALLY EDENTULOUS PATIENTS

A survey and an account of the diverse factors influencing treatment planning is only possible if the are systemized. This is the primary aim of the classification of partially edentulous arches [*Fábián & Fejérdy 1979*] described below. This classification may be referred to as "prosthetic classification" [*Fábián & Fejérdy 1979*]; because its major goal is to enhance treatment planning and denture designing procedures. With regard to this aspect partially edentulous arches can be rendered to five main classes such as 1A, 1B, 2A, 2B and 3, and to one subclass (2A/1) as described below (see also *Figure 1*).

Class 1A

One or more primary fulcrum lines (straight line drawn between two teeth adjacent to the edentulous space) may exist; but none of the primary fulcrum lines is going to become a factual fulcrum line when a denture is inserted. No force of rotation will be generated and the denture may not settle. In case of partially edentulous arches of class 1A fixed dentures are recommended. If still a removable partial denture (RPD) were made, baseplate of RPD can be extremely reduced to a framework.

Class 1B

One or more fulcrum line(s) may exist, which may become a factual fulcrum line when a denture is inserted. The rotational forces, however, will not be very powerful, so that the settling of the denture can be equalized (i.e. compensated due to multiple abutments). In case of partially edentulous arches of class 1B fixed dentures may be recommended. If still a removable partial denture (RPD) were made, baseplate of RPD can be strongly reduced.

Class 2A

Only one primary fulcrum line exists, which may become a factual fulcrum line when a denture is inserted. Rotating around this axis (around the factual fulcrum line) the denture may settle or tip in one direction. In case of partially edentulous arches of class 2A removable partial denture (RPD) is recommended and the baseplate of RPD can be moderately reduced only.

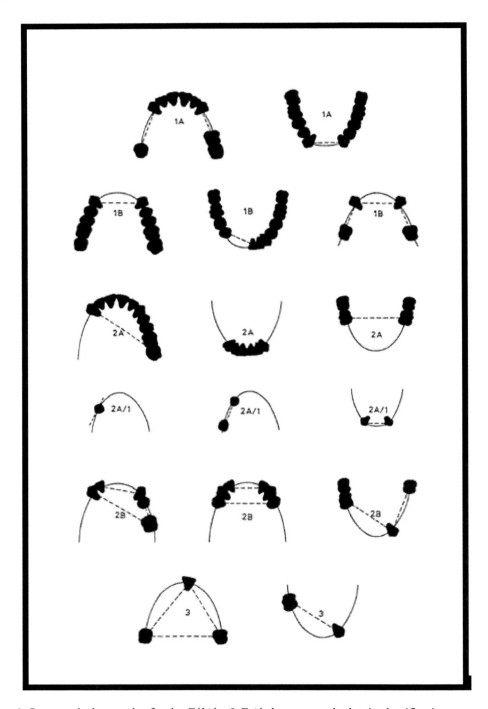

Figure 1. Some typical examples for the *Fábián & Fejérdy* type prosthodontic classification.

Class 2A/1

Only one fulcrum line exists, which may become a factual fulcrum line when a denture is inserted. Rotating around this fulcrum line the denture may settle in one direction. This class is a special case (subclass) of class 2A characterized by very few (maximum one or two) remaining teeth. In case of partially edentulous arches of class 2A/1 removable partial denture (RPD) is recommended and the baseplate of RPD can *not* be reduced.

Class 2B

Several primary fulcrum lines may exist, and one of which may become a factual fulcrum line when a denture is inserted. Rotating around this primary fulcrum line the denture may settle in one direction. In case of partially edentulous arches of class 2B removable partial denture (combined with or without fixed dentures) are recommended and the baseplate of RPD can be moderately reduced only.

Class 3

One or more primary fulcrum line(s) may exist; from which one or more may become a factual fulcrum line when a denture is inserted. Rotating around this/these fulcrum line(s) the denture will tip upward anteriorly and downward posteriorly (i.e. two-directional rotary movements occur). In case of partially edentulous arches of class 3 removable partial denture (RPD) is recommended, the baseplate of RPD can not be reduced and, importantly, *resilient* type telescopes (i.e. delayed type dental support) should be used.

REFERENCE

[1]   Fábián, T. & Fejérdy, P. Prosthetic classification of partially edentulous jaws. *Fogorv Szle*, 1979 72, 310-315.

INDEX

(Related paragraphs are indicated)

A

D

E

F

G

L

M